Introduction to Veterinary Science

Introduction to Veterinary Science

Kian Churchill

Callisto Reference

www.callistoreference.com

Callisto Reference,
118-35 Queens Blvd., Suite 400,
Forest Hills, NY 11375, USA

Visit us on the World Wide Web at:
www.callistoreference.com

ISBN: 978-1-64116-635-5 (Hardback)

Cataloging-in-Publication Data

Introduction to veterinary science / Kian Churchill.
p. cm.
Includes bibliographical references and index.
ISBN 978-1-64116-635-5
1. Veterinary medicine. 2. Animals--Diseases. 3. Animal health. I. Churchill, Kian.
SF745 .I58 2022
636.089--dc23

Table of Contents

Preface

The field of science which deals with different aspects of animal health is known as veterinary science. Some of these aspects are genetics, microbiology, breeding, livestock management, meat products technology, pathology, pharmacology and surgery. Veterinary medicine is a branch of veterinary science which deals with treatment, diagnosis and prevention of injuries, diseases and disorders in animals. There are a wide spectrum of conditions which can affect different animal species, all of which are studied and treated within this discipline. Veterinary science also plays a crucial role in aiding human health through the control and monitoring of zoonotic diseases. This book unfolds the innovative aspects of veterinary science which will be crucial for the progress of this field in the future. Some of the diverse topics covered in this book address the varied branches that fall under this category. It includes contributions of experts and scientists which will provide innovative insights into this field.

A foreword of all chapters of the book is provided below:

Chapter 1 - The branch of science which focuses on the well-being and health of animals is termed as veterinary science. Some of its sub-disciplines include veterinary histology, veterinary virology and veterinary bacteriology. This chapter briefly introduces these sub-fields of veterinary science to provide an extensive understanding of the subject.; **Chapter 2** - The branch of veterinary science which is involved in the study of the form and structure of animals is termed as veterinary anatomy. Some of the different branches of veterinary anatomy are canine anatomy, equine anatomy, cow anatomy and avian anatomy. The topics elaborated in this chapter will help in gaining a better perspective about the anatomy of these types of animals.; **Chapter 3** - There are a wide variety of diseases which can affect animals such as viral diseases, fungal diseases and bacterial diseases. Apart from these, diseases can also be caused by parasites such as helminths. This chapter closely examines these types of animal diseases to provide an extensive understanding of the subject.; **Chapter 4** - The domain of veterinary science which is involved in the study of the behavior of animals in their natural habitat is termed as veterinary ethology. The topics elaborated in this chapter will help in gaining a better perspective about veterinary ethology as well as the different types of animal behavior.; **Chapter 5** - The study of animal parasites which focuses on the relationships between animal hosts and parasites is termed as veterinary parasitology. Some of its sub-disciplines include veterinary entomology and veterinary helminthology. All the diverse aspects related to these branches of veterinary parasitology have been carefully analyzed in this chapter.; **Chapter 6** - There are numerous surgical procedures which are used in the field of veterinary medicine. Some of these are surgical sterilization, cardiac surgery and ophthalmological surgical procedures. This chapter closely examines these key veterinary surgical procedures to provide an extensive understanding of the subject.

At the end, I would like to thank all the people associated with this book devoting their precious time and providing their valuable contributions to this book. I would also like to express my gratitude to my fellow colleagues who encouraged me throughout the process.

Kian Churchill

Chapter 1

Understanding Veterinary Science

The branch of science which focuses on the well-being and health of animals is termed as veterinary science. Some of its sub-disciplines include veterinary histology, veterinary virology and veterinary bacteriology. This chapter briefly introduces these sub-fields of veterinary science to provide an extensive understanding of the subject.

Veterinary science as a subject concerns the treatment of a range of different animals – from domestic pets to farmyard animals – and combines an array of subjects like anatomy and animal behaviour, as well as niche subjects like parasitology (the study of parasites) and gastroenterology (the study of the stomach and intestines).

A veterinarian (sometimes called a vet) is a doctor who works with all types of animals from dogs and cats to cows and sheep, and sometimes even animals like kangaroos. Veterinarians who only work with animals like dogs and cats are known as "small animal vets." Veterinarians who work with animals like cows, sheep, and pigs (livestock) are referred to as "large animal veterinarians. Veterinarians can also specialize in what is considered "exotic" animals like lizards and birds.

A veterinarian can work at an animal clinic. These offices are very similar to a human doctor's office, but vets have some special tools to examine their animal patients better. People can take their animals to the vet for just a check-up, but in special cases for other treatments and surgeries.

A large number of vet clinics offer mobile veterinary care services for farmers. These services are used in emergencies or when it is impractical to take an animal to the vet's office. For example, it is not practical to transport a cow to a vet's office when the cow is giving birth. Instead, the vet will visit the farm and help the cow there. Some livestock farms are so huge that they require a resident veterinarian to care for their animals. A resident veterinarian may live on site and care only for that farm's animals, or a vet might live locally and only work with certain farms in that area.

Currently, there are 22 different veterinary specialty organizations. These are specific skills area that a veterinarian has decided to dedicate their efforts to. Some of these specialties include behavior, dermatology, and anesthesia.

Some veterinarians specialize in pathology and work for diagnostic laboratories. These vets use special equipment to perform biopsies. A biopsy is the surgical removal and examination of tissue obtained from a living animal. Tissues make up the body. Tissues make up everything, even the bones, muscles, and blood. All types of veterinarians send in tissues to be tested, and the diagnostic veterinarians determine whether or not that animal has a disease and sends the results back.

Role of Veterinary Research in Human Society

Virchow's statement is as wise today as it was over a century ago. That all animal species, including *Homo sapiens*, are related and that knowledge gained in one species benefits all lead to the concept of "One Medicine". The One Medicine approach takes advantage of commonalities among species; few diseases affect exclusively one group of animals (wildlife, domestic animals, or humans). On the basis of that view, asserts that veterinary medicine is fundamentally a human health activity. All activities of veterinary scientists affect human health either directly through biomedical research and public health work or indirectly by addressing domestic animal, wildlife, or environmental health. Moreover, veterinary scientists have a responsibility to protect human health and well-being by ensuring food security and safety, preventing and controlling emerging infectious zoonoses, protecting environments and ecosystems, assisting in bioterrorism and agroterrorism preparedness, advancing treatments and controls for nonzoonotic diseases (such as vaccine-preventable illnesses and chronic diseases), contributing to public health, and engaging in medical research. Just as the practice of veterinary medicine contributes to our understanding of all medicine or One Medicine, so must veterinary research. It follows that veterinary research is, at a fundamental level, a human health activity. The centrality of veterinary research and its critical role at the interface between human and animal health are often not understood and undervalued. A vision for veterinary research and its contribution to advancing One Medicine and providing solutions for today's and tomorrow's animal and human health problems is illustrated below.

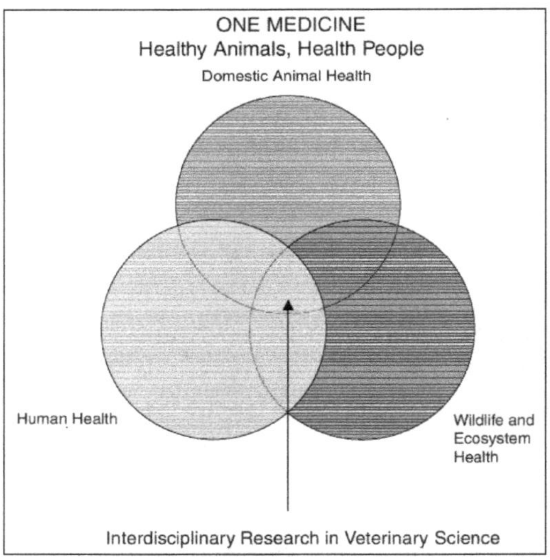

A vision for veterinary research. The One Medicine approach to human and animal health emphasizes the interconnectedness of relationships and the transferability of knowledge in solving health problems in all species.

Veterinary research includes research on prevention, control, diagnosis, and treatment of diseases of animals and on the basic biology, welfare, and care of animals. Veterinary research transcends species boundaries and includes the study of spontaneously occurring and experimentally induced models of both human and animal disease and research at human-animal interfaces, such as food safety, wildlife and ecosystem health, zoonotic diseases, and public policy.

By its nature, veterinary science is comparative and gives rise to the basic science disciplines of comparative anatomy, comparative physiology, comparative pathology, and so forth. Veterinary research occurs in colleges of veterinary medicine, human medicine, dentistry, agriculture, and life sciences; it is done by veterinarians, physicians, and other non-veterinarians in many disciplines. For 2 centuries, responsible public officials have recognized that veterinary research protects our draft animals, our supplies of meat and eggs, and our wildlife. It also advances our ability to maintain the health of all animals, domestic and wild; and informs policy decisions—for example, regulations to prevent and control tuberculosis and brucellosis in dairy cattle. During the same period, scientists have acknowledged the broad and robust contributions of veterinary research to human health.

Veterinary research has the potential to immensely impact the fields of comparative medicine, public health and food safety, and animal health; but its ability to reach its potential relies on adequate infrastructural, financial, and human resources. The National Research Council convened an ad hoc committee to assess the status and future of veterinary research in the United States on the request of the American Animal Hospital Association, the Association of American Veterinary Medical Colleges, the American Veterinary Medical Association, the Centers for Disease Control and Prevention, the National Association of Federal Veterinarians, the National Center for Research Resources (NCRR), and the National Institute of Environmental Health Sciences. Specifically, the committee was asked to identify national needs for research in three fields of veterinary science—comparative medicine, public health and food safety, and animal health; to assess the adequacy of our national capacity, mechanisms, and infrastructure to support the needed research; and, if appropriate, to make recommendations as to how the needs can be met. Specific budgetary or organizational recommendations were not to be included in the report.

The three fields of veterinary science encompass research with domestic animals (such as livestock and poultry), wild animals (such as deer and exotic species), companion animals (such as dogs, cats, and horses), service animals (such as horses and dogs), and laboratory animals. Specifically, future needs for research were assessed in the three fields of veterinary science, which are not limited to science conducted by veterinarians; they include science performed by professionals who have veterinary degrees and professionals who have various other degrees.

The contributions of veterinary research to advancements in medicine are rich. In ancient academic amphitheaters, comparative anatomical and physiological studies provided a basis for our understanding of embryonic development, human blood circulation and lymphatics, the brain and the rest of the nervous system, and the structure of virtually all organs. As modern medicine evolved, Pasteur's experiments on rabies and anthrax vaccination in sheep, Koch's studies of tuberculosis, and Salmon's direction of research in the US Bureau of Animal Industry—all of which depended on the knowledge of comparative or veterinary research—provided the basis of contemporary preventive medical treatments. More recent contributions of veterinary researchers include Brinster's pioneering studies in embryo transplantation and the immunological discoveries of Nobel Prize winner Peter Doherty. In the last half century, the widespread use of animal models in comparative medicine and the improved management of laboratory animals have been integral to the advancement of scientific knowledge in human medicine.

In 1878, Congress appropriated $10,000 for the US Department of Agriculture (USDA) to fund the first research in the United States specifically directed toward veterinary science. This study was "investigating diseases of swine and infectious and contagious diseases which all other classes of domestic animals are subject" and enabled D.E. Salmon to establish that quarantine and disinfection prevent spread of infectious diseases. Salmon's successful research led to an act of Congress on May 29, 1884, that established the Bureau of Animal Industry (BAI) in USDA. The act provided, in part, "that the Commissioner of Agriculture shall organize in this Department a Bureau of Animal Industry, and shall appoint a Chief thereof, who shall be a competent veterinary surgeon." Research in BAI made major scientific advances in the understanding of human diseases. BAI's findings included the isolation of the first species of Salmonella, the discovery of hog cholera and of how the virus and serum provide immunity, elucidation of the life cycle of the cattle tick, and the discovery of the protozoan parasite that caused Texas cattle fever. The latter made possible the scientific approach to conquering yellow fever in the Panama Canal Zone. In 1920, Simon Flexner of Rockefeller Institute of Medical Research noted that "our knowledge of yellow fever would in all likelihood have been delayed if the work of the Bureau of Animal Industry of the US Department of Agriculture on Texas fever had not been done."

BAI was a major contributor to public health, Secretary of Agriculture James Wilson's report for 1909 stated that the BAI "not only deals with the livestock industry, but has an important bearing upon public health through the meat inspection, through efforts for the improvement of the milk supply, and through the investigations, prevention and eradication of diseases which affect man as well as the lower animals. Indeed, the animal and the human phases of the Bureau's work are so closely related and interwoven that they could not be separated without detriment."

At the turn of the twentieth century, the university-based schools of veterinary medicine began to develop research units. Advanced medical institutions included comparative medicine in their structure and used animal disease models to elucidate the basic nature of human disease. Rous, in 1910, was the first to discover a virus that caused cancer (sarcoma in chickens). Other discoveries in comparative medicine include Shope's findings of the viral nature of papillomas in rabbits and Bittner's finding that viruses in milk cause mammary gland tumors in mice. In 1938, the association of a bleeding disorder of cattle with sweet clover stimulated the search for the toxicant; it was found to be dicumarol, which was quickly developed as an anticoagulant for humans and as a rodenticide for public health.

Three factors led to a marked increase in veterinary research in the massive economic growth and academic reformation that followed World War II. First, the number of veterinary schools with specific dedication to veterinary research doubled. Second, veterinarians were specializing; they formed the American College of Veterinary Pathologists, the American College of Veterinary Preventive Medicine, and subspecialties with expertise in fields related to public health and medical science. Third, animal models were being used to make major advances in basic research, and institutions of veterinary science had access to the newly developing federal funding mechanisms. Veterinary scientists made contributions in the pathogenesis of yellow fever, plague, and smallpox. Gross isolated a virus that caused naturally occurring lymphomas in mice, and Jarrett discovered that retroviruses were responsible for the transmission of leukemia among cats. Brinster and Mintz inoculated teratoma cells into normal mouse blastocysts to produce normal but mosaic mice and showed that tumor cells lose malignancy and differentiate normally. Slemons and Easterday discovered that wild ducks were a reservoir of avian influenza viruses.

In recent times, the application of molecular biology to problems in veterinary science has blurred the distinction between medical science and veterinary science in many fields. As microbial and genetic discoveries were made, pathogenesis studies were required to integrate the new knowledge into useful clinical advances. Those advances include a creative model of enteric bacterial disease (Moon), demonstration of the transmissibility and pathogenesis of scrapie, a proposal that human kuru was a transmissible spongiform encephalopathy (Hadlow), and the isolation of bovine leukemia virus (Miller) and bovine immunosuppressive retroviruses (Van Der Maaten) 5 years before AIDS and HIV appeared. Now modern molecular and genetic sciences and their applications in integrative, whole-animal biology make possible exciting advances for the benefit of both animals and people.

Contemporary Issues in Veterinary Science

The historical contributions of veterinary research have been considerable, but its vital role in public health and food safety has been brought into stark reality in the last 2 decades. Concerns have been driven by the recognition that many emerging infectious diseases of humans are zoonotic. Such diseases as Escherichia coli O157:H7 infection, bovine spongiform encephalopathy (BSE), and avian influenza highlight the importance of research to improve veterinary public health and food safety. There is a need for more research on those diseases and many others, such as anthrax and Rift Valley fever that may be used in terrorist attacks through agriculture and the food supply.

The need for research on animal health problems that do not threaten public health or food safety was emphasized by the 2001 outbreak of foot-and-mouth disease in the United Kingdom. The economic consequences of the outbreak— through the loss of domestic and international trade and tourism and the costs of the eradication program—were devastating. Current knowledge and technology for preventing or responding to such a disease do not meet increasing public expectations for food security and are not adequate to mitigate the risks posed by the globalization of agriculture and increasing world travel and trade in animals and animal products or the threat of agricultural bioterrorism.

Veterinary research has evolved to address societal changes. Companion animals play a central role in the quality of life of an increasing proportion of the public; the beneficial psychosocial effects of the human-animal bond are widely accepted. Companion animals are also important sentinels for human disease and toxicant exposure, and companion-animal research improves our understanding of zoonotic diseases and how to address them; diagnostic and therapeutic data from companion animals can often be translated to human medicine. Because the health, well-being, and longevity of companion animals are a growing concern for a substantial portion of society, demand for research on companion animal health and disease has increased; indeed, it is crucial for improving the health and welfare of these animals, which serve not only as companions, but as aides, detectives, and soldiers.

In addition to the health of food and companion animals, the health of wildlife and ecosystems is of special importance to an increasingly urban and affluent society. The countryside is increasingly affected by urban development and industrial agriculture. There is growing concern about wildlife preservation and endangered species and growing recognition of the value of wildlife as sentinels for environmental health generally. The emergence of Lyme disease in the human population of New England partly due to changing land-use patterns and of Chronic Wasting Disease (a transmissible spongiform encephalopathy similar to BSE) in elk and deer in the western United States and Canada highlight the importance of research on wildlife and ecosystem health.

Veterinary Histology

Veterinary Histology is a branch of anatomy concerned with the visual examination of cells, intercellular structures as well as their organization in tissues and organs, by means of the microscope and by using appropriate preparations thin enough to transmit light or electrons. Studying the normal microscopic structure of the animal body is the basis for understanding abnormal microscopic lesions (histopathology), body functions, immunology, clinical pathology and several other disciplines in veterinary medicine. Veterinary Histology deals with the techniques of studying cells and tissues, cell biology and the four basic tissues of the body (epithelium, connective tissue, muscle and nervous tissue).

Methods of Histology

Methods of Direct Observation of Living Cells and Tissues

Generally living cells and tissue are difficult to examine microscopically, because they are relatively transparent and thick. But there are different methods for studying living cells and tissues.

Examination of living cells and tissues without any chemical treatment:

- Fresh, unclosed direct method: Bits of tissues or drops of blood taken from a freshly anaesthesized animal are spread on a glass slide and examined under a microscope. Often saline solution is used to keep the tissue moist. The type of microscope used can be dark – field or phase contrast microscope.
- Cell/tissue culture: Is means the of direct observation of living cells. For this purpose living cells are removed from an organism cultured (i.e. kept alive and allowed to multiply) in septic conditions with appropriate nutrient and environmental conditions. The cultured cells are then examined without any chemical treatment. Culturing techniques permit the continual observation, manipulation and testing of explantes cells without any jeopardy to the donor, cellular differentiation, cellular transformation, cytogenetics, cellular metabolism, cell to cell interaction, host/parasite relationships, and other biological process have been studied by this technique cell culture is indispensible in diagnostic virology, vaccine development and production.
- Transparent viewing chamber: Permit an extended period of observation neuovascularization, cellular differentiation and movement, other vital process are studied by these techniques. In this method, for example, holes are made in rabitis ear and covered with glass discs. Through the glass one can see the growth of blood vessels and nerves directly under the microscope. The anterior chamber of the eye is a naturally occurring viewing chamber that is used in this approach.

Histology of Endocrine System

Histology of Mammals

The pituitaty, pineal, thyroid, parathyroid, and adrenal glands possess certain features that distinguish them as organs of the endocrine system. They are very rich in wide, thin-walled vessels called sinusoids. The sinusoids are intimately associated with parenchymal cells, whose secretory products (hormones) pass directly into the circulatory system. Endocrine glands lack ducts. In contrast, exocrine glands convey their secretions (e.g., enzymes, mucus, and bile) through ducts to a mucosal or skin surface.

Endocrine cells are not limited to the glands. For example, hormones are secreted by interstitial cells of the testes, corpora lutea and ovarian follicles, islets of Langerhans, and enterochromaffin cells of the gastrointestinal epithelium. The pituitary gland (hypophysis) is a major endocrine gland that is suspended from the hypothalamus of the brain. It releases several hormones, many of which influence the activity of other endocrine glands. The glandular portion, the adenohypophysis, forms from an out pocketing of the ectoderm of the dorsal portion of the oral cavity, called Rathke's pouch. The pars distalis, pars tuberalis, and pars intermedia constitute the adenohypophysis. The neural part of the pituitary gland, the neurohypophysis, is derived from a ventral out pocketing of the diencephalon. It is divisible into a median eminence, infundibular stalk, and pars nervosa.

The pars distalis is the largest portion of the pituitary gland. The parenchyma consists of irregular cords of cells separated by sinusoids and sparse connective tissue. There are two main types of parenchymal cells: chromophobes, characterized by a small amount of cytoplasm that stains poorly, and chromophils, with more abundant cytoplasm that is readily stained. The chromophils are classified as acidophils (alpha cells) and basophils (beta cells). Basophils tend to be larger than acidophils. Chromophobes are smaller than chromophils and are most evident in groups, appearing as clusters of closely packed nuclei in tissue sections. The pars intermedia are situated between the pars distalis and the pars nervosa. In the horse these regions are closely apposed. In other domestic mammals the pars intermedia and pars distalis are parrially separared by a small cleft, the hypophyseal cavity, which is the vestigial cavity of Rathke's pouch. The pars intermedia consist predominantly of basophilic cells. Follicles filled with colloid are often present. The pars tubcralis is mainly located around the infundibular stalk. It is composed primarily of cords, clusters, and follicles of small, faintly basophilic cells. The neurohypophys is contains numerous unmyelinated nerve fibers whose cell bodies are located in the supraoptic and para ventricular nuclei of the hypothalamus. Their axons converge at the median eminence (ventral boundary of the third ventricle) and form the hyporhalamohypophyseal tract. They pass through the narrow infundibular stalk to the pars nervosa (infundibular process).

The neurosecretions of these cells move along within the axolls and accumulate at the terminal regions of the nerve fibers as Herring bodies, which are best demonstrated with special staining methods. Overall, the pars nervosa has an unorganized, fibrous appearance, and individual axons are indistinct. Numerous pituicytes (neuroglial cells) are scattered among the nerve fibers. They possess round to oval nuclei and long cytoplasmic processes. Their cytoplasm cannot be distinguished from nerve fibers in routine histologic preparations. The infundibular cavity, which is continuous with the third ventricle and lined by ependymal cells, extends deep into the pars nervosa in the cat and pig and to a lesser extent in the dog and horse. In ruminants the cavity does not reach beyond the infundibular stalk.

These relationships are evident in mid sagittal sections of the pituitary gland. The pineal gland (pineal body; epiphysis cerebri) is a dorsal evagination of the roof of the diencephalon. It is covered by connective tissue of the piamater and divided into lobules by septa of connective tissue. The parenchyma is composed predominantly of pinealocytes, which are arranged as clusrers, cords, or follicles. These epirhelioid cells have a round nucleus and acidophilic cytoplasm. Neuroglial cells are also present. Each lobe of the thyroid gland is surrounded by a thin capsule of connecrive tissue and divided into lobules by thin trabeculae. The latter are continuolls with sparse intralobular connective tissue that contains numerous sinusoids.

In the pig and cow the connective tissue is abundant. Each lobule consists of numerous follicles of various sizes that are frequently filled with colloid. The follicular cells vary in height, depending on the state of activity of the follicle. Their appearance changes from squamous or low cuboidal in the resting stage to cuboidal or columnar in the active stage. In an active follicle the periphery of the colloid adjacent to the apical surface of the follicular cells is vacuolated. In an inactive follicle, the colloid has a smoother peripheral surface and vacuoles are not present. Parafollicular (C) cells occur among the cells that line the thyroid follicles and also between the follicles. They are larger and have a paler cytoplasm than the follicular cells. Their nuclei are relatively large and pale.

Para follicular cells usually occur singly, bur may also appear in groups. In the dog these cells are particularly abundant the parathyroid glands are classified as internal and external. Those that are adjacent to or embedded in the thyroid gland are the internal parathyroids. The external pararhyroids lie a variable distance away from the thyroid gland. The parathyroid glands are surrounded by a thin capsule of connective tissue, which may be absent where the glands are deeply embedded within the thyroid gland. A stroma of connective tissue is well developed in the pig and cow, but is sparse in other domestic mammals. The parenchyma of the parathyroid gland consists primarily of clusters and cords of principal (chief) cells. There are two different functional stages of the principal cell. The light principal cell is inactive and has a large, pale nucleus and pale, acidophilic cytoplasm. The dark principal cell is a smaller, active cell with a small, dark nucleus and a deeply acidophilic cytoplasm. In the sheep and goat, light cells tend to be located peripheral to the more central, dark cells. In the other domestic mammals these cells are distributed randomly.

Oxyphilic cells are large cells with an acidophilic cytoplasm and a pyknotic nucleus. They have been reported to occur in small numbers in the pa rathyroid glands of the horse and cow, particularly older animals. The paired adrenal glands are situated close to the anterior end of the kidneys. The glands are covered by a capsule of dense irregular connective tissue that sometimes contains smooth muscle. Clusters of epithelioid cortical cells also occur in the capsule. Thin trabeculae project partially into the parenchyma.

Each adrenal gland is organized into a peripheral cortex and a central medulla. The adrenal cortex is divided into four zones. The zona glomerulosa (zone multiformis) is the outermost zone. In the carnivore, horse, and pig the parenchymal cells of this region are columnar and arranged into arcs. In the horse the columnar cells are especially tall. In ruminants the zona glomerulosa contains polyhedral cells that form irregular c1usrers or cords. The zona intermedia lie between the zone glomerulosa and the zona fasciculata. It consists of small, closely packed cells. This zone is seen more often in the horse and carnivore than in the other domestic mammals.

The zona fascicuiata, the widest zone of the adrenal cortex, is formed by radially arranged cords of cuboidal or polyhedral cells. The cords are one or two cells thick and separated by sinusoids. The cytoplasm of the cells in this zone frequently appears foamy because of the presence of numerous lipid vacuoles. The zona reticuiaris is the innermost zone of the ad renal cortex. It is arranged as an irregular network of anastomosing cords of cells surrounded by sinusoids. The adrenal medulla is composed mostly of columnar or polyhedral chromaffin cells, which form clusrers and anastomosing cords separated by sinusoids. In domestic mammals an outer and inner zone of the medulla can often be distinguished. The former consists of larger, more darkly stained cells, and the latter contains smaller, more lightly stained cells. Ganglion cells, either individually or in clusters, are scattered through the medulla. Because the cortex and medulla interdigitate at their junction, projections of the zona reticular is may appear within the medulla.

Histology of Chicken

As in mammals, the pituitary gland (hypophysis) of the chicken is attached to the base of the brain below the diencephalon and is encapsulated by the duramater. The adenohypophysis is composed of the pars distal is and pars tuberal is. Pars intermedia are absent. The pars distalis is divided into a cephalic region and a caudal region. Both regions contain cords of acidophils and basophils, and clusters of chromophobes. The acid ophils of the cephalic region are pale, and those of the caudal zone arc more darkly stained. Thus, the cephalic zone appears more basophilic, and the caudal zone appears more acidophilic. The cords of cells of the former are more closely packed than those of the latter. Some parenchymal cells of the pars distal is may be arranged around a lumen filled with colloid, especially in older birds. Cysts lined by ciliated cells and mucous cells also occur in this part of the pituitary gland.

The pars tuberalis surrounds the infundibulu m and spreads dorsally over the ventral surface of the brain for a short distance. Ventrally, it extends to the posterior margin of the cephalic zone of the pars distalis. The pars tuberalis contains small, round to elongated, slightly basophilic cells that are arranged in several layers. The neurohypophysis includes the median eminence of the tuber cinereum, the infundibular stalk, and the pars nervosa (infundibular process). The median eminence and the infundibular stalk consist primarily of nerve fibers, neuroglial cell s, and ependymal cells that line the infundibular cavity. The pars nervosa has an irregular surface and consists of numerous lobules. Each lobule contains a diverticulum of the infundibular cavity that is lined by ependymal cells. The latter are surrounded by irregular masses of tissue consisting of pituicytes and other neuroglial cells, nerve fibers, and Herring bodies. The pineal gland (epiphysis cerebri) is a small, conical body that is situated between the cerebral hemispheres and the cerebellum.

It is surrounded by connective tissue and is composed of a body and a narrow, ventral stalk that is attached to the roof of the third ventricle. The parenchyma of the gland is arranged into lobules separated by thin septa of connective tissue. The lobules contain cells, predominantly pinealocytes that form rosettes or follicles. The thyroid glands are composed of numerous colloid-filled follicles, as in mammals. Cells that are similar in function to the parafollicular cells of mammals, however, occur in the ultimobranchial bodies, rather than the thyroid glands, of the chicken. The parathyroid glands ate each surrounded by a capsule of connective tissue. The parenchyma is composed of irregular cords of chief cells, separated by connective tissue and numerous sinusoids.

The adrenal glands are enclosed within a capsule of dense connective tissue. Unlike mammals, the parenchyma is not organized into a distinct cortex and medulla. Instead, it is composed of intermingled cortical (interrenal) tissue and medullary (chromaffin) tissue. The cortical cells are arranged as irregular cords. These cells have dark nuclei and appear columnar when the cords are sectioned longitudinally. In a cross section of a cord the cells appear all and pyramidal with several cells arranged radially. Medullary tissue is composed of polygonal cells. There are larger than conical cells and possess a large, round nucleus and basophilic cytoplasm. Ganglion cells occur among the medullary cells. Two ganglia (the cranial and caudal suprarenal ganglia) are opposed to the surface of the adrenal glands and ate frequently included in histological sections of this gland. The glands of endocrine system are ductless glands, encapsulated (most), highly vascularized, and secret hormones, (proteins glycoproteins steroids, polypeptides or catecholamines. The endocrine gland include: pituitary, adrenal, thyroid, Islets of langerhans (pancreas), interstitial cells of tests, follicle and colporalutea.

Pituitary Gland Hypohysis Cerebri

It composed of two parts; Adenohypophysis (anterior lobe): consists of pars distalis, pars intermedia, and pars tuberalis and Neurohypophysis (posterior lobe): consists of paranservosa (infundibular process), median eminence of tuber cineraum and infundibular stalk.

1. Adenhypophysis: Pars distalis comprises of the greater bulk of adenohypophysis and covered by fibrous CT (maeninges). The Paracheyma consists of two types of cell groups: Chromophobic cells and chromophilic cells.

- Chromophobic cells (chromophobes): In light microscopy, these cells are agranular and unstained and they forms 50% of the cells of pars distalis. They are small and round with little affinity for stain and also called chief cells, principal cells, reserve cells or and cells.
- Chromophilic cells (chromophils): These cells are divided as acidophils and basophils:
  - Acidophils:
    - Have granules that are easiniphilic;
    - Are 40% of the cells in pars distalis;
    - Larger than the chromophobes;
    - Granule size 300×900nm in diameter;
    - Produce somatotrphic hormones (growth hormones) and prolactin.
  - Basophils:
    - Are large than acidophils;
    - Granules have affinity for hematoxilin (basophilic) and size ranges from 150-200nm in diameter;
    - Are 10% of the total cells in pars distalis;
    - Produce ACTH, FSH, LH, TSH;
    - Pars intermedia consists of weakly basophilic cuboidal cells;
    - Function not well known;

- Pars intermedia is located adjacent to pars nervosa;
- Cells are nonspecific basophils;
- Secrete melanocyte stimulating hormone (MSH).

2. Neurohypophysis: It isn't a true gland but a mass of neurglia & nerve. It is the ventral infagiantion of the nervous tissue of hypothalamus. It includes pars nervosa (infundibular process), median promine ace of tubercinereum and infundibular salk. Numerous unmylinated neurosns which comerise the hypotalamophyseal tract and their cell bodies are located in suproatptic and paraventricular nuclei of the hypatholamus (are neurosecretory neurons). The neurosecretion moves along the axons and accumulation in the nerve fibers as herring bodies. Pituicytes and neuroglial elements are scattered among the nerve fibers. The secretory products of these neurons are:

- From paraventicular nuclei – Oxytocin;
- From supraotic nuclei - ADH or vasopressin;
- From both nuclei- neurophysin - carrier molecules for transporting prohormonal products of the above hormones.

Hypothalamic Connection with Hypophysis

1. Vascular relationship: Adenohypophysis has hypothalamo-hypophyseal portal system through which the secretion (releasing or inhibiting factors from hypothalamus control the release of the homone from adenohypophysis. Rostal hypophyseal arteries (in hypothealamus) – arterioles – primary capillary loops (supply parsdistalis indirectly) – veins – secondary capillary loops supplying the parst distalis. Neural relationship: Neurophophysis has hypotalamo- hypophyseal tract system through the nerve fibers from paraventicular and suprooptic nuclei in the hypothalamus.

2. Thyroid Gland: The gland has lobes and covered by capsules of connective tissues. The structural unit of thyroid gland is thyroid follicle. The follicles are hollow sphres that are variable in size and the center of the follicle is filled with gel – like material called colloid. This is the storage from of the follicular epithelial secretory products. The lining epithedium of follicle varies from low cuboidal to high columnar cuboidal to high columnar. The height of the cells within a given follicle is generally uniform. The thyroid epithelium consists of follicular lining cells (90% of the cellular pop) and parafollicular cells pale stained cells). Follicular cells are acidophilic with basaly positioned nucleus.

Histological Points for Differentiating Active and Inactive Follicle

1. Active follicles: It has high (columnar) epithelium which is usually small in size and the colloid has peripheral irregularities and vacuoles. They are strongacidophilic.

2. Inactive follicles: Has low epithelium (low cuboidal or even squamous). They are large in size and the colloid at the periphery is smooth in profile and vacuoles aren't present. The colloid is slightly basophilic. The storage of the secretory products within the extracellular follicle in the

form of thyroglobulin of colloid is unique to thyroid endocrine gland. The hormone T4 (thryoxine) and T3 (triiodothyronine) are produced from thyroglobulin the colloid.

3. Adrenal gland: Adrenal gland is called suprarenal gland and small organs situated near the cranial poles of the kidneys. They are enclosed in capsule of dense fibrous CT and send trabeculae in to the parenchy of gland. Recticular fibers and collagen fibers form the stroma. Adrenal gland has cortex and medulla (central).

4. Cortex: The adrenal cortex is peripherally located region and subdivided into three distinct zones.

- The outermost, zona glomerulus;
- The middle, zona fasciculate;
- The zone reticularis, which lies adjacent to the medulla.

5. Zonal glomerulosa: In ruminants is formed of irregular clusters and cords of cells. In horse, donkey, carnivores and pig, zone is called the zone arcuate because the cells are arrangenged in aros, with their convexity directed toward the periphery. The cells are all tall columnar in horse but smaller in other animals. It produces minerals corticoids; aldestrone, deoxycorticosterone, cortisole.

6. Zona fasiculate: It consist of radially arranged coids of cuboidal or columnar cell usually with one cell thickness. The cells are polyhedral and have roughey the same morphologic features as the cells of zona fasiculate. They contain fewer lipid droplets and more lipofusion zona fasiculate and reticularis are involved in production of glucocorticoids (cartisol) and corticosterone.

7. Medulla: The endocrine cells (chromaffin cells) of adrenal medulla are modified postoganlioc symphathetic neurons whose secretory activity is regulated by ganglionic symphathetic innervations. Epinephrine and norepinephrine are synthesized in those cells and the cells have large spherical nucleus and argentaffin granules. The cells are also arranged in irregular cords and cluster separated by dense network of sinusoidal capillaries.

8. Pancreatic islets: The endocrine cells of pancreas are clustered in pancreatic islet of langerhans (2%) of pancreatic tissue. This structure has various shapes; spherical to ovoid and found intermingled with exocrine pancreatic tissue. The islet cells are arranged in irregular anastmosing cords composed of two major cells A (α) and B (ß) cells but other cells are also assumed to exist C, D (δ) and F cells. A-cells represent 5-30% of the islet population and are arygrophilic. They produce glucagon and arranged at periphery in cattle. B-cells represent indistinct and nonargyrophilc with polyangulr shape and they are the most numerous cells in islet (60-80% of the population).

In cattle locate mostly in the center. They produce insulin C-cells are immature precursor cells for other types. The D-cells produce somatostatin and relatively are located at periphery of islet. It inhibits the secretion of glucogan and insulin whereas; F-cells in dog produce pancreatic polypeptides and F cells are also assumed to produce gastroentero – pancreatic hormones. For example, pancreatic polypeptide, vaso active, intesunial polypeptides and cholecytos kinin-pancreozymin.

Veterinary Microbiology

Veterinary Microbiology is the branch of study mainly concerned with microbes that are responsible for causing diseases to animals. It is purely concerned with microbial (bacterial, fungal, viral) diseases of domesticated animals (livestock, fur-bearing animals, game, poultry, and fish) that supply food and other useful products. Microbial diseases caused by the wild animals living in captivity and who are the members of the feral and fauna will also considered if the infections are because of their interrelation with humans or domestic animals.

Veterinary Virology

Veterinary virology and prion research has contributed greatly to our understanding of viruses and prions, the infections and diseases that they cause and their epidemiology and ecology. The importance of veterinary virology and prion research to animal health and the quality of our food supply is obvious and widely appreciated. However, the contributions of veterinary virology and prion research are not limited to animal health and the quality of our food supply. Veterinary virology and prion research has also had several major direct impacts in our understanding of human diseases. For example, many important human viruses or prions (or agents very closely related to them) were discovered by veterinarians, veterinary virologists, or prion researchers. Most human viruses and prions originate from animal agents that cross the so-called "species barrier" and became infectious to human beings. Research in animal viruses is therefore directly related to emerging human diseases. Veterinary virology and prion research has also led to many developments that directly impact human health.

For example, both traditional and modern rational vaccines were developed, or heavily influenced, by veterinary research. Veterinary viruses have also been used as surrogates of human viruses in the discovery and development of novel antiviral drugs and vaccines against human pathogens. Moreover, pathogenesis of human viral infections is also often studied by analyzing that of closely related veterinary viruses.

Veterinary virology is of course of paramount importance to animal health, which is in turn essential for the safety of our food supply. The viruses that infect any of the animal species used as major sources of protein in the human diet can all threaten human health and wellbeing. There is a low but concrete probability of viral pandemics in any of these animal species, which would have drastic impacts on the supply of proteins for the human diet. The latest outbreak of foot and mouth disease virus (FMDV) in the UK in 2001 is a good example of a geographically restricted but major disruption to the production of animal protein. In only 10 months, 581,802 heads of cattle (approximately 1 in 20), 3,487,014 of sheep (approximately 1 in 10), and 146,145 pigs in the UK were lost to the outbreak. Veterinary virology is therefore directly pertinent to the security of the food supply, importance which is obvious and widely recognized. However, veterinary virology also has direct impacts in human health, impacts which are not so often equally well appreciated.

Viruses and prions pose a major direct threat to global human health. Many viruses affecting humans are actually zoonotic, that is they infect animals and are maintained in animal reservoirs from which they spread to human beings. Old human viruses such as influenza are continuously re-entering into the human population from their animal reservoirs, with a low but concrete probability of producing another global pandemic. Such threat was just highlighted by the 2009 H1N1 strain, which most likely was recombined in pigs before being transmitted to humans. Other more recently identified viruses, such as hepatitis E (HEV), are most likely periodically transmitted to humans directly from their animal reservoirs. New human viruses or prions such as SARS, Nipah, or bovine spongiform encephalopathy (BSE, also known as "mad cow disease") also periodically enter into the human population from animal reservoirs. It is currently accepted in Public Health that "most new human infections are of animal origin." Before they enter into human populations, most viruses are therefore perpetuated in susceptible animals. Major outbreaks of animal disease can also provide a large source for the introduction of novel viral pathogens in the human population. For example, the large outbreak of BSE eventually resulted in the introduction of a new prion disease to humans, variant Creutzfeldt-Jakob disease (vCJD). Veterinary virology is consequently directly pertinent to emerging and established infectious human diseases.

Several animal viruses are also closely related to human viruses, being transmitted by similar routes, producing similar diseases, and being controlled by similar immune responses. Such animal viruses are therefore excellent models to study pathogenesis of, and therapeutic and preventive approaches against, the equivalent human viruses. This approach has been especially useful in the development of novel vaccines. It has also been useful to understand the pathogenesis of, and even developing drugs against, human viruses that infect no practical animal models, such as HCV or HIV. Veterinary virology is therefore also directly pertinent to our understanding of human disease, and to the development and testing of novel antiviral therapeutics or vaccines.

Scopes in Veterinary Sciences

Viral diseases constitute a continuous threat to human health. Viruses such as influenza continue to produce periodic epidemics and kill scores of human beings. Influenza is estimated to kill more than 36,000 people per year in the USA and 500,000 in the world. The flu pandemic of 1918 is estimated to have killed up to 1 in 20 people living at the time. The recent emergency of a novel H1N1 strain proves that new pandemics are likely to occur in the not so distant future. Viral diarrheas are one of the major causes of infant death in large parts of the world. They are estimated to cause 5 to 20 million infant deaths in Africa and Latin America per year. HIV has already killed more than 25 million people and it currently infects more than 33 million more (23 million of them in Sub-Saharan Africa). Hepatitis C virus (HCV) infects 3 to 4 million more people every year, resulting in 170 million infected people in the world and an estimated 1.7 million cases of liver cancer. New viral diseases are constantly threatening to enter into the human population and produce serious pandemics. Virology research is therefore essential to human health.

Veterinary sciences have played major roles in virology research since the very origins of the discipline. The search for novel infectious agents started immediately after the seminal works by Pasteur, Koch and their contemporaries had established the bases for the microbial theory of infectious diseases. A purely technical development, the Chamberland-Pasteur unglazed porcelain ultrafilter, resulted in the discovery that some infectious agents were much too small to be regular bacteria. Bacteria, parasites or fungi could be identified under the optic microscope, but infectivity was then the only property that allowed the identification and characterization other infectious agents. The infectivity of infectious agents of animals and plants could be readily tested, in contrast to that of human agents. In those early days, therefore, much progress was made on veterinary (and plant) viruses.

Tobacco mosaic virus, TMV, was the first infectious agent identified to be ultra-filterable, by Ivanofsky and Beijerinck Mayer had earlier shown that the disease could be transmitted by the "juice" of ground leaves of infected plants. However, these studies failed to consider the agent as a novel microorganism. Ivanofsky focused on potential technical aspects of ultracentrifugation, which he assumed had allowed bacteria to pass through the filter. Beijerinck instead did realize that the filterable agent was distinct from bacteria, but he considered the infectivity being in an infectious fluid (from which the name "virus" -poison- was derived). For such reasons, many refer to a virus of cattle, foot and mouth disease virus (FMDV), as the first to be discovered. Like Ivanofsky and Beijerinck had found before for TMV, Loeffler and Frosch (in collaboration with Koch) found the agent of FMDV to be ultra-filterable. But Loeffler and Frosch recognized the infection to be transmitted by a novel type of particulate agent much smaller than bacteria. FMDV is therefore often considered as the first virus to be identified. FMDV was without discussion the first mammalian virus identified, and the first virus shown to produce a known infectious disease in organisms other than plants.

Veterinary virology kept on playing a leading role in early virology. While many veterinarian viruses were being discovered, the first human virus, yellow fever virus, was identified only in 1901 and the second one, in 1907. At the end of the first decade after the discovery of FMDV, 13 animal and only 3 human viruses had been identified. Veterinary virology also took the lead in identifying many of the virus families that include the agents of important human diseases. The rabbit myxomavirus was the first poxvirus identified, 22 years before human poxviruses were even observed. Likewise, the swine pseudorabies virus (PRV) was the first herpesvirus identified, 17 years before the first human herpesvirus (herpes simplex type 1). Animal virology also identified the first picornavirus (FMDV), tumor virus, solid tumor virus, influenzavirus, alphavirus, papillomavirus, parvovirus, encephalitis virus, arenavirus, calicivirus and coronavirus, among others. For the first 60 years of virology, there was in fact no discrimination between veterinary and human virology. Such lack of discrimination was in no small part responsible for the explosive growth in virology knowledge during those yearly years.

Even after the early years, veterinary virology has continued playing major roles in the discovery of viruses that infect humans. In more recent years, the focus has been on the identification of emerging human viruses. Perhaps the most dramatic example is the discovery of Hendra virus as the causative agent of an outbreak that killed 14 horses and their trainer in Australia in 1994 (and half of all other human beings infected since then). A related virus, Nipah, caused a first outbreak in Malaysia in 1998-99, which killed 105 of the 265 people infected. Nipah has continued causing repeated outbreaks ever since, mostly in India and Bangladesh, with a mortality rate of approximately 75%. The latest outbreak was in 2007, but others will likely occur.

Hendra virus was discovered by veterinary virologists at the Animal Health Laboratory of CSIRO Livestock (Australia) as the causative agent of an outbreak of respiratory illness that affected an entire stable and killed 14 racing horses (and their trainer). Following on this work, Nipah was promptly identified as so closely related to Hendra that both viruses are commonly considered together. The group at the Animal Health Laboratory identified the ability of these viruses to infect a variety of domestic and laboratory animals and their routes of secretion. Most importantly from a human health perspective, they further progressed to identify fruit bats ("flying foxes" of the genus *Pteropus*) as natural reservoirs for these viruses, and horses and pigs as intermediate reservoirs in close proximity to humans. The more recent identification of the mechanisms whereby these viruses enter into cells may eventually result in the development of novel antiviral strategies to prevent infection with such viruses.

The veterinary virologists at the Animal Health Laboratory of CSIRO Livestock have even developed a potential vaccine that protects against these two pathogens. The vaccine showed solid protection of cats against lethal Nipah challenge. Therefore, veterinary virology was critical in identifying these two new human viruses. It was also critical in characterizing their ecology, thus helping to prevent further human infections, and in developing protective measures against infection with these viruses. Veterinary virology therefore continues to play a major role in the identification and characterization of novel viral pathogens that affect human beings.

Novel viruses are constantly introduced into the human population from their animal reservoirs, as recently shown by SARS and in the more distant past by Junin virus and HIV. In most cases, socio-ecological changes are the most likely cause of the exposure of humans to these new viruses. Deforestation, human settling in remote areas (often to enjoy an "undisturbed" landscape), ecotourism, increases in human population in countries with large previously uninhabited areas, a taste for exotic foods, and climate changes resulting in movement or displacement of wild animals to areas in closer contact with human beings, are all factors contributing to our current enhanced exposure to animal viruses. International travel for business, tourism, or to visit relatives leaving in different countries, is a major factor helping to promptly disseminate any new virus through the world. As none of these factors are likely to drastically change in the near future, our exposure to novel viral pathogens will continue to be exacerbated for the foreseeable future. It is estimated that approximately three quarters of all newly discovered human viruses come from animal reservoirs. Continuous research in veterinary virology is therefore essential to ensure that the required expertise will be available when the next animal virus is introduced into the human population.

Veterinary Bacteriology

The field of Veterinary Bacteriology plays a major role in veterinary medicine, human health, and economics. This overview describes representative bacteria that are pathogenic and can cause infectious diseases to animals. Others are potential infectious agents to humans, and they can threaten public health. In addition, the outcome of a disease may lead to an economic loss, especially for farm animals, wildlife, and companion animals.

Several major groups of bacteria are considered very significant in animal health and welfare. Some of these bacteria are very pathogenic, their severe pathogenicity cause different kinds and levels of infections to livestock, pets and wildlife. Generally, bacteria are classified according to Bergey's Manual into different groups. The classification is based on the specific characteristic features and uniqueness of the bacteria.

In veterinary bacteriology, it is very important to identify the nature of the bacteria that cause the infection in animals. There is a broad range of laboratory protocols, methods, and techniques that facilitate the microbiological analysis. Specimens should be obtained from infected animals. Consequently, the appropriate laboratory analysis will lead to the identification of the unknown bacteria that are the causative agent(s) for the infection.

Specimens for laboratory diagnosis include samples like blood, urine, feces, milk, semen, nasal discharge, wound or abscess swabs, aborted fetus, biopsy specimens and necropsy specimens. Samples for necropsy involve liver, kidney, brain, lymph nodes, spleen, lung, and even intestines. The laboratory methods and techniques start with a good sampling procedure, collection, and transportation of samples to the bacteriology laboratory. In most cases, it is essential to start with a direct microscopic examination for the sample. However, pure culture technique is a must.

In most of the laboratory investigations, *Grams Staining* is the first step to be considered. In this respect, the bacteria can be classified either gram-positive "purple color" or gram- negative "pink color". In certain cases, there is weak or no reaction with gram staining due to the lack of cell wall, as in mycoplasma. The results from gram staining will help to select further tests to identify the pathogen.

Pure culture techniques are very important and they are required to perform different tests. In pure culture, it is possible to obtain a single type of bacterial colony. This will facilitate the identification of the unknown microorganism. Some bacteria such as chlamydia and spirochaetes will not grow in laboratory media, but they require tissue cultures or laboratory animals to propagate their numbers.

The use of biochemical tests in bacterial identification is very helpful, and it is an important segment in the diagnostic laboratory. Biochemical tests involve carbohydrate, amino acid, and lipid metabolisms. In addition, these tests depend on the presence or absence of specific bacterial enzymes.

Oxygen requirements for bacterial growth vary according to the type of bacteria. Therefore, bacteria can be classified either aerobic as Bacillus anthracis, or facultative anaerobic as Escherichia coli, or anaerobic as Clostridium tetani, or microaerophilic as Mycobacterium bovis.

There are numerous immunological tests that are normally used in bacterial diagnostic laboratory. The tests are based on antibody-antigen reactions such as precipitation, agglutination, complement fixation and toxin neutralization. Other examples are fluorescent antibody techniques, and enzyme immunosorbent assay (ELISA). There are other valuable methods which assist in the identification and classification of bacteria; DNA base composition, polymerase chain reaction (PCR), and fatty acid profiles.

Animal Health

There are several bacterial diseases that can infect these animals. Infectious disease could be specific to one organ or system.

Cattle

Mastitis

Mastitis is inflammation of the udder. Udder infection in dairy cattle leads to a major economic impact. Etiology of the disease can be any of the following bacterial species that are potential pathogens. Species like Streptococcus agalactiae, Streptococcus dysgalactiae, and Streptococcus uberis are all gram-positive cocci arranged in chains. On the other hand, Staphylococcus aureus is also gram-positive cocci, but their arrangement is in clusters. Other pathogens that are considered to be causative agents in environmental mastitis are Escherichia coli and Enterobacter aerogenes -both are gram-negative short rods. Mycoplasma mastitis caused by some species belongs to the genus Mycoplasma. It is very contagious.

Collibacillosis

Collibacillosis is also known as calf scours. It is a disease that affects dairy and beef calves. The disease targets the intestinal tract and causes severe diarrhea. It is usually caused by Escherichia coli. Another bacteria that can cause scours is Salmonella spp. Collibacillosis is not limited to calves, but can also occur in piglets and lambs.

Foot Rot

Foot Rot in cattle is caused by *Fusobacterium necrophorum*. This bacterial species is aerobic gram-negative rods with variable lengths. The pathogen is usually acquired from soil and enters the body through skin abrasions and wounds. In addition, *F. necrophorum* can cause liver abscesses and mastitis.

Sheep

Enterotoxaemia

Enterotoxaemia in sheep usually affects lambs. This clinical condition is due to toxins produced by Clostridium perfringens. The bacterial species is anaerobic gram-positive rods, and endospore-forming. Type D affects lambs in feedlots. Other types of C. perfringens cause enterotoxemia in calves, kids, piglets, and foals.

Paratuberculosis

Paratuberculosis is also known as Johne's disease. It is a chronic infectious disease of sheep, goats, and cattle. Infection occurs when the animal ingests feed and water contaminated by fecal material of infected animals. On some farms, it is not unusual for Johne's disease to become endemic. The causative agent for the disease is *Mycobacterium paratuberculosis*. It is very slow growing, non-motile, gram-positive, and acid-fast positive (red in color). The shape of *M. paratuberculosis* is short straight non-branching rods. The bacterial arrangement is either in singles or clumps. Special growth media and lengthy incubation periods are required.

Infectious Necrotic Hepatitis

Infectious necrotic hepatitis in sheep is also known as black disease. It is a fatal disease caused by Clostridium novyi Type B, which are anaerobic gram-positive rods. The bacteria form endospores and produce exotoxins. The transmission of *C. novyi* occurs via ingestion. The infection usually follows initial destruction in the liver tissues. This destruction is mainly caused by young liver flukes, as a predisposing factor for the disease. In this respect, the exotoxins that are produced by *C. novyi* will be absorbed and cause more tissue damage in the liver. The exotoxins can circulate via blood and induce hemorrhages in different organs. Older sheep are most affected with a high mortality rate.

Pigs

Pneumonia

Pneumonia of pigs is also called enzootic pneumonia of swine. It is caused by Mycoplasma hyopneumoniae, a pathogen that lacks a cell wall. The disease is contagious and easily spread among pig farms. Sometimes, it can become complicated with the presence of other bacteria.

Atrophic Rhinitis

Atrophic rhinitis is another infectious disease in swine. The infection is due to the bacterial species Bordetella bronchiseptica. This pathogen is an aerobic gram-negative short rods, and β-hemolytic on blood agar plates. It causes chronic and debilitating disease in pigs. Bronchopneumonia is very common, and in young pigs may cause twisted snout.

Erysipelas

Erysipelas is a disease caused by Erysipelothrix rhusiopathiae. This bacterial species is gram-positive rods or pleomorphic and filamentous pending on its two types of colonies (smooth or rough). The bacteria are found on the mucous membrane of pigs and other animal species, and in contaminated soil and water. They can resist and survive adverse environmental conditions. The infection is transmitted via direct contact. The disease has more than one form; skin form also called diamond skin, the painful arthritic form, and the cardiac form.

Greasy Pig Disease

Greasy pig disease is caused by *Staphylococcus hyicus*, facultative anaerobic gram-positive cocci, producing DNAase enzymes, and forming non-pigmented colonies on plated culture media. In addition, it is non-hemolytic on blood agar plates. The disease is characterized with the formation of exudative and crusty skin lesions that can cover most of the body. It is highly contagious and it is more severe in young pigs. The infection is mainly through wounds or abrasions in the skin due to the fact that *S. hyicus* is always found on the pig's skin.

Critical Needs for Research in Veterinary Science

Research in veterinary science is critical to the protection of public health and the advancement of science that benefits both humans and animals as individuals and populations. Veterinary research includes studies on prevention, control, diagnosis, and treatment of diseases and on the basic biology and welfare of animals. It transcends species boundaries to include the study of spontaneous and experimental models of both human and animal disease and research at important human-animal interfaces, such as food safety, wildlife and ecosystem health, zoonotic diseases, and public policy.

The rich history of veterinary research, which includes studies on infectious disease and in other biomedical sciences, is replete with seminal contributions to the improvement of animal and human well-being. The many contributions of veterinary research were the results of society's recognition of its important role and society's subsequent support in the form of human, fiscal, and infrastructural resources. The current level of support for veterinary research, however, has not kept pace with the challenges posed by new and emerging threats and the nation's growing demands for knowledge in biomedicine and animal health. That society's needs are outgrowing our knowledge base is seen in examples of missed opportunities to safeguard and improve human and animal health and welfare.

The capacity of veterinary research depends on the availability of human and financial resources, research facilities, and infrastructure. Failure to provide the necessary resources could have devastating effects on both human and animal welfare, impede biomedical advances, and harm the economy and society as a whole.

Challenges for Veterinary Research

Veterinary research offers numerous opportunities for improving animal and human health, and unforeseeable challenges can be met best with a competent and properly equipped veterinary research community.

Public Health and Food Safety

Foodborne disease is a major cause of morbidity and mortality in the United States. Animals—both domesticated and wild—are frequent reservoirs of foodborne pathogens that can cause human illness. Human public health is affected not only by foodborne pathogens but also by the security of our food animals. A new awareness of the need for research on food and agricultural biosecurity arose after September 11 and the "anthrax letter" attacks later in 2001 because biosecurity research is closely related to maintaining safe agriculture and the food supply. Veterinary research on public health and food safety can contribute to:

- Improving detection and surveillance of foodborne pathogens associated with livestock and poultry production.
- Developing interventions to reduce their dissemination.
- Understanding the development and mechanisms of antibiotic resistance among foodborne pathogens associated with animals in the food chain.
- Developing preharvest and postharvest surveillance systems, diagnostic and detection systems, vaccines, immunomodulating drugs, animal and product tracking systems, and ecologically sound means of disposal of animal carcasses.
- Improving our ability to detect and identify disease and pathogens in animal populations and our understanding of interactions between pathogens and hosts so that effective preventive measures and countermeasures can be developed.

A concerted research effort can reduce the recurrence of food pathogens associated with livestock and poultry and ensure the security of our food supply.

Animal Health and Welfare

The increasing demand for veterinary research in animal health and welfare has several underlying causes:

- The perspective of the role of animals in human society and in the ecosystem has changed.
- A secure supply of food animals—such as poultry, cows, and fish—depends on their health.
- Some food-animal diseases affect human health directly (for example, some strains of high-pathogenicity avian influenza virus).
- Companion and service animals have an important role in human welfare.
- Laboratory animals are integral to our understanding of basic biology and physiology and are crucial for biological and medical advances.
- Wildlife health is important for the maintenance of the ecosystem and for the economy.
- Some emerging infectious diseases are associated with zoonoses (animal diseases that can be transmitted to humans).

Veterinary research is poised to improve human and animal health further through advances in preventive medicine, enhanced treatment for animal diseases, and a better understanding of transmission of zoonotic and other emerging diseases between wild and domestic animals and humans.

Comparative Medicine

Comparative medicine is the field that compares medical and scientific discoveries and knowledge of more than one animal species, including humans. Research in comparative medicine is invaluable for the overall medical research enterprise and for the improvement of animal health. Animal models used in biomedical research provide a whole-animal perspective that cannot be achieved at the molecular, cellular, or organ-system level. With technological advances, many new fields are emerging in comparative medicine, for example:

- Comparative genetics, which aims to develop reliable molecular markers of specific genetic traits to identify carrier and affected animals.
- Genome and phenome research that identifies specific genotypes associated with phenotypes.
- Stem-cell research and cloning.
- Genetically engineered animal models.
- Biomaterial developed to treat human and animal diseases.

Continuous progress in biomedical research will depend on our ability to develop and refine animal models to advance biomedical research, to preserve valuable models, and to improve methods for developing genetically engineered animal species other than the mouse to advance understanding of select diseases.

Research Agenda and Strategies

The especially compelling scientific opportunities to improve the quality of life of and minimize biological threats to animals and humans include the following:

- Implement the concepts of One Medicine and interdisciplinary and translational research in the broader biomedical research agenda.
    - Substantially improve the integration of molecular biology, genomics, immunology, whole-animal physiology, pathophysiology, and other disciplines in clinical disease research.
    - Encourage scientists, through grant-funding mechanisms and other means, to work collaboratively across disciplines, institutions, and agencies.
    - Encourage research institutions to foster research environments that nurture and reward successful team-oriented investigators and research.
    - Expand veterinary student involvement in ecosystem health and increase their opportunities to work collaboratively to study and understand complex systems and the intricate relationships between humans (individuals, cultures, and societies), animals (domestic and wild), and the environment.
- Set priorities for research to expand our knowledge, detection, and control of infectious diseases.
    - Emphasize classes of disease agents of the highest economic importance, including those most likely to cause massive epizootics or epidemics and new and emerging diseases and candidate bioterrorism agents.
    - Emphasize the study and eradication of laboratory animal diseases that adversely affect the quality of biomedical data.
    - Focus research on the molecular bases of virulence and on how pathogenic organisms replicate and survive in the environment, including studies of vector biology, wild-animal hosts and reservoirs, host defense factors, and host-pathogen interaction.
    - Develop and validate rapid, sensitive, reliable, and where possible quantitative systems for detecting and monitoring disease-causing organisms.
- Expand the study and use of bioinformatics and develop databases and other resources that are readily accessible to the scientific community to enable.
    - A population-level view of disease and research on the interaction between wildlife, domestic animals, and humans.
    - Tracking of pathogen prevalence in animals, including companion, food-producing, and laboratory animals.
    - Tracking of foodborne diseases.

    - Maximizing the sharing and efficiency of developing, preserving, and housing important rodent and other animal models.

- Quantify critical, scientifically based measures of animal health and welfare to optimize efficient, effective, sustainable, and socially responsible food-animal production and laboratory animal research.
- Expand research on the human-animal bond and the overall role of animals in society.

Although the different disciplines of veterinary research are grouped in three categories—public health and food safety, animal health and welfare, and comparative medicine—the disciplines are intertwined. For example, research in comparative medicine contributes to animal health through development of preventive medicine and treatment. Study of wildlife diseases contributes not only to wildlife health and conservation but also to public health because many human diseases are zoonotic. In short, veterinary research has interfaces with human and animal health and is interdisciplinary; therefore, collaborative and interdisciplinary research is crucial in translating scientific advances from one traditional discipline to another. However, such research may be hampered by administrative barriers, cultural barriers, and lack of economic resources. Agencies that support veterinary research have their own missions. When proposed interdisciplinary research is relevant to the mission of several agencies but does not perfectly fit the mission of any one agency, it can be difficult to get funding to support it.

The veterinary research community should facilitate and encourage collaborative research across disciplines, institutions, and agencies by reducing administrative barriers and by nurturing and rewarding successful team-oriented investigators. The community should encourage the development of a long-term national interagency strategy for veterinary research. The strategy could include a specific focus at the National Institutes of Health (NIH) on integrated veterinary research via the Roadmap initiative. NIH should consider having a veterinary liaison like the veterinary-medicine and public-health liaison at the Centers for Disease Control and Prevention (CDC) to help to ensure integration of veterinary and human medical research. Other federal agencies, state agencies, private foundations, and supporters of veterinary research should recognize and provide long-term support for collaborative, integrated veterinary research.

Addressing critical issues in veterinary science requires adequate human, infrastructure, and financial resources. The infrastructure and financial resources for the conduct of veterinary research in institutions that play a major role were examined and compared with the resources needed to do the research proposed to meet societal needs.

The National Research Council report "National Needs and Priorities for Veterinarians in Biomedical Research" projected a deficit of 336 veterinary pathologists in the United States and Canada in 2007, and the American College of Veterinary Pathologists reported needs for 149 veterinary pathologists in 2004. Similar human resource needs have been reported by the US Department of Agriculture (USDA), CDC, and the American College of Laboratory Animal Medicine. The shortage of veterinary researchers is due partially to declining interests in research among veterinary students, which in turn could be attributed to the following:

- The long period required to attain a DVM, a PhD, and postdoctoral training.

- The substantial tuition debt accrued during DVM training.
- The sparse financial support for graduate students in veterinary science.
- The brief exposure of veterinary students to basic science and research throughout their academic curriculum and internships.

The extended training could be partially addressed by establishing more combined-degree programs, and financial incentives could be provided to veterinary students interested in research through grants, fellowships, and possibly a loan-forgiveness program. However, stimulating students' interest in veterinary research may require a substantial change in the culture of colleges of veterinary medicine (CVMs). Academic faculties are driven to incorporate clinical learning processes into the early years of veterinary education and may not adequately integrate basic science and research in veterinary curricula. The capacity of academic veterinary curricula to incorporate and demand teaching of evidence-based medicine, including the use of research data and statistical analyses, will have a great impact on animal health and the mind-set of those who support it. A consequence of failure to train the next generation of veterinary researchers adequately is that opportunities for veterinary science to address public-health needs and to improve animal and human health will be missed. A strong workforce of veterinary researchers is needed to provide the data required for informed decisions in matters that govern day-to-day activity in animal health and welfare—decisions that underlie the economic stability necessary for adequate national animal health care. Veterinary research is essential to informed decision-making by policy-makers who aim to develop effective legislation and regulations based on sound science.

Additional veterinary researchers must be trained to alleviate the demands and to meet societal needs for veterinary research. A debt-repayment initiative similar to the NIH Clinical Research Loan Repayment Program could address concerns about the large debt burden faced by graduates of CVMs. If NIH's Center for Cancer Research training initiative in comparative pathology and biomedical sciences and USDA's Agricultural Research Service PhD training program for veterinarians prove to be successful in recruiting and retaining veterinary researchers, they could be expanded and used as models for other agencies and companies.

To meet the nation's needs for research expertise in veterinary science, changes in recruitment and programming for graduate and veterinary students will be required. Changes would involve enhancing research cultures in veterinary colleges and strengthening of summer research programs, combined DVM/PhD degree paths, and the integration of basic science into clinical curricula. The AVMA Council on Education, which is charged to review colleges of veterinary medicine for accreditation and publishes guidelines for the process, should strengthen the guidelines for assessment of research in regard to opportunities for research experiences for veterinary students. Research scientists in training should be made aware of national problems in animal health and welfare be given the opportunity to incorporate cutting-edge science into experimental design, and develop programs of high quality that compete nationally with other disciplines of science.

Increasing the veterinary research workforce requires an enlarged training capacity of educational institutions. The last major federal program to support construction of facilities for CVMs ended nearly 40 years ago. AAVMC has documented that 1,641,000 ft^2 of new and 611,000 ft^2 of renovated facilities are needed to train additional veterinary and graduate students to meet the demands of public practice. Space for classrooms, teaching, and research laboratories at all biosafety levels and housing for research animals is needed. Existing funding sources, such as state and university funds and gifts from foundations and private donors, are unlikely to meet the needs of the nation.

AAVMC and its members should identify ways in which the CVMs' facility needs can be met financially and logistically. They should consider mounting an extensive outreach effort to educate policy-makers in federal and state governments about the necessity of additional facilities to train adequate veterinary researchers.

The recommendations of the 1999 Strategic Planning Task Force on USDA Research Facilities and the provisions of HSPD-9 should be implemented immediately. Bio containment laboratories should receive special attention. Adequacies and shortfalls in facilities—federal and non-federal—needed to support veterinary research should be documented and quantified. Other research resources for veterinary research include libraries, databases, animal health monitoring and surveillance systems, electronic communication systems for sharing data and clinical information, specialized populations of animals, and collections of research materials, such as tissue samples. Effective communication among the various entities involved in veterinary research is needed to maximize the value of studies and to leverage the resources of the relatively small veterinary research community. In particular, databases with clinical records that can be exchanged among teaching hospitals, private practices, and diagnostic laboratories would provide data that could serve as valuable cost-efficient tools for retrospective and prospective research. Likewise, tissue samples and other specimens (for example, serum, DNA, and microorganisms) from both healthy and diseased animals offer exciting opportunities to study animal diseases and epidemiology if they are archived properly for research with client or owner confidentiality protected and made available to the research community. Of equal importance, surveillance systems that effectively and efficiently integrate animal health, food-product safety, and human health monitoring findings into user-friendly and easily accessed networks are needed.

The American Animal Hospital Association, AAVMC, and AVMA should address the need for more effective communication among the federal, university, and private sector entities involved in veterinary research. The need for databases, animal health monitoring and surveillance systems, specimen collections, and other sharable research tools to support veterinary research should receive special attention. Organization of a working task force or national workshop to devise an operating plan for developing and managing these clinical and research databases and collections and to identify methods for their support would be an important first step toward the formation of national databases and archives (such as specimen banks and clinical databases) for veterinary research.

In addition to databases and tissue samples, many disciplines in veterinary research have benefited substantially from access to well-characterized animal colonies with known diseases. Preserving the genomes of those unique model animals is critical to facilitate research in animal diseases. The genetic similarity between humans and other animals is a compelling argument that studies with such animals would reveal both normal and abnormal pathways and mechanisms. Those animal colonies are imperative for integrative physiology and pathophysiology studies.

NIH and USDA should address the importance of engineered and spontaneous model colonies of animals and ensure that these valuable resources are not lost. This can be accomplished for some species by cryopreservation and preservation of their germ plasma in tissue banks until it is needed for funded, targeted research or by transfer of their genetic mutations into smaller laboratory species. For other species, maintenance of the whole animal may be necessary.

A review of the organizations that are most likely to fund veterinary research reveals that some research disciplines do not have an identifiable source of financial support from government agencies. Those disciplines include ecological research on zoonotic emerging diseases, dynamics of select agent, biodefense pathogens in wildlife, companion-animal and equine research, wildlife and conservation research, and zoo animal and exotic-pet research. Those disciplines contribute to animal health and welfare and to important elements of human health research or have direct human social impact, but they do not have dependable, permanent financial resources that would ensure their continuing advancement in research.

The veterinary research community should actively engage NIH, USDA, the Department of the Interior, the National Science Foundation, and other federal agencies and urge them to recognize and address the need for financial support for the disciplines of veterinary research that lack identifiable sources of federal funding despite their contributions to public health, comparative medicine, and animal health and welfare.

Chapter 2

Veterinary Anatomy

The branch of veterinary science which is involved in the study of the form and structure of animals is termed as veterinary anatomy. Some of the different branches of veterinary anatomy are canine anatomy, equine anatomy, cow anatomy and avian anatomy. The topics elaborated in this chapter will help in gaining a better perspective about the anatomy of these types of animals.

Veterinary anatomy is the study of the internal biological structures and systems of animals, including the respiratory, cardiovascular, reproductive and neurological systems. Veterinary physiology is the scientific investigation of animals' biological systems, along with how these systems operate.

Imaging Technology within Anatomy and Physiology

In the days of the first anatomists and physiologists discussed above, fewer tools and techniques were available to allow visualisation of the body. Over the years many techniques have been developed by scientists that have been essential for veterinary and human anatomists and physiologists alike. Dissection and drawing were always essential skills and are still used today. As the first microscopes were developed the ability to see within the tissue and cell both anatomy and physiology were advanced, alongside medical practice. The first modern microscope developed by Hans and Zacharias Janssen in 1590 has certainly changed over the years. There is also much evidence to suggest the use and theories on early microscopes and lens magnification from early China 4000 years ago and even the ancient Greeks and Romans. Hooke also designed a microscope and wrote the now famous 'Micrographia' and Antonie van Leeuwenhoekthe Father of the Microscope developed this work and his publications to the Royal Society were validated by none other than Hooke. The modern microscope has advanced greatly with optical microscopy utilising a nonlinear optical phenomenon, electron microscopy, confocal microscopy and even hand held microscopes now available for the pursuit of anatomical, physiological and medical research and diagnosis.

Since the discovery of X-rays, developments in medical imaging have provided a powerful tool of investigation allowing visualisation of the body in detail never before seen. The combination of postmortem cadaveric dissection and imaging techniques of live patients has proven to be an important technique in understanding the anatomy and physiology of the live animal.

1895 saw X-rays observed for the first time by German physicist Wilhelm Roentgen. By imaging his wife's hand, Roentgen deducted that bone and metal were opaque on radiographs and medical uses of the technology quickly followed. Marie Curie used a portable X-ray unit to visualise skeletal trauma in soldiers on French battlefields. Whilst, the use of X-ray crystallography was vital in understanding the genetic code, which in turn has had an enormous impact upon the understanding of physiology.

In later years, Godfrey Hounsfield expanded the use of X-rays by developing computer software that could integrate multiple radiographic images to give a three-dimensional view inside the body. This was the discovery of computed tomography (CT). CT had a significant advantage over radiographs alone as it allowed the distinction of different soft tissue types to be visualised. In 1971 the first CT scan of patient took place, successfully scanning the brain for a tumour in the frontal lobe. The invention of CT had vital practical applications, and as a result, Hounsfield was awarded the Nobel Prize for Physiology or Medicine in 1979.

The risks of using ionising radiation were acknowledged, particularly regarding imaging of the foetus, and as such, a reduction in use of X-rays was seen and replacement with ultrasonography and magnetic resonance imaging occurred. Ian Donald pioneered the use of ultrasound in obstetrics and gynaecology in a paper published in 1958. Since this time, two-dimension ultrasound techniques have been significantly developed and three-dimension ultrasound can map and quantify blood flow. Ultrasound has been a critical milestone for medical imaging and a fundamental method of non-invasive research.

However, the breakthrough of magnetic resonance imaging (MRI) has become a vital diagnostic and research tool in recent years. Nuclear magnetic resonance was originally discovered by Felix Bloch and Edward Purcell in 1946 and formed a foundation for the development of modern day MRI. The use of NMR was developed by Paul Lauterbur when he applied gradients to magnetic fields to create a two-dimensional image and Sir Peter Mansfield developed methods of slice selection and creating and interpreting images. These advance resulted in the development of MRI as we know it now and the men shared the Nobel Prize in Medicine or Physiology in 2003. MRI is an important medical imaging tool, using no ionising radiation and providing a practical alternative to invasive procedures.

A recent development in imaging is that of imaging mass spectrometry that allows tissue samples to be visualised on a molecular level without labelling with chemicals or antibodies. The mass spectrometry imaging technology was developed by a group of physicists, including Caprioli and the technique is particularly sensitive for use on proteins and peptides. This technology however cannot map the transcriptome and a new technique, mass spectrometric imaging, has been developed as a result.

Moving forwards, it is predicted that radiography will progress to tomography based methods as opposed to projection based and molecular imaging may become more popular. It is also very likely that the field of imaging will continue to develop and give us deeper insights into anatomy and physiology. Imaging is a key part of both anatomy and physiology but by no means the only tool used. We can see the advances made in imaging but many tools have either developed over the years or been discovered in more recent years. Genetics has revolutionised the worlds of anatomy and physiology for example. Understanding cellular and molecular biology alongside anatomy and physiology has become essential in the research we undertake today. Anatomy seeks to understand the structure, location and composition of the parts within organisms and their relationships with each other. Physiology seeks to understand the functions and processes of organisms, how they work and ultimately assist with understanding and treating diseases and disorders. Therefore whilst imaging is essential for both of these practices, the continued development and discovery of more tools are needed in order to further our research. Much of the work in this book uses these techniques, or a combination of them in the pursuit of advancing anatomical and physiological knowledge and understanding.

Respiratory System in the Animals

The respiratory systems from different groups of animals, although morphologically different, have in common the following characteristics: they have a large capillary network, the gas exchange surfaces are thin and moist; constant renewal of oxygen-rich fluid (air or water) order to provide oxygen and remove carbon dioxide; free movement of blood within the capillary network. According to Atwood, the assumptions stated above, are present either external respiration is carried out by: 1) cutaneous diffusion (earthworm and some amphibians), 2) by thin tubes called tracheae (some insects), 3) by gills, the respiratory system of fish or 4) by diffusion through the lungs, respiratory organs present in amphibians, reptiles, birds and mammals.

Respiratory Organs in Vertebrates

The steps of the evolution of terrestrial vertebrates are: change from anaerobic to aerobic life, accretion of unicells into multicellular organs, formation of a closed circulatory system, evolution of metal-based carrier pigments that improved oxygen uptake, formation of invaginated respiratory organs, physical translocation from water to land, development of a double circulation and progression from ectothermic-heterothermy to endothermic-homeothermy. In vertebrates, the blood performs the task of transporting oxygen to the cells and carbon dioxide to the external environment.

The development of the respiratory organs of vertebrates is closely related to the primitive pharynx, since the gills of aquatic vertebrates and the lungs of terrestrial vertebrates and aquatic mammals have pharyngeal embryology origin.

In all vertebrates, at a certain stage of their development, arise bilaterally in craneo-caudal direction from the inner side of the pharynx, a series of diverticula, which evaginate towards the outer surface, forming the pharyngeal pouches. The number of pharyngeal pouches is greater in lower vertebrates, reaching fourteen in cyclostomes and only four or five in birds and mammals. The pharyngeal pouches are separated by masses of mesenchyme that have the designation of pharyngeal arches, in which is located an arterial structure, called the aortic arch, which extends from the ventral aorta to the dorsal aorta.

During the ontogenesis of higher vertebrates, the pharyngeal pouches fail to open to the outside, contrarily to what happens in fish and, temporarily, in amphibians. Thus, in higher vertebrates, the pharyngeal pouches just remain during the embryonic period, where they undergo several changes, but very few or none of their initial characteristics are presented in adults. In amniotes, as in humans, only the first pair of pharyngeal pouches remains, giving origin bilaterally, the eustachian tube and middle ear.

Respiratory System in Fish

The fish gill adapted a structure for extraction of oxygen from water that is formed by a large number of filaments spaced out along the gill arches on either side of the pharynx. Each filament has a series of plates projecting at right angles from its upper and lower surfaces, the secondary lamellae, which are extremely numerous, are the site of gaseous exchange and form a fine sieve which ensures that all the water comes into close contact with the blood.

The gills are multifunctional organs that are responsible for the gas exchange (respiration) but also for the osmoregulation, acid-base regulation, and excretion of nitrogenous waste.

The epithelial surface of a gill arch is structurally and functionally zoned. The filaments are covered by two distinct epithelial surfaces, the lamellar and filament epithelia, also termed the secondary and primary epithelia respectively. Gas exchange occurs through the secondary lamellae, and the non-respiratory functions of the gills take place in the primary epithelium.

The primary epithelium contains the chloride cells, which vary in morphology and number according to the milieu where the fish lives. The presence of an accessory cell beside the chloride cell is characteristic of seawater or seawater- adapted fish. The secondary epithelium that covers the free part of the secondary lamellae has an exclusive relationship with the arterioarterial vasculature, i.e., the pillar cells. This epithelium consists of an outermost layer of pavement cells that exhibits structural characteristics suggestive of cell coat secretion and an innermost layer of less differentiated cells. In contrast to the primary epithelium, the secondary epithelium does not exhibit any obvious differences between freshwater and seawater fish.

The lamellar structure helps to increase the surface area but depends on the following complex anatomy to maintain the flat space necessary for circulation: separation between epithelial sheets (by pillar cells) and connection between the basal lamina of epithelial sheets by groups of strands (collagen columns).

To prevent ballooning and to ensure the sheet-flow dynamics of blood, the two layers of respiratory epithelium are connected by many strands of extracellular matrix (ECM) materials, which are called collagen columns. These columns, made of collagen fibers, are essential for reinforcing the lamellae structure and the internal force of blood pressure. Since collagen triggers the coagulation cascade when exposed to blood, the collagen columns are surrounded by the plasma membrane of pillar cells, which isolate them from circulation.

In the interface between pillar cells and collagen columns, exist adhesion junctions termed as "column junctions" and "autocelullar junctions", both of which are essential constituents of the gill lamellae. The "column junctions" is a cell-ECM adhesion and "autocelullar junctions" a membrane-membrane adhesion, both involved in maintaining structural integrity and hemodynamic of branchial lamellae.

The pillar cells have a spool-shape and possess a cylindrical cell body connecting two parallel sheets of respiratory epithelium. They also enfold 5 to 8 collagen columns and have numerous myofilaments, parallel to the collagen columns, which consist of actin and myosin, which form the contractile apparatus of the cell.

The pillar cells are a type of endothelial cells that delimits a network of vascular compartments within the lamellae of gill fish, but since they share characteristics with smooth muscle cells, we can say that these cells are specialized vascular cells with characteristics of both endothelial and smooth muscle cells.

The contractile apparatuses of the pillar cells possibly prevent collagen columns from being stretched and provide plasticity to the vascular network of the lamella against changes in blood pressure. Other possible function for the contractile structures of the pillar cells is that they can change the diameter of the vascular channels, and therefore contribute to the regulation of blood flow through the lamellae. Besides the pillar cells, the gill epithelium of freshwater fishes have pavement cells (also termed as respiratory cells in older literature), mucus cells, neuro-epithelial cells and chloride cells.

The neuroepithelial cells are isolated or clustered on the internal side of the primary lamellae facing the respiratory water flow. They are probably involved in local and central modulation of the branchial functions by interacting with the branchial nervous system and by paracrine secretion of substances such as serotonin. These cells share several morphofunctional features with the cells of the neuroepithelial bodies in the lungs of air-breathing vertebrates.

The chloride cells are described as large, granular, acidophilic and mitochondria-rich cells and exhibit an extensive tubular system emanating from the basolateral membrane, an array of sub-apical vesicles, large ovoid nucleus and abundance of Na^+, K^+ -ATPase enzyme. There is a marked difference between species in the structure of the apical membrane of chloride cells which precludes their absolute identification.

They are located in the primary epithelium in close proximity to the blood vessels and are sites of active chloride secretion and high ionic permeability, performing an integral role in acid-base regulation. As in other vertebrates, fish must maintain homeostasis of intra and extracellular pH and therefore use the parallel strategies of buffering and excretion to defend against pH changes. During alkalosis conditions, the area of exposed chloride cells is increased, which serves to enhance base equivalent excretion as the rate of Cl^-/ HCO_3- exchange is increased. Conversely, during acidosis, the chloride cells surface area is diminished by an expansion of the adjacent pavement cells, and this response reduces the number of functional Cl^-/HCO_3- exchangers.

Under softwater or toxic conditions, chloride cells proliferate on both surfaces of the gill and might impair gas transfer owing to a thickening of the lamellar blood-to-water diffusion barrier. Water enters through the fish's mouth and out through the gill, slits in a direction that is opposite to the blood flow in the gill, providing a constant renewal of the oxygen supply in contact with the respiratory organ.

The exchange of oxygen and carbon dioxide takes place by diffusion from the surrounding water and the blood that flows within the capillary network of the gills, and because of this countercurrent flow fish can extract 80 to 90% of dissolved oxygen in water.

During the larval development of fish, the teleosts in particular, the skin is the cutaneous surface that ensures gas exchange, and only in the final stage of this period begins the hematosis through the gills, when the muscle-skeleton structure of the oral cavity becomes able to coordinate food intake with the flow of water through the branchial system.

Lungfishes

Changing conditions of life imposed new requirements on the morphology and physiology of the organisms. One of these changes is the evolutionary transition from aquatic to terrestrial life, leading to adaptations in locomotion, breathing, hearing, mechanism for food capture and other functions.

The first air-breathing vertebrates were fishes, and a Devonian air-breathing sarcopterygian (lobe-fin) occupies the basal position in the lineage extending from the Paleozoic fishes to the most derived tetrapods.

The evolution of tetrapods from sarcopterygian fish is one of the major transformations in the history of life and involved numerous structural and functional innovations. The Styloichthys changae, one fossil of sarcopterygian fish, exhibits the character combination in a stem group close to the last common ancestor of tetrapods and lungfish.

The recent discovery of a well-preserved species of fossil sarcopterygian fish form in the late Devonian of Arctic Canada, that represents an intermediate between fish with fins and tetrapods with limbs, provides unique insights into how and in what order important tetrapod characters arose. The morphological features and geological setting of this new animal are suggestive of life in shallow-water, marginal and subaerial habitats.

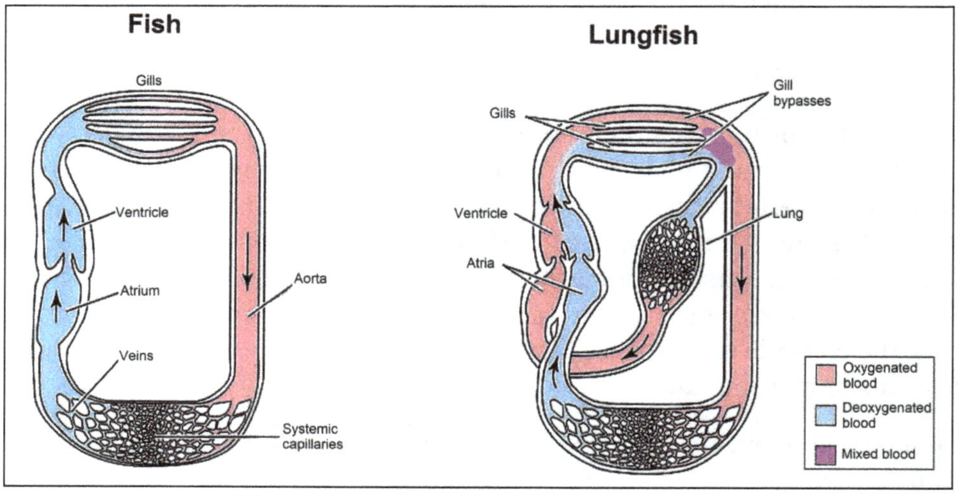

Blood flow in oxygenation system in fish and lungfish.

The relevance of the extant air-breathing fishes as models for events in the Paleozoic has been a recurring theme for more than one century. The lungfish is considered homologous to the lungs of all higher vertebrates and the precursor of the enteleost gas bladder.

In our days the lungfish are represented by three genera, the Australian lungfish, Neoceratodus forsteri, and the other two genera: the African (Protopterus) and South American (Lepidosiren) lungfish. The Australian Neoceratodus differ from the other lungfish because they breathe air for short periods and for this reason the lung is an accessory organ which is only used during periods of high activity in its natural habitat. They have efficient gills and possess only a single lung, unlike both Protopterus and Lepidosiren which have paired lungs and much reduced gills.

The lung of N. forsteri consists of a single elongated chamber compartmentalized by a thick cartilaginous structural framework. The epithelial lining of these supporting structures comprised abundant capillaries interspersed with cells resembling alveolar type II and type I cells. These epithelial cells which appear to be the only cell type lining the gas-diffusing surface, have long cytoplasmic plates bearing microvilli, which form part of the gas-exchange membrane. The cells contain large numbers of osmiophilic bodies resembling mammalian lamellar bodies, and it is possible that these lungfish cells may be the common ancestral cell for the alveolar type I and II found in the mammalian lung. They also have a surfactant-like material containing both SP-A and SP-B like proteins, suggesting that even in this primitive lung, these proteins are still involved in surfactant homeostasis.

To breathe air the Neoceratodus may raise to surface, exhale through the mouth, inhale and dive forward or rise to the surface, breathe and reverse back into the water.

Protopterus and Lepidosiren are bimodal breathers, that use both gills and lungs for respiratory gas transfer, but they are obligate breathers because they die if denied access to air. The Protopterus occupy a variety of habitats both lentic (standing water) and lotic (running water) and possess the capacity to aestivate, reducing their metabolic rate, which allow them to survive to extreme heat or for long dry periods. In the Protopterus, the gills and skin uptake only 10% of the total O_2 uptake and these structures are much more effective in removing the CO_2.

The reedfish Calamoichthys calabaricus is one of the phylogenetically most primitive extant air-breathing fishes, and represents an animal successfully adapted not only for air breathing but also for making short-term use of terrestrial environments. In this primitive living actinopterygian fish the oxygen uptake is achieved by the gills, skin and a paired lungs and in the total volume oxygen uptake, the lungs account for 40%, the gills 28%, and the skin 32%.

In the Lepidosiren 99.15% of the total diffusing capacity lies in the lungs, 0.85% in the skin and only an insignificant 0.0013% in the gills, which shows that the gills don't have any importance as a gas exchange organ in this species. Oxygen uptake is accomplished by the lungs and dioxide carbon is eliminated by the skin.

The structure of the gills lamellae of Lepidosiren consists of a stratified epithelium that rests on the basal membrane and has at least three layers of cuboidal cells with large nuclei. Close to the epithelium there are numerous capillaries.

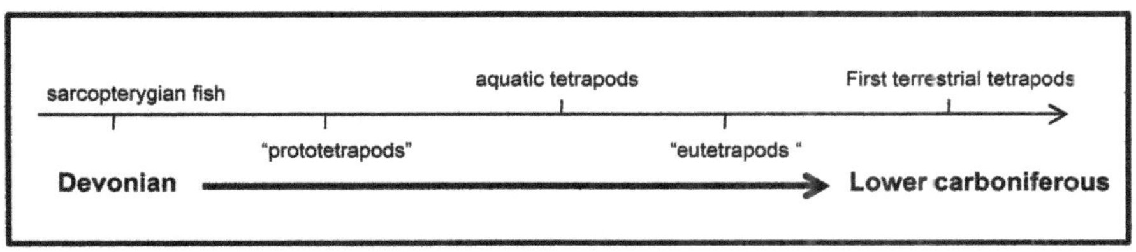

Tetrapods evolution

Each lung of these lungfish has a main duct and numerous chambers of different sizes, which decrease in size as they progress caudally. The honeycomb-like edicular parenchyma is disposed in these chambers and most chambers contain a central lumen, which connects with the air duct. The duct, the chambers and edicular parenchyma consist of connective tissue septa held upright by smooth muscular/elastic trabeculae and are supplied and drained by branches of the pulmonary artery and vein. Most interedicular septa have a double capillary net. The air-blood barrier consists of three layers: a simple squamous epithelium made up of a single type of cell, the endothelial cells of the blood capillaries and the combined basal lamina of the epithelial and endothelial cells.

The skin of these fish has two layers, the epidermis and the dermis. The epidermis consists of a stratified epithelium with six to ten layers of diverse cell types. Most prominent are superficially located cuboidal cells with a large central nucleus and the mucous cells that are dispersed among the other cell layers. The dermis is a dense connective tissue, with blood vessels and small ossified scales. Numerous blood capillaries and melanophores lie beneath the basal membrane and between the subjacent layers.

In the Protopterus and Lepidosiren the ventilation of the gills occurs through the action of a positive pressure buccal pump anterior to the gills and an opercular suction pump posterior to the gills. These pumps generate a nearly continuous water pressure gradient favouring a water flow in the mouth, through the gills and out the opercular opening. The ventilation of the lungs in Protopterus is achieved by the same musculoskeletal elements involved in aquatic ventilation, the buccal force pump mechanisms.

Early in their history, fish developed supplementary air breathing organs in two taxonomic lines – Actinopterygians and Sarcopterygians. The onset of aerial respiration in primitive fish was an important milestone in the evolution of terrestrial vertebrates.

The fish-tetrapod transition was one of the greatest events in the vertebrate evolution. Tetrapods first appeared in the late Devonian about 360 million years ago, but appear to have been primarily aquatic animals. For some investigators the freshwater origin of tetrapods remains the most likely scenario, but several recent findings raise the possibility that the tetrapod land invasion could come from a marine habitat.

The evolution of tetrapods occured under environmental influences and presumption that hypoxia habitat conditions were similar to those commonly encountered in tropical lowland habitats during dry seasons.

The sequence of evolution begun with sarcopterygian fish, followed by the appearance of a "prototetrapods" (e.g. Elginerpeton), the emergence of aquatic tetrapods (e.g. Acanthostega), the appearance of "eutetrapods" (e.g. Tulerpeton) and the first truly terrestrial tetrapods (e.g. Pederpes) in the lower Carboniferous. Several morphological changes were observed during the evolution process, developing specialized features that allowed land locomotion and air breathing.

The sudden change from gill respiration to lung breathing would pose considerable physiological problems. One of the consequences of gill loss, would be the concentration of respiratory CO_2 within the body, which required buffering by bicarbonate ion and affected processes such as acid-base balance, O_2 binding by haemoglobin, ventilation rate, respiratory control and also affected nitrogen excretion, ion regulation and water balance, vital processes that would need to be assumed by others organs.

The advantages of tetrapod gill loss included head mobility, development of hearing and the origin of different ventilatory and feeding mechanisms.

In the primitive pure buccal pumping, found in most air- breathing fishes, including lungfishes, the axial musculature does not contribute to expiration or inspiration. In fact, the buccal pump breathing has been proposed to constrain the evolution of tongue morphology and head shape.

The aspiration breathing was present in some early tetrapods, but it only arised when the early amniotes appeared. Aspiration breathing evolved in two steps: first, from pure buccal pump breathing to the use of axial muscles for expiration and buccal pump for inspiration; second, to pure aspiration-breathing, in which axial muscles are used for both expiration and inspiration.

The musculoskeletal units responsible for breathing also serve other functions such as feeding or locomotion, and the conflicting mechanical requirements of multiple functions possibly constrain the performance and evolution of one or both functions. The evolution of aspiration breathing may have allowed the musculoskeletal systems of the head and tongue of amniotes to diversify, but the ribs and intercostal musculature became constrained by their dual function in aspiration breathing and high speed locomotion.

The loss of gills is also in connexion to the cutaneous respiration as a site gaseous exchange which can function in water and land.

So, the possible evolution of the respiratory mechanisms maybe begun with an ancestral fish adapted for oxygen uptake and CO_2 elimination in aquatic medium, but under conditions of low oxygen, developed adaptations that allowed the fish to come to the surface to obtain extra oxygen from the air, but the gills still functioned for CO_2 elimination.

At this stage of evolution, the skin would function mainly for CO_2 elimination and, as the lung became more efficient and more involved, not only in uptake of oxygen but also in elimination of carbon dioxide, the skin became less important and probably covered with hardened scales to reduce water loss and the animal could now remain away from water for longer periods. It seems possible to accept that the cutaneous respiration was important for the earliest land vertebrates.

Respiratory Organs in Amphibians

Based on paleontological criteria, the first amphibians have arisen by evolution of fish Crossopterígeos ripidistios, extinct in the late Devonian period.

Modern amphibians occupy a central position in understanding the fundamental changes that have occurred in the evolution of air breathing. Dual subsistence in water and land has required development of certain respiratory adaptations.

The transition from aquatic to land environment exposed the gas exchange organ to a much richer oxygen ambience, which allowed a drastic reduction in the ventilation requirements, but at the same time created problems for the disposal of carbon dioxide, because at 20 °C the water solubility of this gas is 28 times greater than that of oxygen.

To prevent a severe respiratory acidosis, the Terran animal began to use the skin as an important respiratory organ, designed especially for the removal of carbon dioxide, which required a substantially reduction of the barrier represented by the scales that covered the surface of their aquatic ancestors. At the same time there must have occurred an increased bicarbonate concentration in plasma, in order to compensate the increase of carbon dioxide.

These animals are mainly characterized for presenting an aquatic larval form, the tadpole stage, where hematosis takes place through the gills. Next they suffered a metamorphosis that allowed them to reach adulthood in terrestrial habitat and in which the breathing air was carried out by the lungs, skin and mouth. The amount of cutaneous and buccal gas exchange and its percentage in the total gas exchange, varied from species to species and also during seasons.

Amphibians have the simplest lungs, rudimentary lungs that are adequate for ectothermic and low aerobic metabolism animals.

The paired lungs of recent amphibians are unicameral lying in the dorsal pleuroperitoneal cavity. In the various amphibian species the lungs differ greatly in size, their topographic extension and the dimension of exchange surface by the development of interconnected folds with highly varying number of subdivisions and height of their folds. The highly varying extent in lung exchange is due to differences in the amount of gas exchange performed by via lungs in concert with cutaneous and buccal cavity exchange.

Moreover, the absence of an individualized chest well, with no ribs or diaphragm, the amphibian's pulmonary ventilation is mainly accomplished at the expense of swallowing air, carried out by rising of the oral cavity floor.

The remarkable heterogeneity of the morphology of the amphibian gas exchangers matches that of the diversity of the environments in which the animals live, the lifestyle they pursue, and their pattern of interrupted development. The skin is the main pathway for gas transfer in aquatic species while in terrestrial ones; it has been relegated or rendered redundant.

In the salamanders (Plethodontidae), some of which live in cold well-aerated waters, gas exchange occurs across the skin and buccal cavity. Skin breathing is important in all extant amphibians but is the only means of gas exchange in those salamanders (terrestrial and aquatic) which possess neither lungs nor gills. Gas exchange takes place in the dense subepithelial capillary network, the inflow to which is in part from the arterial system and in part from a branch of the pulmonary arch carrying venous blood. The oxygenated cutaneous blood flows into the venous system. This is in contrast to the arrangement of pulmonary outflow in tetra- pods and lungfish which allows (complete or partial) separation of oxygenated from venous blood.

The caecilians (Apoda) possess long, tubular lungs, but in some species the left lung is remarkably reduced or totally missing. The lungs of caecilians are internally sub- divided, forming air cells that are supported by diametrically placed trabeculae.

In the newts (Urodela), animals that are mostly aquatic, the lungs are poorly vascularised with the internal surface being smooth. Lungs of most amphibians such as Amphiuma tridactum and the cane toad, Bufo marinus, have an abundance of smooth muscle tissue, a feature that may explain the high compliance of the lungs. In Amphiuma, during expiration, the lung virtually collapses, producing an almost 100% turn-over of inspired air. Amphiuma is aquatic but has very well developed lungs.

The lungs of terrestrial species are highly elaborate pre- senting a series of stratified septa that divided the lung into small air cells and the lungs of Anura and Apoda are more complex than those of Urodela.

Respiratory Organs in Reptiles

It is assumed that reptiles made their appearance on Earth about 310 million years ago, and their adaptation was so perfect that they dominated the planet for over a hundred million years. The innumerous fossils that have been dis- covered allow us to group them in a numerous orders capable for living in different habitats, such as land, air or aquatic environment.

Reptilians are the first vertebrates adequately adapted for terrestrial habitation and utilization of lungs as a sole pathway for acquisition of oxygen. The skin that was no longer necessary for gas exchange became an armor to protect against dehydration, being waterproof, dry, covered with keratinized epidermal scales or developing dermal bone plates.

Compared with their gigantic prehistoric ancestors, cur- rent reptiles are small and insignificant and can be grouped in four orders: chelonians, such as turtles and tortoises; rincocéfalos, like Sphenodon of New Zealand; crocodiles (crocodiles and caimans) and squamata order (lizards and snakes).

The reptilian display great pulmonary structural heterogeneity and there is no single model of reptilian lung. Based on complexity of internal organization, different classification suggested that the turtles, monitor lizard, crocodiles and snakes have a profusely subdivided (multicameral) lung, the chameleons and iguanids have a simpler (paucicameral) lung and the teju lizard (Tupinambis nigropunctatus) have a saccular, smooth-walled, transparent (unicameral) lung.

Division of the lumen of the lung into a number of chambers, by septation, enlarges the exchange area, fact that is observed in turtles, lizards and crocodiles.

The lungs are localized in the pleuroperitoneal cavity and there is no diaphragm separating the thoracic from the abdominal cavity. Presence of ribs and intercostal muscles in reptiles, allow the development of more effective pulmonary ventilation than that of the amphibians which do not have these anatomical structures.

Generally, the pattern of organization of the respiratory system of reptiles is identical to mammals, with the lungs coated externally by a serosa. The conducting portions are supported by complete cartilaginous rings, which continue through the extra and intrapulmonary bronchi. The branching of the bronchial intrapulmonary tree in reptiles is similar to mammals, however they have specific designations, which appear sequentially bronchus, tubular chambers, niches and aedicules.

The intrapulmonary bronchi of the reptiles that give immediate access to respiratory areas correspond to the mammalian respiratory bronchioles, the tubular chambers, according to their position and morphofunctional structure, are equivalent to the alveolar channels in mammals, and the niche are similar to alveolar sacs. By its position in the respiratory system and anatomical constitution the aedicules are equivalent to the alveoli of mammals, however they have an oblong structure compared with the spherical form of mammal's alveoli.

The intrapulmonary bronchi of turtles that live essentially in aquatic environment have a reinforcement that extends to or near the respiratory areas, characteristic that is similar to the aquatic mammals that have the ability to dive to great depths, such as seals, dolphins and whales. This reinforcement, along with the presence of a smooth muscle, appears to be adaptations that allow these animals to support the high pressures to which they are subjected during the immersion to great depths.

The epithelium of the trachea and bronchi is pseudo- stratified columnar ciliated, with non-ciliated secretory cells and basal cells, all in direct contact with the basal membrane. Isolated or groups of neuroendocrine cells were also identified within the conducting portion of the lung of turtles and crocodiles.

The epithelial cells lining the respiratory surface of reptilian lungs are differentiated into type I and type II cells and it is possible to observe multilamellar bodies similar to those present in mammals. These suggest that also in reptiles occurs the synthesis of surfactant lipo-protein material responsible for the stability of their respiratory unit, the aedicula.

The role of surfactant in reptiles, which are not highly susceptible to collapse from surface tension forces, is obscure, and may have other important functions such as prevention of transendothelial transudation of blood plasma across the blood-gas barrier, immune suppression and attraction of macrophages. Reptilian lungs have preponderance of smooth muscle tissue and this tissue has been associated with intrapul- monary connective movement of air.

Respiratory System in Birds

Birds' respiratory system, the lung – air sac system, is the most complex and efficient gas exchanger that has evolved in air-breathing vertebrates. The compact and virtually constant-volume avian lung has been totally uncoupled from the compliant, avascular air sacs.

The main properties that impart high respiratory efficiency on the lung–air sac system of birds are a cross-current design and inbuilt multicapillary serial arterialisation system; auxiliary counter-current system; large tidal volume; large cardiac output; continuous and unidirectional parabronchial ventilation; short pulmonary circulatory time; superior morphometric parameters; a particularly large respiratory surface area and a remarkably thin blood-gas (tissue) barrier.

Their respiratory system allows them to breathe at altitudes that can reach nine thousand meters without acclimatization, fact that is impossible for humans and other mammals, in which the barometric pressure of high altitudes can at least induce a comatose state.

To maintain physiological function at high altitude, under reduced environmental oxygen availability, the capacity to transport O_2 must increase. The exposure to hypoxia causes an immediate increase in breathing due to stimulation of arterial chemoreceptors and changes in metabolic state. The ability to adjust peripheral heat dissipation to facilitate the depression of body temperature during hypoxia, which reduced the metabolic demand, allows birds to fly high and for long periods, and is a result of an evolutionary adaptation. The bar-headed goose, a typical high altitude bird, depresses metabolism less than low-altitude birds during hypoxia and breathes substantially more than birds that fly at low altitudes. The bar-headed goose has haemoglobin with higher O_2 affinity and may be capable of generating higher inspiratory airflows.

The respiratory system of birds is separated into lung (the gas exchanging part) and a series of airs sacs (non respiratory) with anastomosing air capillaries and pneumatized bones, that allow unidirectional flow of air, compared to the blind sac and tidal flow in mammalian lungs.

Lack of diaphragm displaced the lungs to the coelomic cavity where they are closely attached to the ribs. Intercalated between the sacs, the lungs are largely continuously ventilated back-to-front by a concerted action of the cranial and caudal groups of air sacs.

There are fundamental differences in the breathing mechanics of different birds, driven in part by the morphological differences of the rib cage and sternum associated with skeletal adaptations to locomotion. The uncinate processes are bony projections that extend from the vertebral ribs, providing attachment sites for respiratory muscles.

The elongation of ribs, rib cage and sternum associated with diving species, as well as longer uncinates, maybe important upon resurfacing when inspiration occurs against the pressure of water against the body. The reduction in the sternum and the shortest uncinate length found in the walking species, suggests that they may play a reduced role during breathing in these species.

The circular lumen of the trachea has a cartilaginous or partially ossified support ring, whose number varies according to species and is lined by a cilindric pseudociliated epithelium with goblet cells. The trachea bifurcates into two primary bronchi, with an epithelial lining similar to the trachea but with incomplete cartilaginous rings, which disappear or are reduced when they reach the bronchial lung parenchyma. The pair of lungs of the birds are relatively small, non- compliant, localized in the dorsal thorax region and with little moving during breathing, as air is driven unidirectionally though the lung, via the system of air sacs.

The connection between the primary bronchus and the secondary and tertiary bronchi is labyrinthic, markedly opposed to the monopodic branch of mammal. The primary bronchus gives rise to four craneo-medium secondary bronchus and to seven caudal-dorsal secondary bronchus. In the secondary bronchus the mucosa is lined by a simple cuboidal or columnar epithelium, without goblet cells. Tertiary bronchus or parabronchus are arranged in a series of parallel lines, whose ends are open to the secondary bronchus. All the way through the parabronchus have recurrent anastomoses between them. The number of parabronchus varies from species to species, but is higher in the birds that fly better, has been estimated in Gallus domesticus between 300 and 500 parabronchus. Parabronchus have an average diameter of 500 μm, and are lined by a simple squamous epithelium, just like the mammals' alveolar channels. Along the inner surface of parabronchus, small vesicular structures with hexagonal shape emerge, with 100 to 200 μm in diameter. These structures called atria are separated from each other by septa mainly consisting of smooth muscle cells located in the freeboard, and collagen and elastic fibers, located at the base. The atria epithelium has two types of cells, one of which are the granular cells that are confined to the atria, have a cytoplasm that contains multilamellar bodies and are considered analogous to the cells of type II pneumocytes of the mammal's lungs. The other are the squamous cells, which line the inner surface of the atria and are based on a continuous basal membrane, forming the simple squamous epithelium. From the deepest area of each atria arise 2 to 4 infundibula that continue with the air capillaries with 3 to 10 μm diameter. They are lined by squamous cells, that are similar to the cells of the atria, but they are not based on the basal membrane. The infundibula and air capillaries of adjacent atria form anastomosis to one another.

The blood capillaries are surrounded by extremely small air capillaries and other capillaries, which give an appearance of a dense network. The blood capillaries are embedded in a rigid structure with numerous cross-braces that provide mechanical support of the small vessels at numerous points. This feature contributes to mechanical strength of blood capillaries and allows them to have a remarkably thin blood-gas barrier (BGB) that is uniformly arranged all around the circumference of the blood capillary.

The diameters of the air capillaries are comparable to those of blood capillaries and as a consequence of the very small diameter, the surface tension of these air capillaries is so high, despite their very well-differentiated surfactant, that they can only remain patent as rigid structures in a volume- constant lung. The surfactant of these rigid air capillaries lowers the high air capillary surface tension to such an extent that the remaining surface tension cannot suck fluid from the blood into the air capillary, thus preventing edema and maintaining gas exchange.

Together with the extensive network of blood capillaries, the air capillaries form the gas exchange surface of the bird's lungs. Unlike those observed in lung alveoli of mammals, the air capillaries are not terminal fund sacs formations, and therefore allow a unidirectional air flow through the lungs of birds.

The lung air sacs are pair formations, and their total number for the two lungs varies between 6 and 14 depending on the species, are generally referred to as cranial group and caudal group, and all cranial bags communicate with all secondary bronchi, fact that does not occur with caudal bags. The oxygen concentration is higher inside the caudal bags whereas the concentration of carbon dioxide reaches higher values inside the cranial bags. This qualitative difference is explained by the particular pattern of unidirectional airflow that occurs in the lungs of birds.

The inhaled air moves into the respiratory system, when- ever the chest cavity expands by the action of inspiratory muscles, and during expiration the air is expelled by action of the expiratory muscles. Although the birds do not have diaphragm, the entry and exit of air in to the respiratory system is a process similar to the observed in mammals.

During inhalation, air flows through the mesobronchus in to the posterior air sacs, and at the same time, the air enters the anterior air sacs via the dorsal secondary bronchus and parabronchus. During exhalation, the air leaves the posterior air sacs and passes through the parabronchus, and to a lesser extent, through the mesobronchus, to the trachea. At the same time in the anterior air sacs, the air moves through the secondary ventral bronchus towards the trachea. There is thus, during the two phases of the respiratory cycle, a continuous unidirectional flow through the parabronchus.

The flow inside the air capillaries and inside the blood capillaries occurs in opposite directions, i.e., in the blood capillaries the flow goes from the most peripheral areas of the parabronchus into its axis, while in the air capillaries move away from the axis of parabronchus. It is established a counter-current system of gas exchange between air capillaries and blood capillaries.

Briefly we can say that the anatomical and physiological features that have just been summarily exposed, such as a continuous and unidirectional ventilation of parabronchus, lower capacity of the air sacs, large surface for gas exchange and a very thin air-blood barrier, explain the unique characteristics of the respiratory system of birds, allowing them to extract oxygen from the highly rarefied air atmosphere.

Respiratory System in Mammals

Some 300 million years ago, the ancestors of modern reptiles finally emerged completely from water and made a commitment to air breathing. From them, developed the two great classes of vertebrates with high maximal oxygen consumption: the mammals and the birds. A remarkable feature of these two groups is that although the cardiovascular, renal, gastrointestinal, endocrine and nervous systems show many similarities, the lungs are radically different. The distinct morphology of avian and mammalian lungs reflects not only an increased demand for gas exchange, but is historically correlated with the divergent modes of locomotion that facilitate higher rates of ventilations.

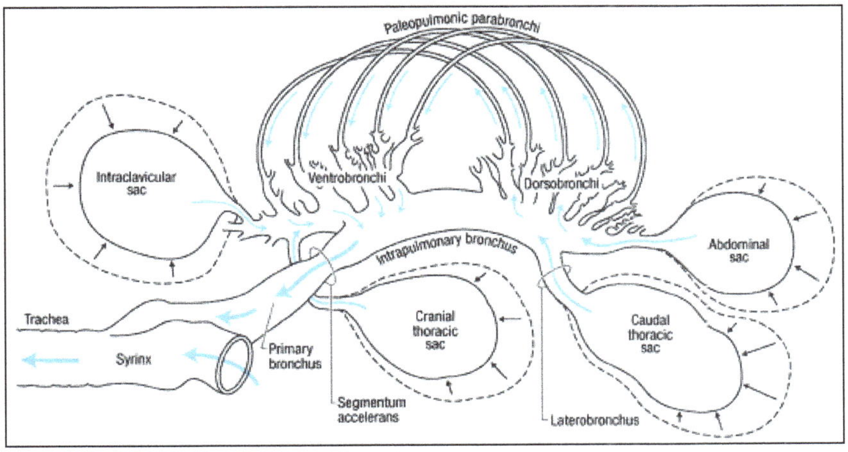

Birds respiratory systems.

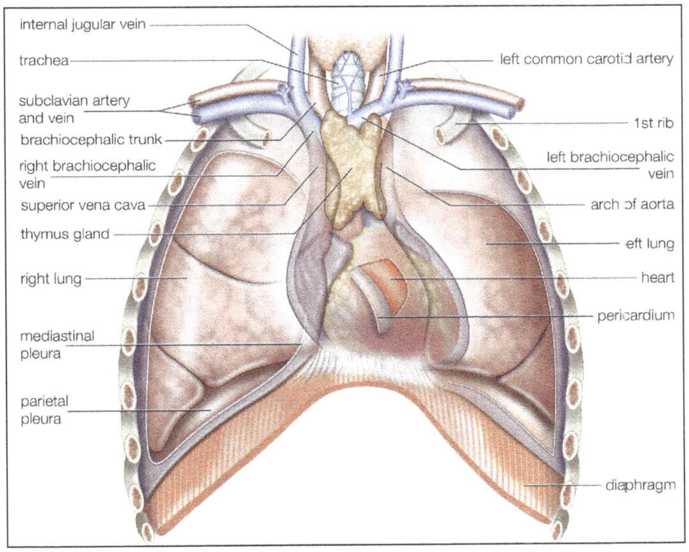

Mammals respiratory systems.

It is thought that mammals made their appearance on Earth during the Jurassic Period, the age of reptiles, when the process of divergence of the continents begun. Mammals evolved homoiothermy independently from birds, but in a very similar way. For the mandatory increased metabolism, they required a correspondingly increased gas exchange surface, which became available by the development of the broncho-alveolar lung.

The nearest ancestors of mammals appear to have been same group of reptiles and the lung of the mammals derived from a multicameral reptilian lung with three rows of lung chambers. The branched conducting bronchial system originated by stepwise further subdivision of these lung chambers, terminating in the branched respiratory bronchioli and ductus, covered with alveoli.

Of all tetrapods' breathing systems, the mammals' respiratory system has been the most extensively studied, often with the aim to acquire knowledge with medical relevance.

In mammals there is no dissociation between locomotion and respiratory movements and both are closely coupled especially during exercise.

The strong musculature of the diaphragm does not only act as a forceful inspiratory muscle together with the intercostals musculature, but is also responsible for maintaining a pressure gradient between the pleural and the peritoneal activity during strong exercise. During respiration at rest, expiration is performed by elastic retractile forces of the extended rib cage and by the retraction forces of the lung itself out of the surface tension of the alveoli together with their extended elastic fibre systems. During exercise, expiratory movement of the intercostals musculature is strongly supported by the muscles of the abdominal wall, which is also the case for all sound productions, speech and singing.

In mammals the lungs do not empty completely during the expiration, and the result is that convective flow alone cannot take the inspired gas to the periphery of the lung where some of the gas-exchanging alveoli are located. Instead the last part of the distance is accomplished by a relatively large peripheral airways to allow mixing of the inspired air with that already in the lung, and the resulting large alveoli cause additional problems.

In the mammalian lung, the airway and vascular systems form a complex multigenerational dichotomous branching tree-like arrangement. Transported by bulk-flow (convention) in the initial (large) parts of the bronchial system and mainly by diffusion in the terminal (fine) sections of the airway system, the inspired air ultimately reaches the alveoli where it is exposed to capillary blood across a thin, extensive tissue barrier.

The alveolar surface is mainly lined by type I and type II cells. Type II cells secrete surfactant.

In mammals the capillaries are located in the alveolar walls which are widely separated from each other. Thus the BGB has to withstand the full transmural pressure. The capillary is typically polarized with one side having very thin BGB whereas on the other side the barrier is thicker and contains strands of type collagen which provides support for the alveolar wall and maintains the integrity of the alveoli. In contrast to an uniform thin BGB in the birds, in mammals half of the surface area of the capillaries provides inefficient gas exchange due to its increased thicknes.

Animal Cell Structure

Animal cells are typical of the eukaryotic cell, enclosed by a plasma membrane and containing a membrane-bound nucleus and organelles. Unlike the eukaryotic cells of plants and fungi, animal cells do not have a cell wall. This feature was lost in the distant past by the single-celled organisms that gave rise to the kingdom Animalia. Most cells, both animal and plant, range in size between 1 and 100 micrometers and are thus visible only with the aid of a microscope.

The lack of a rigid cell wall allowed animals to develop a greater diversity of cell types, tissues, and organs. Specialized cells that formed nerves and muscles—tissues impossible for plants to evolve—gave these organisms mobility. The ability to move about by the use of specialized muscle tissues is a hallmark of the animal world, though a few animals, primarily sponges, do not possess differentiated tissues. Notably, protozoan's locomote, but it is only via nonmuscular means, in effect, using cilia, flagella, and pseudopodia.

The animal kingdom is unique among eukaryotic organisms because most animal tissues are bound together in an extracellular matrix by a triple helix of protein known as collagen. Plant and fungal cells are bound together in tissues or aggregations by other molecules, such as pectin. The fact that no other organisms utilize collagen in this manner is one of the indications that all animals arose from a common unicellular ancestor. Bones, shells, spicules, and other hardened structures are formed when the collagen-containing extracellular matrix between animal cells becomes calcified.

Animals are a large and incredibly diverse group of organisms. Making up about three-quarters of the species on Earth, they run the gamut from corals and jellyfish to ants, whales, elephants. Being mobile has given animals, which are capable of sensing and responding to their environment, the flexibility to adopt many different modes of feeding, defense, and reproduction. Unlike plants, however, animals are unable to manufacture their own food, and therefore, are always directly or indirectly dependent on plant life.

Most animal cells are diploid, meaning that their chromosomes exist in homologous pairs. Different chromosomal ploidies are also, however, known to occasionally occur. The proliferation of animal cells occurs in a variety of ways. In instances of sexual reproduction, the cellular process of meiosis is first necessary so that haploid daughter cells, or gametes, can be produced. Two haploid cells then fuse to form a diploid zygote, which develops into a new organism as its cells divide and multiply.

The earliest fossil evidence of animals dates from the Vendian Period (650 to 544 million years ago), with coelenterate-type creatures that left traces of their soft bodies in shallow-water sediments. The first mass extinction ended that period, but during the Cambrian Period which followed, an explosion of new forms began the evolutionary radiation that produced most of the major groups, or phyla, known today. Vertebrates (animals with backbones) are not known to have occurred until the early Ordovician Period (505 to 438 million years ago).

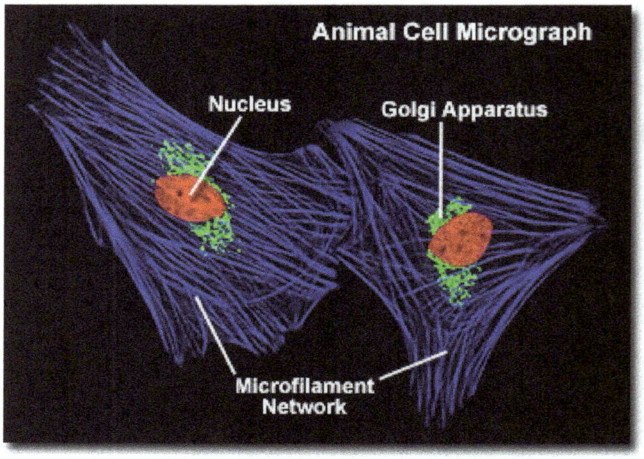

Cells were discovered in 1665 by British scientist Robert Hooke who first observed them in his crude (by today's standards) seventeenth century optical microscope. In fact, Hooke coined the term "cell", in a biological context, when he described the microscopic structure of cork like a tiny, bare room or monk's cell. Illustrated in figure are pair of fibroblast deer skin cells that have been labelled with fluorescent probes and photographed in the microscope to reveal their internal structure. The nuclei are stained with a red probe, while the Golgi apparatus and microfilament actin network are stained green and blue, respectively. The microscope has been a fundamental tool in the field of cell biology and is often used to observe living cells in culture.

- Centrioles: Centrioles are self-replicating organelles made up of nine bundles of microtubules and are found only in animal cells. They appear to help in organizing cell division, but aren't essential to the process.
- Cilia and Flagella: For single-celled eukaryotes, cilia and flagella are essential for the locomotion of individual organisms. In multicellular organisms, cilia function to move fluid or materials past an immobile cell as well as moving a cell or group of cells.
- Endoplasmic Reticulum: The endoplasmic reticulum is a network of sacs that manufactures, processes, and transports chemical compounds for use inside and outside of the cell. It is connected to the double-layered nuclear envelope, providing a pipeline between the nucleus and the cytoplasm.
- Endosomes and Endocytosis: Endosomes are membrane-bound vesicles, formed via a complex family of processes collectively known as endocytosis, and found in the cytoplasm of virtually every animal cell. The basic mechanism of endocytosis is the reverse of what occurs during exocytosis or cellular secretion. It involves the invagination (folding inward) of a cell's plasma membrane to surround macromolecules or other matter diffusing through the extracellular fluid.
- Golgi Apparatus: The Golgi apparatus is the distribution and shipping department for the cell's chemical products. It modifies proteins and a fat built in the endoplasmic reticulum and prepares them for export to the outside of the cell.
- Intermediate Filaments: Intermediate filaments are a very broad class of fibrous proteins

that play an important role as both structural and functional elements of the cytoskeleton. Ranging in size from 8 to 12 nanometers, intermediate filaments function as tension-bearing elements to help maintain cell shape and rigidity.

- Lysosomes: The main function of these microbodies is digestion. Lysosomes break down cellular waste products and debris from outside the cell into simple compounds, which are transferred to the cytoplasm as new cell-building materials.
- Microfilaments: Microfilaments are solid rods made of globular proteins called actin. These filaments are primarily structural in function and are an important component of the cytoskeleton.
- Microtubules: These straight, hollow cylinders are found throughout the cytoplasm of all eukaryotic cells (prokaryotes don't have them) and carry out a variety of functions, ranging from transport to structural support.
- Mitochondria: Mitochondria are oblong shaped organelles that are found in the cytoplasm of every eukaryotic cell. In the animal cell, they are the main power generators, converting oxygen and nutrients into energy.
- Nucleus: The nucleus is a highly specialized organelle that serves as the information processing and administrative center of the cell. This organelle has two major functions: it stores the cell's hereditary material, or DNA, and it coordinates the cell's activities, which include growth, intermediary metabolism, protein synthesis, and reproduction (cell division).
- Peroxisomes: Micro bodies are a diverse group of organelles that are found in the cytoplasm, roughly spherical and bound by a single membrane. There are several types of micro bodies but peroxisomes are the most common.
- Plasma Membrane: All living cells have a plasma membrane that encloses their contents. In prokaryotes, the membrane is the inner layer of protection surrounded by a rigid cell wall. Eukaryotic animal cells have only the membrane to contain and protect their contents. These membranes also regulate the passage of molecules in and out of the cells.
- Ribosomes: All living cells contain ribosomes, tiny organelles composed of approximately 60 percent RNA and 40 percent protein. In eukaryotes, ribosomes are made of four strands of RNA. In prokaryotes, they consist of three strands of RNA.

In addition the optical and electron microscope, scientists are able to use a number of other techniques to probe the mysteries of the animal cell. Cells can be disassembled by chemical methods and their individual organelles and macromolecules isolated for study. The process of cell fractionation enables the scientist to prepare specific components, the mitochondria for example, in large quantities for investigations of their composition and functions. Using this approach, cell biologists have been able to assign various functions to specific locations within the cell. However, the era of fluorescent proteins has brought microscopy to the forefront of biology by enabling scientists to target living cells with highly localized probes for studies that don't interfere with the delicate balance of life processes.

Circulatory Systems in Animals

The circulatory systems of animals differ in the number of heart chambers and the number of circuits through which the blood flows.

Simple Circulatory Systems

The circulatory system varies from simple systems in invertebrates to more complex systems in vertebrates. The simplest animals, such as the sponges (Porifera) and rotifers (Rotifera), do not need a circulatory system because diffusion allows adequate exchange of water, nutrients, and waste, as well as dissolved gases. Organisms that are more complex, but still have only two layers of cells in their body plan, such as jellies (Cnidaria) and comb jellies (Ctenophora), also use diffusion through their epidermis and internally through the gastrovascular compartment. Both their internal and external tissues are bathed in an aqueous environment and exchange fluids by diffusion on both sides. Exchange of fluids is assisted by the pulsing of the jellyfish body.

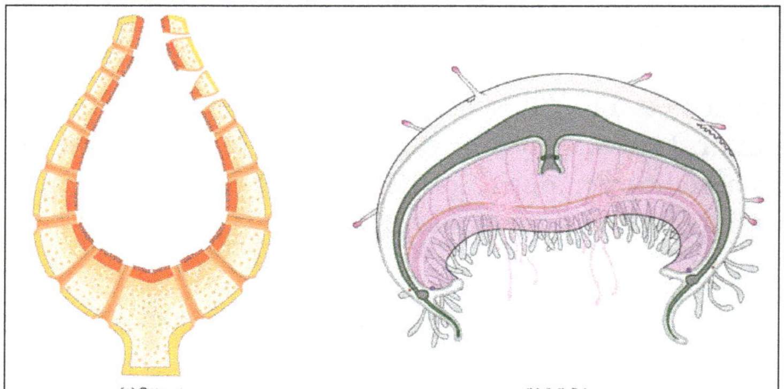

Animals without circulatory systems: Simple animals consisting of a single cell layer, such as the (a) sponge, or only a few cell layers, such as the (b) jellyfish, do not have a circulatory system. Instead, gases, nutrients, and wastes are exchanged by diffusion.

For more complex organisms, diffusion is not efficient for cycling gases, nutrients, and waste effectively through the body; therefore, more complex circulatory systems evolved. Closed circulatory systems are a characteristic of vertebrates; however, there are significant differences in the structure of the heart and the circulation of blood between the different vertebrate groups due to adaptation during evolution and associated differences in anatomy.

Fish Circulatory Systems

Fish have a single circuit for blood flow and a two-chambered heart that has only a single atrium and a single ventricle. The atrium collects blood that has returned from the body, while the ventricle pumps the blood to the gills where gas exchange occurs and the blood is re-oxygenated; this is called gill circulation. The blood then continues through the rest of the body before arriving back at the atrium; this is called systemic circulation. This unidirectional flow of blood produces a gradient of oxygenated to deoxygenated blood around the fish's systemic circuit. The result is a limit in the amount of oxygen that can reach some of the organs and tissues of the body, reducing the overall metabolic capacity of fish.

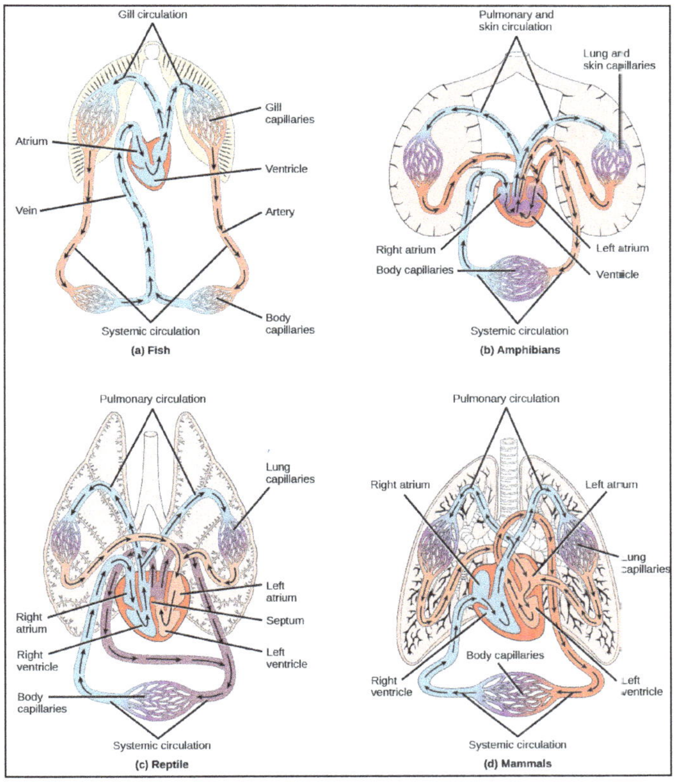

Examples of animal circulatory systems.

Figure shows: (a) Fish have the simplest circulatory systems of the vertebrates: blood flows unidirectionally from the two-chambered heart through the gills and then to the rest of the body. (b) Amphibians have two circulatory routes: one for oxygenation of the blood through the lungs and skin, and the other to take oxygen to the rest of the body. The blood is pumped from a three-chambered heart with two atria and a single ventricle. (c) Reptiles also have two circulatory routes; however, blood is only oxygenated through the lungs. The heart is three chambered, but the ventricles are partially separated so some mixing of oxygenated and deoxygenated blood occurs, except in crocodilians and birds. (d) Mammals and birds have the most efficient heart with four chambers that completely separate the oxygenated and deoxygenated blood; it pumps only oxygenated blood through the body and deoxygenated blood to the lungs.

Amphibian Circulatory Systems

In amphibians, reptiles, birds, and mammals, blood flow is directed in two circuits: one through the lungs and back to the heart (pulmonary circulation) and the other throughout the rest of the body and its organs, including the brain (systemic circulation).

Amphibians have a three-chambered heart that has two atria and one ventricle rather than the two-chambered heart of fish. The two atria receive blood from the two different circuits (the lungs and the systems). There is some mixing of the blood in the heart's ventricle, which reduces the efficiency of oxygenation. The advantage to this arrangement is that high pressure in the vessels pushes blood to the lungs and body. The mixing is mitigated by a ridge within the ventricle that diverts oxygen-rich blood through the systemic circulatory system and deoxygenated blood to the pulmocutaneous circuit where gas exchange occurs in the lungs and through the skin. For this reason, amphibians are often described as having double circulation.

Reptile Circulatory Systems

Most reptiles also have a three-chambered heart similar to the amphibian heart that directs blood to the pulmonary and systemic circuits. The ventricle is divided more effectively by a partial septum, which results in less mixing of oxygenated and deoxygenated blood. Some reptiles (alligators and crocodiles) are the most primitive animals to exhibit a four-chambered heart. Crocodilians have a unique circulatory mechanism where the heart shunts blood from the lungs toward the stomach and other organs during long periods of submergence; for instance, while the animal waits for prey or stays underwater waiting for prey to rot. One adaptation includes two main arteries that leave the same part of the heart: one takes blood to the lungs and the other provides an alternate route to the stomach and other parts of the body. Two other adaptations include a hole in the heart between the two ventricles, called the foramen of Panizza, which allows blood to move from one side of the heart to the other and specialized connective tissue that slows the blood flow to the lungs. Together, these adaptations have made crocodiles and alligators one of the most successfully-evolved animal groups on earth.

Mammal and Bird Circulatory Systems

In mammals and birds, the heart is also divided into four chambers: two atria and two ventricles. The oxygenated blood is separated from the deoxygenated blood, which improves the efficiency of double circulation and is probably required for the warm-blooded lifestyle of mammals and birds. The four-chambered heart of birds and mammals evolved independently from a three-chambered heart.

Animal Reproductive System

Animal reproductive system is any of the organ systems by which animals reproduce. The role of reproduction is to provide for the continued existence of a species; it is the process by which living organisms duplicate themselves. Animals compete with other individuals in the environment to maintain themselves for a period of time sufficient to enable them to produce tissue nonessential to their own survival, but indispensable to the maintenance of the species. The additional tissue, reproductive tissue, usually becomes separated from the individual to form a new, independent organism.

Unlike most other organ systems, the reproductive systems of higher animals have not generally become more complex than those of lower forms. Asexual reproduction (i.e., reproduction not involving the union of gametes), however, occurs only in the invertebrates, in which it is common, occurring in animals as highly evolved as the sea squirts, which are closely related to the vertebrates. Temporary gonads are common among lower animals; in higher animals, however, gonads are permanent organs. Hermaphroditism, in which one individual contains functional reproductive organs of both sexes, is common among lower invertebrates; yet separate sexes occur in such primitive animals as sponges, and hermaphroditism occurs in animals more highly evolved—e.g., the lower fishes. Gonads located on or near the animal surface are common in the lowest invertebrates, but in higher animals they tend to be more deeply situated and often involve intricate duct systems. In echinoderms, which are among the highest invertebrates, the gonads hang directly into the sea and spill their gametes into the water. In protochordates, gametes are released into a stream of respiratory water that passes directly into the sea. Duct systems of the invertebrate flatworms (Platyhelminthes) are relatively complex, and those of specialized arthropods (e.g., insects, spiders, crabs) are more complex than those of any vertebrate. Copulatory organs occur in flatworms, but copulatory organs are not ubiquitous among vertebrates other than reptiles and mammals. The trend toward fewer eggs and increased parental care in higher animals may account for the relative lack of complexity in the reproductive systems of some advanced forms. Whereas trends toward increasing structural complexity have often been reversed during evolution, reproductive behaviour patterns in many phylogenetic (i.e., evolutionary) lines have become more complicated in order to enhance the opportunity for fertilization of eggs and maximum survival of offspring.

A direct relationship exists between behaviour and the functional state of gonads. Reproductive behaviour induced principally but not exclusively by organic substances called hormones promotes the union of sperm (spermatozoa) and eggs, as well as any parental care accorded the young. There are a number of reasons why behaviour must be synchronized with gonadal activity. Chief among these are the following.

Individuals of a species must congregate at the time the gonads contain mature gametes. This often entails migration, and some members of all major vertebrate groups migrate long distances to gather at spawning grounds or rookeries.

Individuals with gametes ready to be shed must recognize members of the opposite sex. Recognition is sometimes by external appearance or by chemical substances (pheromones), but sex-linked behaviour is often the only signal. Geographical territories frequently must be established and aggressively defended. The building of nests, however simple, is essential reproductive behaviour in many species.

When fertilization of aquatic forms is external, sperm and eggs must be discharged at approximately the same time into the water, since gametes may be quickly dispersed by currents. Courtship, often involving highly intricate behaviour patterns, serves to release the gametes of both mating individuals simultaneously.

When fertilization is internal, willingness of the female to mate is often essential. Female mammals not in a state of willingness to mate not only will not mate but may injure or even kill an aggressive male. The unwillingness of a female mammal to mate when mature eggs are not present prevents loss of sperm needed to preserve the species.

Parental care of fertilized eggs by one parent or the other has evolved in many species. Parental behaviour includes fanning the water or air around the eggs, thereby maintaining appropriate temperature and oxygen levels; secretion of oxygen from a parent's gills; transport of eggs on or in the parental body (including the mouth of some male parents); and brooding, or incubation, of eggs.

Some species extend parental care into the postnatal period, feeding and protecting the offspring.

Such behaviour patterns are adaptations for survival and thus are essential; all are induced by the nervous and endocrine systems and are typically cyclical, because gonadal activity is cyclical.

Reproductive Systems of Invertebrates

Gonads, Associated Structures and Products

Although asexual reproduction occurs in many invertebrate species, most reproduce sexually. The basic unit of sexual reproduction is a gamete (sperm or egg), produced by specialized tissues or organs called gonads. Sexual reproduction does not necessarily imply copulation or even a union of gametes. As might be expected of such a large and diverse group as the invertebrates, many variations have evolved to ensure survival of species. In many lower invertebrates, gonads are temporary organs; in higher forms, however, they are permanent. Some invertebrates have coexistent female and male gonads; in others the same gonad produces both sperm and eggs. Animals in which both sperm and eggs are produced by the same individual (hermaphroditism) are termed monoecious. In dioecious species, the sexes are separate. Generally, the male gonads ripen first in hermaphroditic animals (protandry); this tends to ensure cross-fertilization. Self-fertilization is normal, however, in many species, and some species undergo sex reversal.

Sponges, Coelenterates, Flatworms and Aschelminths

Sponges are at a cellular level of organization and thus do not have organs or even well-developed tissues; nevertheless, they produce sperm and eggs and also reproduce asexually. Some species of sponge are monoecious, others are dioecious. Sperm and eggs are formed by aggregations of cells called amoebocytes in the body wall; these are not considered gonads because of their origin and transitory nature.

In hydrozoan coelenterates, temporary gonads are formed by groups of cells in either the epidermis (outer cell layer) or gastrodermis (gut lining), depending on the species; scyphozoan and anthozoan coelenterates generally have gonads in the gastrodermis. The origin and development of gonads in coelenterates, particularly freshwater species, are often associated with the seasons. Freshwater hydrozoans, for example, reproduce asexually until the onset of cold weather, which stimulates them to form testes and ovaries. Colonial hydrozoans asexually produce individuals known as polyps. Polyps, in turn, give rise to free swimming stages (medusae), in which gonads develop. The body organization of sponges and coelenterates is such that most of their cells are in intimate contact with the environment; consequently, gametes are shed into the water, and no ducts are necessary to convey them to the outside.

In contrast to sponges and coelenterates, platyhelminths generally have well-developed organ systems of a permanent nature and, in addition, have evolved secondary reproductive structures to convey sex products. One exception is the acoels, a group of primitive turbellarians; they lack permanent gonads, and germinal cells develop from amoebocytes in much the same manner as in sponges. The majority of flatworms, however, are monoecious, the primary sex organs consisting of one or more ovaries and testes. The tube from the ovary to the outside is called the oviduct; it often has an outpocketing (seminal receptacle) for the storage of sperm received during copulation. In many species the oviduct receives a duct from yolk (vitelline) glands, whose cells nourish the fertilized egg. Beyond the entrance of the duct from the yolk glands the oviduct may be modified to secrete a protective capsule around the egg before it is discharged to the outside. The male organs consist of testes, from which extend numerous tubules (vasa efferentia) that unite to form a sperm duct (vas deferens); the latter becomes an ejaculatory duct through which sperm are released to the outside. The sperm duct may exhibit expanded areas that store sperm (seminal vesicles), and it may be surrounded by prostatic cells that contribute to the seminal fluid. The sperm duct eventually passes through a copulatory organ. The same basic structural pattern, somewhat modified, is found in higher invertebrates.

Aschelminthes (roundworms) are mostly dioecious; frequently there are external differences between males and females (sexual dimorphism). The males are generally smaller and often have copulatory spicules. Nematodes have relatively simple reproductive organs, a tubular testis or ovary being located at the end of a twisted tube. The portion of the female tract nearest the ovary forms a uterus for temporary storage of fertilized eggs. Some species lay eggs, but others retain the egg in the uterus until the larva hatches. The sperm are released into a cavity called the cloaca. A number of free-living nematodes are capable of sex reversal—if the sex ratio in a given population is not optimal or if environmental conditions are not ideal, the ratio of males to females can be altered. This sometimes results in intersexes; i.e., females with some male characteristics. Hermaphroditism occurs in nematodes, and self-fertilization in such species is common.

Annelids and Mollusks

Annelids have a well-developed body cavity (coelom), a part of the lining of which gives rise to gonads. In some annelids, gonads occur in several successive body segments. This is true, for example, in polychaetes, most of which are dioecious. Testes and ovaries usually develop, though not invariably, in many body segments; and the sperm and eggs, often in enormous numbers, are stored in the coelom. Fertilization is external. In oligochaetes (all of which are monoecious) on the other hand, the gonads develop in a few specific segments. Sperm are stored in a seminal vesicle and eggs in an egg sac, rather than in the coelom. A portion of the peritoneum, the membrane lining the coelom, becomes a saclike seminal receptacle that stores sperm received from the mate. The earthworm, Lumbricus terrestris, is an example of a specialized annelid reproductive system. Female organs consist of a pair of ovaries in segment 13; a pair of oviducts that open via a ciliated funnel (i.e., with hairlike structures) into segment 13 but open to the exterior in segment 14; an egg sac near each funnel; and a pair of seminal receptacles in segment 9 and another in segment 10. Male organs consist of two pairs of minute testes in segments 10 and 11, each associated with a ciliated sperm funnel leading to a tiny duct, the vas efferens. The two ducts on each side lead to a vas deferens that opens in segment 15. Testes and funnels are contained within two of three pairs of large seminal vesicles that occupy six body segments. Leeches (Hirudinea), also monoecious, have one pair of ovaries and a segmentally arranged series of testes with duct systems basically similar to those of earthworms.

Although mollusks have a close evolutionary kinship to annelids, they have reduced or lost many structures characteristic of segmented worms. The coelom persists only as three regional cavities: gonadal, nephridial (kidney), and pericardial (heart). In ancestral forms these were interconnected so that gametes from the gonad passed through the pericardial cavity, the nephridial cavity, then to the outside through a nephridial pore. The various groups of mollusks have tended to modify this arrangement, with the result that gonads have their own pore; among amphineurans, for example, the sexes are usually separate, and there is one gonad with an associated pore. Gastropods show considerable variability, but generally one gonad (ovary, testis, or ovotestis—a structure combining the functional gonads of both sexes) is located in the visceral hump and connected to the outside by a remnant of the right kidney. In hermaphroditic forms, one duct carries sperm as well as eggs. The gonadal ducts of gastropod females often secrete a protective capsule around the fertilized eggs; in males, the terminal portion of the duct is sometimes contained in a copulatory organ. Pelecypods may be either monoecious or dioecious, but the gonads are usually paired. In mussels and oysters, the gonads open through the nephridial pore, but in clams the reproductive system opens independently. The cephalopods are all dioecious. The single testis or ovary releases its products into the pericardial cavity and this, in turn, leads to a gonopore, the external opening. The oviduct of the squid is terminally modified to form a shell gland. The male system is more complex—the gonoduct leads into a seminal vesicle where a complicated torpedo-shaped sperm case (spermatophore) is secreted and contains the sperm. Spermatophores are then stored in a special structure (Needham's sac) until copulation occurs.

A remarkable characteristic of some mollusks is the ability to alter their sex. Some species are clearly dioecious; however, among the monoecious species there is considerable variability in their hermaphroditic condition. In some species, male and female gonads, although in the same individual, are independent functionally and structurally. In others, an ovotestis produces both sperm and eggs. Oysters display a third condition; young oysters have a tendency toward maleness, but, if water temperature or food availability is altered, some individuals develop into females. Later, a reversal to the male condition may occur. The sexual makeup of an entire oyster population also has a seasonal aspect; in harmony with the group, an individual may undergo several alterations in the course of a year. A similar phenomenon, called consecutive sexuality, occurs in limpets. These gastropods stack themselves in piles, with the younger animals on top. The animals on top are males with well-developed testes and copulatory organs; those in the middle are hermaphroditic; those on the bottom are females, having lost the testes and copulatory organ (penis) by degeneration. A decrease in the number of females in a stack induces males to assume female characteristics, but the transition is retarded when an excess of females is present. The degree of maleness or femaleness is probably controlled in part by environmental and internal factors.

Arthropods

The phylum Arthropoda includes a vast number of organisms of great diversity. Most arthropods are dioecious, but many are hermaphroditic, and some reproduce parthenogenetically (i.e., without fertilization). The primary reproductive organs are much the same as in other higher invertebrates, but the secondary structures are often greatly modified. Such modifications depend on whether fertilization is internal or external, whether the egg or zygote (i.e., the fertilized egg) is retained or immediately released, and whether eggs are provided some means of protection after they have left the body of the female. The mandibulate arthropods (e.g., crustaceans, insects) include more species than any other group and have invaded most habitats, a fact reflected in their reproductive processes.

Crustaceans (e.g., crabs, crayfish, and barnacles) are for the most part dioecious. The primary reproductive organs generally consist of paired gonads that open through paired ventral (bottom side) gonopores. Females often have a seminal receptacle (spermatheca) in the form of an outpocketing of the lower part of the female tract or as an invagination (inpocketing) of the body near the gonopore. Males have appendages modified for clasping the female during copulation or for guiding sperm. A number of groups have members that reproduce parthenogenetically. Branchiopods (e.g., water fleas, fairy shrimp) have simple paired gonads. The female gonopore often opens dorsally (on the back side) into a brood chamber; the male gonopore opens near the anus. Males have appendages for clasping females during copulation. Ostracods, or seed shrimp, have paired tubular gonads. The eggs may be brooded by the female, or they may be released into the water via a gonoduct and gonopore. The terminal portion of the male gonoduct is enclosed in a single or paired penis. Many species reproduce parthenogenetically. Some experts contend that this is the only method employed, even though functional males may be present in the population. Copepods (e.g., Cyclops) have paired ovaries and an unpaired testis. The terminal portion of the oviduct constitutes an ovisac for storage of eggs. The male deposits sperm in a spermatophore that is transferred to the female. Sexual dimorphism is particularly evident among parasitic copepods. Frequently, parasitic females can hardly be recognized as copepods except for the distinctive ovisacs. Males, on the other hand, are free-living and are recognizable as copepods.

The hermaphroditic Cirripedia (e.g., barnacles) are among the exceptions to the generalization that crustaceans are dioecious. It has been suggested that hermaphroditism in barnacles is an adaptation to their sessile, or stationary, existence, but cross-fertilization is more common than self-fertilization. The ovaries lie either in the base or in the stalk of the animal, and the female gonopore is near the base of the first pair of middle appendages (cirri). The testes empty into a seminal vesicle through a series of ducts; from the vesicle extends a long sperm duct within a penis that may be extended to deposit sperm in the mantle cavity of an adjacent barnacle. The terminal portion of the oviduct secretes a substance that forms a kind of ovisac within the mantle cavity, where fertilized eggs undergo early development. Although most barnacles are hermaphrodites, some display a peculiar adaptation in that they contain parasitic dwarf or accessory males. Dwarf males are much smaller than the host barnacle in which they live and are degenerate, except for the testes. In some species they live in the mantle cavity of hermaphroditic forms and produce accessory sperm; in other species only the female organs persist in the host animal and the accessory male is a necessity.

Amphipods and isopods (e.g., pill bugs, sow bugs), like most crustaceans, are dioecious and have paired gonads. Females of both groups have a ventral brood chamber (marsupium) formed by a series of medially directed (i.e., toward the body midline) plates (oostegites) in the region of the thorax, the region between head and abdomen. Many isopods are parasitic and have developed unusual sex-related activities. Certain species are parasitic on other crustaceans. After a series of molts (i.e., shedding of the body covering) a parasitic larval (immature) isopod attaches to the shell of a crab. If it is the only larva to do so, it increases in size and develops into an adult female. If another larva subsequently attaches, the new arrival becomes a male. It has been demonstrated that the testes of the functioning male larva will change to ovaries if the larva is removed to a new, uninfected host. Thus, the larvae of these species apparently are intersexual and can develop into either sex. This phenomenon, reminiscent of that in mollusks, demonstrates the way in which similar adaptations have evolved in diverse groups of organisms.

The gonads of crabs and lobsters are paired, as are the gonopores. The females of many species have external seminal receptacles on the ventral part of the thorax; those of other species have internal receptacles in the same region. In some species, seminal receptacles are absent, and the male simply attaches a spermatophore to the female. Thus, males either have appendages (gonopods) by which sperm are inserted in the body of the female or produce spermatophores for sperm transfer. The sexual dimorphism of many decapods can be altered by parasitism. An example of this is the crab that is parasitized by a barnacle. A barnacle infection in male crabs induces the secondary sex characters of the crab to resemble those of a female; however, masculinization does not occur in parasitized females. At each molt a parasitized male crab increasingly resembles a female even though the testes may be completely unaffected. Feminization results from a hormonal alteration of the parasitized crab.

Insects are rarely hermaphroditic, but many species reproduce parthenogenetically (without fertilization). The insect ovary is composed of clusters of tubules (ovarioles) with no lumen, or cavity. The upper portion of each ovariole gives rise to oocytes (immature eggs) that mature and are nourished by yolk from the lower portion. The oviduct leads to a genital chamber (copulatory bursa, or vagina), with which are often associated accessory glands and a seminal receptacle. Some accessory glands form secretions by which eggs become attached to a hard surface; others secrete a protective envelope around the egg. The eighth and ninth body segments are often modified for egg-laying. The paired testes consist of a series of seminal tubules that form primary spermatogonia (immature spermatozoa) at their upper ends. As the spermatogonia mature a covering is secreted around them. Eventually they enter a storage area (seminal vesicle). The terminal portion of the male system is an ejaculatory duct that passes through a copulatory organ. A pair of accessory glands, often associated with the ejaculatory duct, contributes to the semen (fluid containing sperm) or participates in spermatophore formation. The ninth body segment and sometimes the tenth bear appendages for sperm transfer. Scorpions and spiders have tubular or saclike gonads; the female system is equipped to receive and store sperm, and, in some species, the female retains the eggs long after fertilization has occurred. Male spiders may have a cluster of accessory glands associated with the terminal portion of the reproductive system for the manufacture of spermatophores, or they may have expanded seminal vesicles for the retention of sperm until copulation takes place. Often specific appendages are adapted for sperm transfer.

Echinoderms and Protochordates

Echinoderms (e.g., sea urchins), hemichordates (including acornworms), urochordates (e.g., sea squirts), and cephalochordates (amphioxus) are restricted to a marine habitat. As with many other marine animals, their gametes are shed into the water. In echinoderms, the gonads are generally suspended from the arms directly into the sea; with few exceptions, the sexes are separate. Female starfishes have been known to release as many as 2,500,000 eggs in two hours; 200,000,000 may be shed in a season. Males produce many times that number of sperm. Acornworms reproduce only sexually, and the sexes are generally separate. The gonads lie on each side of the gut as a paired series of simple or lobed sacs. Each opens to the exterior, either directly or via a short duct. The eggs, when shed, are in coiled mucous masses, each of which contains 2,500 to 3,000 eggs.

In urochordates and cephalochordates the gonads develop in the wall of a cavity (atrium) that receives respiratory water after it passes over the gills. Gametes are released into the cavity, and then carried into the sea by the water flowing from the cavity. Most urochordates are hermaphroditic. One ovary and one testis may lie side by side, each with its own duct to the atrium; some species have many pairs of ovaries and testes. The eggs develop in so-called ovarian follicles consisting of two layers of cells, as in many vertebrates. The inner layer remains with the ovulated, or shed, egg, and the cells become filled with air spaces, which apparently help the eggs to float. Amphioxus, the highest animals lacking vertebral columns, are dioecious. They have 24 or more pairs of ovaries or testes lacking ducts. When ripe, the gonads rupture, spilling their gametes directly into the atrium.

Mechanisms that Aid in the Union of Gametes

Sponges, Coelenterates, Flatworms and Aschelminthes

The processes of sperm transfer and fertilization have been documented for only a few species of sponges. Flagellated (i.e., bearing a whiplike strand) sperm are released from the male gonad and swept out of the body and into the water by way of an elaborate system of canals. A sperm that enters another sponge, or the one from which it was released, is captured by a flagellated collar cell (choanocyte). The choanocyte completely engulfs the sperm, loses its collar and flagellum (or "whip"), and migrates to deeper tissue where the egg has matured. The choanocyte containing the sperm cell fuses with the egg, thus achieving fertilization. In freshwater coelenterates, sperm are also released into the water and carried by currents to another individual. Unlike the mechanism in sponges, however, coelenterate eggs arise in the epidermis, or surface tissue, and are exposed to sperm that may be nearby in the water; thus, no intermediate transport cell is needed. Many species of marine coelenterates expel both sperm and eggs into the water, and fertilization takes place there. Some medusoid coelenterates (jellyfish), however, offer some protection to the egg. After leaving the gonad, the egg becomes temporarily lodged in the epidermis on the underside of the organism, where fertilization and early development occur.

In all flatworms, fertilization is internal. Among species with no female duct, sperm are injected, and fertilization occurs in the inner layer of tissue. Most flatworms, however, have an elaborate system of male and female ducts. Generally, the male gonoduct passes through a penis-like organ, and sperm are transferred during copulation. In parasitic species, which often cannot find a mate, self-fertilization serves as the means for reproduction. Sperm and ova unite in the oviduct, which then secretes yolk around the zygote.

Male nematodes (roundworms) are usually equipped with a pair of copulatory structures (spicules) that guide the sperm during copulation. The posterior end of some males also exhibits a lateral (sideward) expansion (copulatory bursa) that clasps the female during copulation. Other males loop their tail around the female in the region of her gonopore. Unlike many other aschelminthes, nematodes have sperm cells that are amoeboid; i.e., their cell contents seem to flow. Some male rotifers have a copulatory organ.

In some species of annelid polychaetes (marine worms) reproductive activity is synchronized with lunar cycles. At breeding time the body of both sexes differentiates into two regions, an anterior atoke and a posterior epitoke, in which gonads develop. When the moon is in a specific phase, the epitoke separates from the rest of the body and swims to the surface. The female epitoke apparently stimulates the male epitoke to release sperm, and sperm release, in turn, evokes expulsion of eggs. Fertilization is external. So well-coordinated is this phenomenon that tremendous numbers of epitokes appear on the surface at about the same time.

Sexually mature oligochaetes have a clitellum, which is a modification of a section of the body wall consisting of a glandular, saddlelike thickening near the gonopores. During copulation, the clitellum secretes mucus that keeps the worms paired while sperm are being exchanged. Following copulation, the clitellum secretes substance for a cocoon, which encircles the worm and into which eggs and sperm are deposited. The worm then manipulates the cocoon until it slips off over the head. Thereupon, the ends of the cocoon become sealed, and fertilization and development take place inside. Many leeches also form a cocoon; but the males of some species have a penis that can be inserted into the female gonopore. In other leeches, a spermatophore is thrust into the body of the mate during copulation.

Union of gametes among mollusks is affected in a number of ways. Marine pelecypods synchronously discharge sperm and eggs into the sea; some freshwater clams are apparently self-fertilizing. One of the more unusual types of reproductive diversity occurs in marine gastropods of the family Scalidae that produce two kinds of sperm cells. A large sperm with a degenerate nucleus acts as a transport cell for carrying numerous small fertilizing sperm through the water and into the oviduct of another individual. Cephalopod males have modified arms for the transfer of spermatophores. The right or left fourth arm of the squid, for example, is so modified. Following an often elaborate courtship, the male squid uses the modified appendage to remove spermatophores from their storage place in his body and place them in the mantle cavity of the female. A cementing substance, which is released from the spermatophore, firmly attaches the spermatophore to the female's body near the oviduct. In some species, the male loses the arm. Manipulation of the eggs by the female's arms may also occur.

Some unusual behaviour patterns have evolved in conjunction with sperm transfer in mollusks. Prior to copulation of certain land snails, a dart composed of calcium carbonate is propelled forcefully from the gonopore of each of the mating individuals and lodges in the viscera of the mate. Even though the snails have assumed a mating posture, sperm transfer cannot occur until each snail has been stimulated by a dart.

Arthropods

Arthropods are as varied as mollusks in their methods of effecting union of sperm and eggs. They have relatively few devices for sperm transfer, but many display a high degree of behavioral complexity.

The male and female scorpion participates in a courtship ritual involving complicated manoeuvres. In some species the male produces spermatophores that are anchored to the ground. In the course of the ritual dance the female is positioned over the spermatophore. The male then presses her down until the sperm packet is forced into her genital chamber, where it becomes attached by means of small hooks. Thus, ultimately, fertilization takes place internally.

Among some spiders the male's pedipalp, a grasping or crushing appendage, contains a bulb and an extensible, coiled structure (embolus). As mating begins, the male dips the pedipalp into semen from his gonopore. The embolus is then placed in the female gonopore, and the sperm are transferred to her seminal receptacle. The female deposits the sperm along with her eggs into a silken cocoon, which she attaches to her body or to an object such as a rock or a leaf.

Sperm transfer in copepods, isopods, and many decapods, often preceded by courtship, is affected by modified appendages, gonopods, or spermatophores. Copepods clasp the female with their antennae while placing a spermatophore at the opening of the seminal receptacle. In some decapods fertilization occurs as eggs are being released into the water.

Fertilization among insects is always internal; there is much variation in the manner in which sperm are transferred to the female. Males of some species form spermatophores that are deposited in a copulatory bursa (vagina) of the female; the wall of the spermatophore breaks down, and the sperm swim to the seminal receptacle. In other species, sperm are introduced directly into the seminal receptacle by an intromittent organ. In still others, sperm, but no spermatophores, are deposited in the copulatory bursa and migrate to the seminal receptacle. In all instances, sperm are retained in the seminal receptacle until after fertilization. An exception to the usual route of sperm transfer occurs in insects that inject sperm into the female's hemocoel (i.e., the space between the body organs). The sperm then migrate to the ovary and oviduct and unite with eggs before the eggshell is formed.

Parthenogenesis

Most frequently, parthenogenesis is the development of a new individual from an unfertilized gamete. Often referred to as unisexual reproduction, it has been observed in almost every major invertebrate group, with the exception of protochordates (including hemichordates), and frequently occurs alternately with bisexual reproduction (reproduction by union of gametes). Some species, in which males are completely unknown, apparently reproduce only by parthenogenesis. Species that alternate between parthenogenesis and bisexual reproduction (heterogenetic species) often do so in response to changes in population density, food availability, or other environmental conditions.

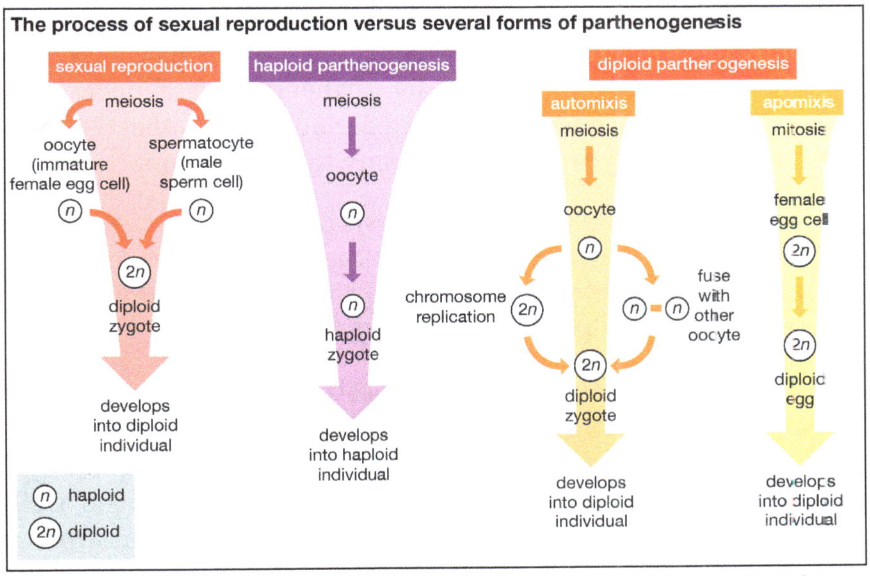

Sexual reproduction: The process of sexual reproduction and several forms of parthenogenesis.

The best known examples of parthenogenetic reproduction are found among rotifers. Males are completely unknown in some genera; in others, they appear in the population only for brief periods and more or less seasonally. Females are the dominant form or are the only sex present in a population throughout most of the year. Because no reductional division (meiosis) occurs in the course of egg maturation, the eggs are diploid-that is, they have the full number of chromosomes; they give rise to new diploid individuals with no chromosomal contribution from a male gamete (diploid parthenogenesis). Even if males were present, sperm could not fertilize the eggs because the latter are already diploid. Under conditions of environmental stress such as seasonal changes, some females form eggs that undergo reductional division, resulting in eggs with the haploid number of chromosomes; such eggs must be fertilized by a male gamete to produce a new female. When the new individual matures, it will probably reproduce parthenogenetically. If, however, there are no males in the population, the haploid eggs can develop into haploid males (haploid parthenogenesis), which then participate in bisexual reproduction. Bisexually produced eggs are often referred to as winter eggs since they have a thick covering that protects the embryo during adverse environmental conditions. Summer eggs, produced parthenogenetically, are thin shelled. Bisexual reproduction occurs, therefore, only often enough to ensure survival of the species.

Nematodes, especially free-living species such as some dioecious soil nematodes, exhibit a type of parthenogenesis known as gynogenesis. In this type of reproduction, the sperm produced by males do not unite with the haploid female egg but merely activate it to begin development. The result is haploid females.

Parthenogenesis, which apparently occurs only rarely in the annelids and mollusks, is found more frequently among the arthropods. The cladocerans (e.g., water fleas), for example, have a reproductive cycle much like that of rotifers—so long as environmental conditions are optimal and food is plentiful, females produce other females by diploid parthenogenesis. When conditions become adverse, males begin to appear in the population, and bisexual reproduction follows. The precise trigger for the appearance of males is not yet known. Fertilized eggs, covered with a highly resistant case, enter a resting stage (ephippium) and can withstand severe temperatures and drying out. The return of favourable conditions leads to the emergence of females that reproduce parthenogenetically. The ability to form a resting stage regulates population density. Whenever the food supply becomes short because of overpopulation by parthenogenetic females, bisexual reproduction is induced, and a dormant stage ensues. During periods of food shortage, the excess females die from lack of food, but the ephippia remain to restore the population.

Insects provide numerous examples of parthenogenesis of varying degrees of complexity. One of the most notable is that of the honeybee. Unfertilized eggs develop into drones, which are males. Fertilized eggs become worker females, which are kept in a nonreproductive state by secretions from the reproductive female, the queen bee.

Life cycles involving alternation between parthenogenesis and bisexual reproduction can be found in many species of Homoptera and Diptera (flies). Aphids (Homoptera) have a seasonal cycle consisting of a bisexual winter phase and a parthenogenetic summer phase; some species spend each phase on a different host plant. Temperature change, length of day, and food availability play major roles in initiating the phases. In the midge, a type of fly, the bisexual phase occurs in adults, and parthenogenesis takes place among the larvae (paedogenesis). Adult female midges deposit fertilized eggs, from which hatch larvae whose ovaries develop while the rest of the body retains a larval form. The ovaries of the larvae release eggs that enter the larval hemocoel (the space between body organs), where they undergo development while feeding on larval tissue. When sufficiently developed, the parthenogenetically produced young emerge either as larvae that continue parthenogenetic reproduction, forming larvae like themselves, or as male or female larvae that mature to become bisexually reproducing adults.

Provisions for the Developing Embryo

Invertebrates have developed a great many methods for protecting the fertilized egg and young embryo and for providing nutrients for the developing young. This is especially true of freshwater and terrestrial forms. Sponges and freshwater coelenterates, exposed to seasonal drying out, provide a tough covering for the eggs that prevents water loss. Many turbellarians envelop the eggs with a capsule and attach it to a hard surface, where it remains until the young emerge. Other turbellarians retain encapsulated eggs in the body until development is complete and the young emerge. All parasitic flatworms enclose their eggs in a protective capsule within which development occurs after it has left the parent's body. Most nematodes and rotifers do likewise, but a few species are ovoviviparous; i.e., the egg hatches in the mother's body. In many forms the amount of yolk provided in the egg and the nature of the egg capsule are correlated with annual seasons—summer eggs generally have less yolk and thinner capsules than do winter eggs. This is true also in a number of crustaceans. Freshwater and terrestrial annelids provide a cocoon for their young and often deposit it in a moist place. One group of leeches, however, does not form a cocoon; instead, the egg, surrounded by a protective membrane, is attached to the underside of the parent. As the young develop, the adult leech undulates its body so that water currents flow over the young. Presumably this serves as a means of aeration. Mollusks that live in freshwater may provide a protective covering for the eggs, or the eggs may be brooded by the female. Some pelecypods (bivalves) release mature eggs into their gill chambers; here the eggs are fertilized, and embryonic development is completed in a protected location. Cephalopods (e.g., squid, octopus) attach the eggs to a surface, then continuously force jets of water over the egg masses, thereby keeping them free of debris and perhaps aerating them. Some echinoderms also brood the eggs until the young emerge.

Arthropods have a particularly wide range of methods for ensuring offspring survival. Brood pouches, common in branchiopods, isopods, and amphipods, are sometimes part of the carapace, or back plate. In other instances, expanded plates on the lower side (sternum) form the pouches. Crayfish cement the fertilized eggs to their swimmerets (modified appendages) and carry them about as they are brooded by the female. The most elaborate provisions for the embryo are found among terrestrial arthropods, especially insects. Although some species simply deposit their eggs and abandon them, many retain the encapsulated egg within the body during early development. Some are viviparous; that is, they bear living young. The eggs of certain species of scorpions have little or no yolk; the embryo is nourished by the parent in a manner similar to that in mammals—part of the scorpion oviduct becomes modified as a uterus for the embryo; another part lies close to the female's gut and absorbs nutritive substances that are conveyed to the developing young. A similar arrangement has evolved in some insects. Other viviparous insects nourish the larvae by glandular secretions from the uterine lining.

Reproductive Systems of Vertebrates

Gonads, Associated Structures and Products

The reproductive organs of vertebrates consist of gonads and associated ducts and glands. In addition, some vertebrates, including some of the more primitive fishes, have organs for sperm transfer or ovipository (egg-laying) organs. Gonads produce the gametes and hormones essential for reproduction. Associated ducts and glands store and transport the gametes and secrete necessary substances. In addition to these structures, most male and female vertebrates have a cloaca, a cavity that serves as a common terminal chamber for the digestive, urinary, and reproductive tracts and empties to the outside. In lampreys and most ray-finned fishes in which the cloaca is small or absent, the alimentary canal has a separate external opening, the anus. In some teleosts the alimentary, genital, and urinary tracts open independently. Hagfishes, which are closely related to the lampreys, have a short cloaca. In many vertebrates other than mammals, especially reptiles and birds, the cephalic, or head, end of the cloaca is partitioned by folds into a urinogenital chamber (urodeum) and an alimentary chamber (coprodeum) that open into a common terminal chamber (proctodeum). Above monotremes (e.g., platypus, echidna) the embryonic cloaca becomes completely partitioned into a urinogenital sinus conveying urine and the products of the gonads, and an alimentary pathway; the two open independently to the exterior.

Gonads arise as a pair of longitudinal thickenings of the coelomic epithelium and underlying mesenchyme (unspecialized tissue) on either side of the attachment of a supporting membrane, the dorsal mesentery, to the body wall. At first, gonadal ridges bulge into the coelom and are continuous with the embryonic kidney. The germinal epithelium covering the gonadal ridges gives rise to primary sex cords (medullary cords) that invade the underlying mesenchyme. These cords establish within the gonadal blastema (a tissue mass that gives rise to an organ) a potentially male component, the medulla. Secondary sex cords grow inward, spreading just beneath the germinal epithelium to form a cortex. If the gonad is to become a testis, only the medullary component differentiates. If the gonad is to become an ovary, only the cortex differentiates.

The length of an adult gonad depends, in part, upon the extent of gonadal-ridge differentiation. In cyclostomes (lampreys and hagfish), elasmobranchs (sharks, skates, and rays), and teleosts most of it differentiates, and the gonads extend nearly the length of the body trunk. In tetrapods (amphibians, reptiles, birds, and mammals), the cranial portion, at the anterior end, generally does not differentiate; in toads only the more caudal, or posterior, portion does so. The middle segment in toads of both sexes gives rise to a Bidder's organ containing immature eggs. In anurans (frogs and toads) and some lizards of both sexes, one segment of the gonadal ridge gives rise to yellow fat bodies that, especially in anurans, diminish in size just prior to the breeding season. In mammals, only the middle portion of the gonadal ridge differentiates.

Some vertebrate species have only one gonad, which may lie in the midline or on one side; the condition is more common among females. Adult cyclostomes of both sexes have one gonad. In lampreys it is in the middle of the body; in hagfishes it is on the right side. Birds are the only other major group of vertebrates in which most females have one gonad, the right ovary being typically absent. Male birds have a pair of testes, however. Exceptions to the condition of single ovaries among birds include members of the falcon family, in which more than 50 percent of mature hawks have two well-developed ovaries. In all bird species a small percentage of females probably have two ovaries; reported instances include owls, parrots, sparrows, and doves, with estimates for doves ranging from 5 percent to 25 percent. A few teleosts and viviparous elasmobranchs have only one ovary; in sharks the right one is usually present, in rays, the left. In amniotes (i.e., reptiles, birds, and mammals) unpaired gonads are unusual. Some lizards have one testis, and some female crocodiles have one ovary. Among mammals, the platypus usually has only a left ovary, and some bat species (family Vespertilionidae) have only the right.

One of two explanations may account for unpaired gonads: the paired embryonic gonadal ridges may fuse to form a median gonad—as in lampreys and the perch—or only one gonadal ridge may receive immigrating primordial germ cells (immature sperm or eggs), with the result that the opposite gonad does not develop—as in chickens and ducks. Both gonadal ridges have been reported to exhibit an equal number of primordial germ cells in embryonic hawks, and these typically have two ovaries.

Among lower vertebrates, mature gonads sometimes produce both sperm and eggs. Hermaphroditism is more general in cyclostomes and teleosts than in other fishes. A teleost may function as a male during the early part of its sexual life and as a female later. In some teleost families sperm and eggs mature simultaneously but in different regions of the gonad. These fish normally function as males during one season and as females the next. Cyclostomes generally are ambisexual during juvenile life—i.e., immature male and female sex cells exist side by side, or, as in Myxine, the anterior part of the immature gonad may be ovary and the caudal part, the testis. It is thought that cyclostomes normally become unisexual at maturity. Hermaphroditism is uncommon among amphibians, although it frequently occurs as an anomaly. In vertebrates above amphibians, true hermaphroditism probably does not exist.

Both male and female duct systems are occasionally absent. In cyclostomes, a few elasmobranchs, and some teleosts, such as salmon, trout, and eels, the gametes are propelled toward the posterior within the coelom, often by cilia (minute hairlike structures), and exit via a pair of funnel-like genital pores near the base of the tail. In cyclostomes, the pores lead to a sinus, or cavity, within a median papilla (i.e., a fingerlike structure) and are open only during breeding seasons.

Male Systems

Testes

In anurans, amniotes (reptiles, birds, and mammals), and even some teleosts, testes are composed largely of seminiferous tubules—coiled tubes, the walls of which contain cells that produce sperm—and are surrounded by a capsule, the tunica albuginea. Seminiferous tubules may constitute up to 90 percent of the testis. The tubule walls consist of a multilayered germinal epithelium containing spermatogenic cells and Sertoli cells, nutritive cells that have the heads of maturing sperm embedded in them. Seminiferous tubules may begin blindly at the tunic, or outermost tissue layer, and pass toward the centre, becoming tortuous before emptying into a system of collecting tubules, the rete testis. Such an arrangement is characteristic of frogs. In certain amniotes—the rat, for example—the tubules may be open ended, running a zigzag course from the rete to the periphery and back again. The average length of such tubules is 30 centimetres (12 inches), and they seldom communicate with each other. In many mammals the tubules are grouped into lobules separated by connective-tissue septa, or walls. The arrangement permits the packing of an extensive amount of germinal epithelium into a small space. In immature males and in adult males between breeding seasons, the tubules are inconspicuous and the epithelium is inactive; in some species, however, spermatogenesis, or production of sperm, proceeds at a variable pace throughout the year. An active epithelium may exhibit all stages of developing sperm. The lumen, or tubule cavity, contains the tails of many sperm (the heads of which are embedded in Sertoli cells), free sperm, and fluid that is probably resorbed. In mammals, in any single zone along a tubule, all sperm are at the same stage of maturation; adjacent zones contain different generations of sperm, and a period of sperm formation and discharge is followed by an interval of inactivity.

In cyclostomes, most fishes, and tailed amphibians the germinal epithelium is arranged differently. Instead of seminiferous tubules there are large numbers of spermatogonial cysts (also called spermatocysts, sperm follicles, ampullae, crypts, sacs, acini, and capsules) in which sperm develop, but in which the epithelium is not germinal. Spermatogenic cells migrate into the cysts from a permanent germinal layer, which, depending on the species, may lie among cysts at the periphery of the testes or in a ridge along one margin of the testis. After invading the thin nongerminal epithelium of a cyst, spermatogenic cells multiply, producing enormous numbers of sperm. The cysts become greatly swollen and whitish in colour; the entire testis also swells and has a granular appearance. As sperm mature, they separate from the epithelium and move freely in the cystic fluid. Finally, the cysts burst, and the sperm are shed into ducts. In the case of cyclostomes and a few teleosts the sperm are shed into the coelom. The cysts, totally emptied, collapse. Then either they are replaced by new ones, or they become repopulated by additional spermatogenic cells. It is not yet known which of these processes occurs.

Testicular stroma, which fills the spaces between seminiferous tubules or spermatogenic cysts, consists chiefly of connective tissue, blood and lymphatic vessels, and nerves; it is more abundant in some vertebrates than in others. Glandular Leydig (interstitial) cells are also present in most, if not all, vertebrates. Thought to be a primary source of androgens, or male hormones, Leydig cells are not always readily distinguishable, and, in some bird species, they may be seen only with the electron microscope. The capillary system of the rat testis, and probably that of many other vertebrates, is such that blood that has bathed the Leydig cells flows to the tubules; it is thus probable that Leydig cell hormones have an immediate effect on the germinal epithelium.

Testes in vertebrates below mammals lie within the body. This is also true of many, sometimes all, members of the mammalian orders Monotremata, Insectivora, Hyracoidea, Edentata, Sirenia, Cetacea, and Proboscidea. Some male mammals—most marsupials, ungulates, carnivores, and primates after infancy—have a special pouch (scrotum) that the testes occupy permanently. A few mammals have a pouch into which the testes descend and from which they can be retracted by muscular action. These include a few rodents such as ground squirrels; most, if not all, bats; and some primitive primates (loris, potto). The scrotum consists of two scrotal sacs, each connected to the abdominal cavity by an inguinal canal lined with the peritoneal membrane. The canals are the path of descent (and retraction) of the testes to the sacs. In descending, the testes carry along a spermatic duct, blood and lymphatic vessels, and a nerve supply wrapped in peritoneum and constituting, collectively, the spermatic cord. Rabbits, most rodents, and some insectivores, which lack scrotal sacs, have instead a wide inguinal canal into which the testes may be drawn and from which they are retracted when in danger of injury. In these mammals, descended testes cause a temporary bulge in the perineal region (i.e., between the anus and the urinogenital opening). In a small number of mammals, the testes permanently occupy the perineal location.

The scrotum is a temperature-regulating device. Warm blood approaching the testis comes close to the vessels carrying cool blood leaving the testis, so that the blood approaching the testis is cooled; the vessels form an intricate vascular network (pampiniform plexus) within the spermatic cord. Failure of both testes to enter the scrotal sacs (cryptorchidism) results in permanent sterility.

In cold weather two sets of muscles, the dartos and cremasteric, pull the testes close to the body. The dartos lies between the two scrotal sacs and is attached to the scrotal skin. The cremaster, wrapped around the spermatic cord, is an extension of the abdominal wall musculature. It retracts the testis. Birds, like mammals, are homoiothermic (warm-blooded), and their testes are near air sacs (extensions of incurrent respiratory tubes). Air in the sacs may help regulate the temperature of the testes.

Ducts

The male duct system begins as the rete testis, a network within the testis of thin-walled ductules, or minute ducts that collects sperm from the seminiferous tubules. The rete is drained by a number of small ducts—usually fewer than ten—called the vasa efferentia, which are modified kidney tubules. In some fishes and amphibians the vasa efferentia connect the testes with the cranial (anterior) end of the kidneys. In anamniotes (e.g., fish and amphibians), therefore, except teleosts, the ducts that drain the kidneys usually drain the testes also. In most amphibians these ducts pass caudad, or posteriorly, to empty independently into the cloaca; in some fishes they pass through a median urinogenital papilla.

Although drainage of the testis and the kidney by the same duct is a basic pattern, there has been a tendency in many vertebrates toward separate spermatic and urinary ducts. This tendency is manifested in one of two ways among anamniotes. In many sharks and in some amphibians (Plethodontidae, Salamandridae, Ambystomatidae), the embryonic kidney duct ultimately drains the testis, and one or more new ducts (ureters) drain the adult kidney. On the other hand, in the primitive fish Polypterus and in most teleosts, the embryonic kidney duct drains the adult kidney, and a new duct arises to drain the testis. Many degrees of separation of the two ducts occur in anamniotes, from the condition of the sturgeon, in which the spermatic duct unites with the urinary duct far toward the head, to the condition in Esox (a pike), in which spermatic and urinary ducts empty independently to the exterior.

In amniotes, the mesonephric kidney is a temporary structure confined to the embryo, but the mesonephric duct persists in the adult male as a sperm duct. A separate ureter drains the adult kidney. The spermatic and urinary ducts empty independently into the cloaca except in mammals above monotremes, in which they are confluent with the urethra. The epididymis of amniotes, a highly tortuous duct draining the vasa efferentia, usually serves as a temporary storage place for sperm; it is small in birds and large in turtles. In mammals, the first part of the epididymis consists of a head, body, and tail that wrap around the testis; it gradually straightens to become the spermatic duct. The epididymis secretes substances that prolong the life of stored sperm and increase their capacity for motility.

In all vertebrates certain regions of the spermatic duct are lined by cilia and a variety of secretory epithelial cells. One end may enlarge to form a sperm reservoir or secrete seminal fluid. In the catfish Trachycorystes mirabilis secretions of the spermatic duct form a gelatinous plug in the female similar to the vaginal plug of mammals. A seminal glomulus in birds functions as a sperm reservoir. In some mammals an enlargement of the spermatic duct called the ampulla contributes to the seminal fluid and stores sperm. Small mucous glands (of Littre) and other glandular structures open into the urethra along its length. Cloacal glands in basking sharks and many salamanders form a jelly that encloses sperm in a spermatophore. Cloacal glands of some lizards produce secretions called pheromones. The siphon sac of elasmobranchs is one of the few accessory sex glands that are a separate organ in animals below mammals. It extends as an elongated pocket into the pelvic fin and secretes nutritive mucus that enters the female reproductive tract with sperm.

Accessory Glands

Accessory sex glands that are conspicuous outgrowths of the genital tract are almost uniquely mammalian. The major mammalian sex glands include the prostate, the bulbourethral, and the ampullary glands, and the seminal vesicles. All are outgrowths of the spermatic duct or of the urethra and all four occur in elephants and horses and in most moles, bats, rodents, rabbits, cattle, and primates. A few members of these groups lack ampullary glands, or ampullary glands and seminal vesicles. Cetaceans (whales, porpoises) have only the prostate, as do some carnivores, including dogs, weasels, ferrets, and bears.

The prostate, the most widely distributed mammalian accessory sex gland, is absent only in Echidna (a marsupial) and a few carnivores. It empties into the urethra by multiple ducts. Many rodents, insectivores, and lagomorphs have three separate prostatic lobes; in a few mammals (some primates and carnivores) the prostate is a single mass with lobules and encircles the urethra at the base of the bladder. In a few mammals (e.g., opossum), the prostate is not a compact mass but a partly diffuse gland. In many rodents (e.g., rat, guinea pig, mouse, and hamster) and some other mammals, the semen coagulates quickly after ejaculation as a result of a secretion from a male coagulating gland, which is usually considered part of the prostatic mass. Coagulated semen forms a vaginal plug that temporarily prevents copulation.

Bulbourethral (Cowper's) glands arise from the urethra near the penis and are surrounded by the muscle of the urethra or penis. Typically, there is one pair, but as many as three (marsupials) may be found. The glands, small in man, large in rodents, elephants, and some ungulates including pigs, camels, and horses, are absent in cetaceans, mustelids (e.g., mink, weasel), sirenians (manatees, dugongs), pholidotans (pangolins), some edentates, and carnivores such as walrus, sea lion, bear, and dog.

Although many mammals have an ampullary swelling on the spermatic duct near the urethra, only a small number form a separate ampullary gland as an outgrowth of the duct. It is very large in some bats, absent in many mammalian orders, and variable in the rest. Although common in rodents, it is absent in guinea pigs and some strains of mice.

Seminal vesicles are paired, typically elongated and coiled fibromuscular sacs that empty into either the spermatic duct or the urethra. Absent in monotremes, marsupials, carnivores, cetaceans, and in some insectivores, chiropterans, and primates, seminal vesicles are exceptionally large in rhesus monkeys and small in man. They are absent in domesticated rabbits, small or rudimentary in cottontails, large in armadillos, and variable in sloths. They contribute the sugar fructose and citric acid to the semen but do not serve as sperm reservoirs.

Female Systems

Ovaries

Ovaries lie within the body cavity and are suspended by a dorsal mesentery (mesovarium), through which pass blood and lymph vessels and nerves. Primitive vertebrate ovaries occur in the hagfish, in which a mesentery-like fold of gonadal tissue stretches nearly the length of the body cavity. Unique in the hagfish is the fact that functional ovarian tissue occupies only the forward half of the gonadal mass, the rear part containing rudimentary testicular tissue. In most fishes except very primitive forms, the ovaries are similarly elongated. In tetrapods other than mammals, the ovaries are usually confined to the middle third or half of the body cavity, particularly during nonbreeding seasons. The ovaries of mammals undergo moderate caudal displacement, finally coming to lie between the kidney and the pelvis.

The appearance of an ovary depends on many factors-e.g., whether one egg or thousands are discharged (ovulated); whether the eggs are immature or ripe; whether mature eggs are small or large; or whether pigments occur in the egg cytoplasm, such as those responsible for yellow yolk. Other factors also affect the appearance of the ovary: the season of the year in seasonal breeders (the ovary enlarges during breeding seasons, diminishes in size between seasons); the age of the animal (whether juvenile, reproductively active, or senile, particularly in birds and mammals); and the fate of ovulated, or discharged, egg follicles, or sacs.

The ovaries are covered with a germinal epithelium that is continuous with the peritoneum lining the body cavity. The term germinal epithelium is inappropriate because in most adults it contains no germ cells, these having moved deeper into the ovary. In hagfishes and amphibians, cells that give rise to eggs are known to occur in the germinal epithelium, and it may be that the germinal epithelium in a few other vertebrates contains similar cells. The germinal epithelium undergoes cell division, however. This is particularly true of species in which enormous expansion of the ovary occurs each breeding season. Beneath the epithelium is a layer of connective tissue, the tunica albuginea, which is much thinner than that surrounding the testes.

A typical vertebrate ovary consists of cortex and medulla. The cortex, immediately internal to the tunica albuginea, contains future eggs and, at one time or another, eggs in ovarian follicles (i.e., developing eggs); it undergoes fluctuations in size and appearance that correlate with stages of the reproductive cycle. The cortex also contains remnants of ovulated follicles and, in mammals, clusters of interstitial cells that, in some species, are glandular. The cortical components are embedded in a supportive framework of connective, vascular, and neural tissue constituting the stroma. Internal to the cortex is the medulla, consisting of blood and lymph vessels, nerves, and connective tissue. The medulla, which contains no germinal elements, exhibits no significant cyclical activity, is usually inconspicuous, is continuous with the dorsal mesentery and, in cyclostomes, is hardly distinguishable from the latter. The mammalian medulla, on the contrary, is almost completely surrounded by cortex and converges on the mesovarium (i.e., the part of the peritoneum that supports the ovary) at a narrow hilus, at which nerves and vessels enter the ovary. In the medulla of the mammalian ovary near the hilus are small masses of blind tubules or solid cords—the rete ovarii—which are homologous (i.e., of the same embryonic origin) with the rete testis in the male. The microscopic right ovary of birds usually consists only of medullary tissue.

Ovaries are characterized as saccular, hollow, lacunate (i.e., compartmented), or compact. The ovary of many teleosts, especially viviparous ones, contains a permanent cavity, which is formed during ovarian development when an invagination of the ovarian surface traps a portion of the coelom. The cavity is therefore unique in that it is lined by germinal epithelium. The lining develops numerous ovigerous folds that project into the lumen and greatly increase the surface area for proliferation of eggs. In most other teleosts, a temporary ovarian cavity develops after each ovulation, when the shrinking cortex withdraws from the outside ovarian wall along one side of the ovary. The resulting cavity is obliterated as eggs of the next generation enlarge. The permanent and temporary cavities of teleost ovaries and a similar cavity in garfish ovaries are continuous with the lumen of the oviduct, and eggs are shed into them. The ovaries of other fishes lack cavities and are characterized as compact. The amphibian ovary, which contains six or more central, hollow sacs that give it a lobed appearance, is characterized as saccular. The sacs are formed when the embryonic medullary and rete cords become hollow and coalesce. Maturing eggs bulge into the sacs but are not shed into them. The ovaries of reptiles, birds, and monotremes have cavities homologous to those in amphibians; the number of medullary spaces in the adults is considerably larger, however, so that the ovaries contain an extensive network of fluid-filled cavities (lacunae). Such ovaries are characterized as lacunate. The ovaries of mammals above monotremes are compact, having no medullary cavities.

An ovarian follicle consists of an oocyte, or immature egg, surrounded by an epithelium, the cells of which are referred to variously as follicular, nurse, or granulosa cells. In cyclostomes, teleosts, and amphibians, the epithelium is one layer thick. In the hagfish and those vertebrates in which the oocyte receives heavy deposits of yolk (elasmobranchs, reptiles, birds, and monotremes), the epithelium appears to be two cells thick, apparently the result of layering of nuclei in a simple columnar epithelium (i.e., epithelium consisting of relatively "tall" cells). Above monotremes the follicular epithelium appears to be many cells thick; in at least one species, however, this is considered an artifact, and all granulosa cells are said to extend between the outer boundary of the epithelium and the oocyte.

The follicular epithelium originates as a few flattened cells derived from the germinal epithelium. Primary follicles are usually situated just under the tunica albuginea; secondary follicles lie deeper in the cortex. The primitive role of the follicular cells appears to be the secretion of the yolk-forming material onto or into the oocyte. Evidence from mammals indicates that the follicular cells may also have a role in converting substances produced elsewhere into female hormones, or estrogens. In some hibernating bats the granulosa cells are filled with glycogen, or animal starch, which may be a source of energy. Mammalian follicles above monotremes are unique in that they develop a fluid-filled cavity (antrum) within the granulosa layer. During antrum formation cell division of the granulosa cells increases, and fluid-filled spaces develop among the cells. The spaces coalesce to form the antrum. Under the influence of pituitary gonadotropic hormones, many antral follicles thereafter continue to grow, forming large so-called Graafian follicles—less than 400 microns, or 0.4 millimetre (0.16 inch), in diameter in large mammals, 150–200 microns, or 0.15–0.2 millimetre (0.006–0.008 inch), in small ones. Graafian follicles contain mature eggs and appear as large blisters on the ovary. At this stage the ovum, suspended within the fluid of the antrum (liquor folliculi) by a slender stalk of granulosa cells, is surrounded by a cluster of these cells, the cumulus oophorus, or discus proligerus. The remaining follicular cells form a thin wall surrounding the antrum. Antra are lacking in a few insectivores (Hemicentetes, Euriculus) because the granulosa cells swell and multiply to form corpora lutea, masses of yellow tissue. In the bat Myotis the antrum is likewise compressed and disappears just before discharge of the egg, or ovulation.

In all vertebrates, oocytes that have begun to grow and mature may, at any time until just before ovulation, cease development and undergo atresia, or degeneration. This is a normal process that reduces the number of eggs ovulated. In small laboratory rodents, atresia takes place in 50 percent of the Graafian follicles in each ovary one or two days before ovulation, thus reducing the number of ovulatable eggs by 50 percent. A similar reduction takes place in hagfish prior to ovulation. Atretic follicles eventually become lost in the stroma of the cortex of the ovary. In mammals especially, follicles lacking oocytes and antra, called anovular follicles, as well as polyovular follicles (i.e., containing more than one oocyte), occasionally occur.

The ovarian follicle of vertebrates, commencing with hagfish, is surrounded by a theca, or sheath, composed of two concentric layers of stromal cells. The outer layer (theca externa) is chiefly connective tissue but may contain smooth muscle fibres. The inner layer (theca interna) has more blood vessels and, in vertebrates that produce heavily yolked eggs, the largest vessels carry venous blood. In these species the cell membranes of the oocyte and granulosa cells have many microvilli (i.e., fingerlike projections), which probably facilitate transport of substances important in yolk formation from the blood vessels to the egg. Mature follicles in the marsupial Dasyatus are said to lack theca, and in some bats only one thecal layer.

During the growth phase, eggs in species with massive amounts of yolk may increase in size 10^6 (1,000,000) or more times as a result of vitellogenesis (deposit of yolk). In goldfish, on the other hand, when vitellogenesis commences, the egg has a diameter of 150 microns (0.15 millimetre [0.006 inch]); that of the mature egg is only 500 microns (0.5 millimetre [0.02 inch]). Mammalian eggs contain little yolk and very little in size. Oogonia (i.e., cells that form oocytes) of the golden hamster average 15 microns (0.015 millimetre [0.0006 inch]) in diameter, and eggs in Graafian follicles average 70 microns (0.07 millimetre [0.003 inch]). The mature eggs of horses and humans are approximately the same size—somewhat less than 150 microns. In seasonally breeding oviparous fishes and amphibians, all eggs are usually in the same stage of development, and the ovary grows to a mature state quite rapidly as a result of growth of the eggs, which frequently number more than 1,000,000. Such ovaries distend the body wall when mature; following spawning, the ovaries shrink rapidly to inconspicuous bodies consisting mainly of oogonia, immature oocytes, and a few stromal cells. In reptiles and birds, ovarian weight also is high in proportion to body weight during egg-laying seasons. The weight of the ovary of the starling, for example, may increase from eight milligrams in early winter to 1,400 milligrams immediately before ovulation. The mature eggs of reptiles and birds are unique in that they are suspended from the ovary by a short stalk (pedicle). The stalk contains a cortex with additional oocytes in various stages of development and extensions of vessels and nerves. Full growth of the follicle in reptiles and birds requires only a few days or weeks (nine days in the domestic hen). In mammals, the ratio of ovarian weight to body weight varies insignificantly throughout the reproductive life of the female, and follicles in many stages of development are constantly present.

Vertebrate eggs are almost universally shed into the coelom or into a subdivision thereof, from which they enter the female reproductive tract. Even in those teleosts in which the eggs are shed into an ovarian cavity, the latter is often of coelomic origin. In many mammals a membranous sac of peritoneum, the ovarian bursa, traps part of the coelom in a chamber along with the ovary. The bursal cavity (periovarian space) may be broadly open to the main coelom, completely closed off from the coelom, or in communication with the coelom by a narrow, slitlike passage. The bursa, moderately developed in lower primates and catarrhines (Old World monkeys), is poorly developed in man. In horses, one edge of the ovary contains a long grooves (ovulation fossa) into which all eggs are shed; the groove is found in a cleftlike ovarian bursa. The ovarian bursa increases the probability that all ovulated eggs will enter the oviduct.

The process of ovulation has been described for all vertebrate classes. Elasmobranchs, reptiles, and birds have massively yolked eggs. As ovulation approaches, the fimbria (i.e., frills, or fringes) of the membranous and muscular funnel surrounding the entrance to the oviduct wave in a gentle, undulating motion. An egg that is nearly free of the ovary is grasped and partially encompassed by the fimbria; when the egg is freed, the fimbria draws the egg into the funnel. At this time, the egg has little shape and is partly squirted and partly flows into the oviduct; never completely free in the coelom, its chances of not entering the oviduct are small. In the case of moderately or poorly yolked eggs cilia help to sweep the eggs into the ostium, or opening, of the oviduct. During ovulation in Japanese rice fish, Oryzias latipes, a tiny papilla, or fingerlike process, develops on the surface of a bulging mature follicle in the centre (stigma) of the follicle. The follicle becomes thin at the stigma, an aperture appears, and the egg rolls out. In rabbits this process differs only in detail. During the final 20 minutes before ovulation in rabbits, some of the tiny blood vessels surrounding the stigma rupture, and a small pool of blood forms under the apex of the cone-shaped papilla. The follicular wall shortly gives way at the apex, and follicular fluid oozes from the opening, followed soon after by the egg. The ovulated mammalian egg typically is surrounded by a layer of columnar follicular cells, the corona radiata; but it is naked in some insectivores and some marsupials. Following ovulation in all vertebrates, the ovary may become smaller, become modified for maintenance of pregnancy, or proceed to form additional eggs.

The process of ovulation in vertebrates has been documented, but the immediate causes remain to be clarified. It is almost certain that an ovulatory hormone is secreted by the pituitary gland (i.e., the so-called master endocrine gland) of all vertebrates. It is highly probable that breakdown of very small fibres that bind the follicular cells together may occur at the stigma, weakening the follicular wall at that location. Hormones from the ovary and other sources may play a role, as may neurohormones, which are hormones released at nerve endings. Rhythmic contractions of the entire ovary occur at ovulation in many vertebrates and have been described in rabbits. The role of mechanical pressure within the follicle, however, is not understood. Ovulation in most mammals (spontaneous ovulators) occurs cyclically as a result of the spontaneous release of the ovulatory hormone. In a few mammals (reflex ovulators) the stimulus of copulation is essential for release of the ovulatory hormone.

Striking postovulatory changes take place in the follicles of mammals and, to lesser degrees, of lower vertebrates. Blood vessels from the theca interna invade the ovulated follicles; the granulosa cells divide, enlarge, accumulate fats, and obliterate any remnants of the collapsed antra. Thereafter, they are known as lutein cells. Theca interna cells undergo changes identical to those of the granulosa cells. The result in mammals is the formation of solid masses called corpora lutea, recognizable as prominent reddish-yellow bulges on the ovary. Corpora lutea produce the hormone progesterone, which is essential for the maintenance of pregnancy. The conversion of postovulatory follicles into structures more or less resembling mammalian corpora lutea has been demonstrated in numerous viviparous reptiles, amphibians, and elasmobranchs; in certain other fishes, including cyclostomes; and in some oviparous amphibians and reptiles. In birds, the postovulatory follicle shrinks, and identifiable corpora lutea do not develop, although some granulosa cells accumulate lipids of unknown significance.

Tracts

The female reproductive tract consists of a pair of tubes (gonoducts) extending from anterior, funnel-like openings (ostia) to the cloaca, except as noted below. The gonoducts are specialized along their length for secretion of substances added to the eggs; for transport, storage, nutrition, and expulsion of eggs or the products of conception; and, in species with internal fertilization, for receipt, transport, storage, and nutrition of inseminated sperm. The predominately muscular tracts are lined by a secretory epithelium and ciliated over at least part of their length. Fusion of the caudal (tail) ends of the paired ducts may occur. Gonoducts are absent in cyclostomes and a few gnathostome fishes that have abdominal pores. A few vertebrates have only one functional gonoduct.

Gonoducts in lungfishes and amphibians are coiled muscular tubes that are ciliated over most of their length. Only occasionally do they unite caudally in a genital papilla before opening into the cloaca. During breeding seasons their diameter increases severalfold because of the highly active secretory epithelium. Between breeding seasons they are small. In some anurans (frogs, toads), such as Rana, the lower end of each gonoduct is expanded to form an ovisac, in which ovulated eggs are stored until spawning; the tube between the ostium (funnel-like opening) and ovisac is the oviduct. In viviparous amphibians the young develop in the ovisac. In amphibians, numerous multicellular glands extend deep into the lining of the female tract. Six successive glandular zones have been described in some urodeles, and these secrete six different gelatinous substances upon the egg. Female urodeles often have convoluted tubular outpocketings of the cloaca called spermatheca; they temporarily store sperm liberated from the male spermatophore.

The two gonoducts of elasmobranchs share a single ostium, a trait found only in Chondrichthyes. The ostium is a wide caudally directed funnel supported in the falciform ligament, which is attached to the liver. The role of the fimbria of the ostium at ovulation has been described. Two oviducts pass forward from the ostium to the septum transversum (i.e., between the heart and abdominal cavities), curve around one end of the liver, then pass posteriorly on each side. Approximately midway between ostium and uterus each oviduct has a shell (nidamental) gland. Fertilization takes place above the shell gland, which may be immense or almost undifferentiated. Half of the shell gland secretes a substance high in protein content (albumen), and the other half secretes the shell—delicate in viviparous forms, thick and horny in most oviparous species. Horny shells may have spiral ridges and many long tendrils, which entwine about an appropriate surface after the egg is deposited. In the viviparous shark Squalus acanthias several eggs pass one after the other through the shell gland, where they are enclosed in one long delicate membranous shell that soon disintegrates. Beyond the shell gland the oviducts terminate in an enlargement, which, in viviparous species, serves as a uterus. An oviducal valve may be found at the junction of oviduct and uterus. Although the two uteri usually open independently into the cloaca, they occasionally unite to form a bicornuate (two-horned) structure. In immature females, the uterus may be separated from the cloaca by a hymen, or membrane. The tract enlarges enormously during the first pregnancy and does not thereafter fully regress to its original size.

The gonoducts of lower ray-finned fishes resemble those of lungfish, but those of gars and teleosts are exceptional in that the oviducts are usually continuous with the ovarian cavities. A median genital papilla receives the oviducts in teleosts, and the papilla is sometimes elongated to form an ovipositor. European bitterlings deposit their eggs in a mussel by means of the ovipositor, and female pipefish and sea horses deposit them in the brood pouch of a male.

With certain modifications, the gonoducts of reptiles and birds are comparable to those of lower vertebrates. Crocodilians, some lizards, and nearly all birds have one gonoduct; the other is not well developed. Even in birds of prey having two functional ovaries, the right oviduct is sometimes undeveloped. The tracts of reptiles generally show less regional differentiation than do those of birds. The oviduct funnel (ostium) in birds forms the chalazae—two coiled, springlike cords extending from the yolk to the ends of the egg. In both reptiles and birds, much of the length of the female tract is oviduct. This region, called the magnum in birds, secretes albumen; lizards and snakes do not form albumen. Behind the albumen-secreting region is a shell gland. In lizards, the gland is midway along the tract. In birds, the shell gland is at the posterior end, has thick muscular walls, and is often inappropriately called a uterus. It is preceded by a narrow region, or isthmus, which secretes the noncalcareous, or soft, membranes of the shell. The shell gland leads to a narrow muscular vagina that empties into the cloaca. The vagina secretes mucus that seals the pores of the shell before the egg is expelled. Special vaginal tubules (spermatheca) store sperm over winter in some snakes and lizards; seminal receptacles have been described in the oviduct funnel in some snakes. In birds, sperm storage glands (sperm nests) often occur in the funnel and at the uterovaginal junction. In lizards and birds, ovulation does not usually occur into a tract already containing an egg. Some lizards shed very few eggs per season; the gecko, for example, sheds only two.

The female reproductive tracts of monotremes, the egg-laying mammals, consist of two oviducts, the lower ends of which are shell glands. These open into a urinogenital sinus, which, in turn, empties into a cloaca. Marsupials have two oviducts, two uteri (duplex uterus), and two vaginas. The upper parts of the vaginas unite to form a median vagina that may or may not be paired internally. Beyond the median vagina, the vaginas are again paired (lateral vaginas) and lead to a urinogenital sinus. The posterior end of the pouchlike median vagina is separated from the forward end of the urinogenital sinus by a partition. When the female is delivering young, the fetuses are usually forced through the partition and into the urinogenital sinus, bypassing the lateral vaginas. The ruptured partition may remain open thereafter, resulting in a pseudovagina. It closes in opossums, and in kangaroos both the median and lateral routes may serve as birth canals. The lateral vaginas in marsupials receive the forked tips of the male penis. Fertilization in all mammals takes place in the oviducts (Fallopian tubes).

In eutherian mammals (i.e., all mammals except monotremes and marsupials), with exceptions noted below, female reproductive tracts beyond the ostia (oviduct funnels) consist of two narrow and somewhat tortuous Fallopian tubes, two large uterine horns (each of which receives a Fallopian tube), a uterine body, and one vagina. Fallopian tubes often have a short dilated ampulla, or saclike swelling, just beyond the ostium. Implantation of the egg occurs only in the uterine horns; the embryos become spaced equidistant from one another in both horns even if only one ovary has ovulated. In some species one horn is rudimentary—the left in the impala (an African antelope)—and the embryos become implanted in the other horn, even though both ovaries ovulate. The body of the uterus in some mammals (e.g., rabbits, elephants, aardvarks; some rodents, bats, insectivores) contains two separate canals (bipartite uterus). In other mammals (ungulates, many cetaceans, most carnivores and bats) the body of the uterus has one chamber into which the two horns empty (bicornuate uterus). There are numerous intermediate conditions between the bipartite and bicornuate condition. Apes, monkeys, and man have no horns, and the Fallopian tubes empty directly into the body of the uterus (simplex uterus). In all mammals, the uterine body tapers to a narrow neck (cervix). The opening (os uteri) into the vagina is guarded by fleshy folds (lips of the cervix). The vagina in eutherian mammals other than rodents and primates terminates in a urinogenital sinus that opens to the exterior by a urinogenital aperture. In some rodents and in higher primates the vagina opens directly to the exterior. In the young of many species a membrane, the hymen closes the vaginal opening. In guinea pigs the hymen reseals the opening after each reproductive period. Sperm are stored over winter in the uterus of some bats and in vaginal pouches in others.

Accessory Glands

Female mammals have fewer accessory sex glands than males, the most prominent being Bartholin's glands and prostates. Bartholin's (bulbovestibular) glands are homologues of the bulbourethral glands of males. One pair usually opens into the urinogenital sinus or, in primates, into a shallow vestibule at the opening of the vagina. Prostates develop as buds from the urethra in many female embryos but often remain partially developed. They become well developed, however, in some insectivores, chiropterans, rodents, and lagomorphs, although their function is obscure. A variety of glands (labial, preputial, urethral) are found in the mucosa, or mucous membrane. Glands in the uterine mucosa provide nourishment for embryos before implantation. Cervical uterine glands secrete mucus that lubricates the vagina, which has no glands.

Adaptations for Internal Fertilization

Fertilization among vertebrates may be external or internal, but internal fertilization is not always correlated with viviparity or the presence of intromittent (copulatory) organs. The latter, uncommon among fishes, amphibians, and birds, are present in all reptiles (except Sphenodon) and mammals.

A considerable number of fishes are viviparous; in them, fertilization is internal, and the males have intromittent organs. The claspers of most male elasmobranchs are usually paired extensions of pelvic fins that are inserted into the female's uterus for transfer of sperm. The clasper, supported by modified fin cartilages, contains a groove along which sperm are conveyed into the uterus and is raised, or erected, by muscles at its base. Gonopodia of male teleosts are fleshy, often elongated modifications of pelvic or anal fins that are directed posteriorly, have a genital pore at the end, and often serve as intromittent organs. In some teleosts, a large penis-like papilla located under the throat is supported by bones. The spermatic duct opens on one side of the papilla. In a few teleosts, hemal spines (ventral projections of vertebrae) form the skeleton of an intromittent organ. Occasionally, the intromittent organ is an asymmetrical tube that matches the asymmetrical genital opening of the female. Still other teleosts have uncomplicated fleshy genital papillae that can be erected. In at least one teleost species, the female has a copulatory organ that she inserts into the genital pore of the male for receiving sperm.

Certain amphibians have internal fertilization but no intromittent organs. The muscular cloaca of the male caecilian, however, can be everted (turned outward) to protrude into that of the female. The male urodele deposits a spermatophore that the female picks up with the lips of her cloaca. Among anurans, Nectophrynoides (a viviparous frog) and Ascaphus (a toad) have internal fertilization, but only Ascaphus has an intromittent organ. It is a permanent tubular extension of the cloaca and resembles a tail. Other anurans have external fertilization and no intromittent organs.

The provision of an eggshell in reptiles requires that fertilization be internal, and all reptiles have intromittent organs except Sphenodon. Reptilian intromittent organs are of two types. Crocodilians and chelonians (turtles) have a penis (phallus), a median thickening in the floor of the cloaca consisting of two cylinders of spongy vascular erectile tissue, the corpora spongiosa. The caudal tip of the penis protrudes into the cloaca as a genital tubercle, or glans penis. The penis is held in the cloacal floor by retractor muscles. When the blood vessels within the spongy bodies are filled with blood, the penis swells, the retractor muscle relaxes, and the genital tubercle protrudes from the vent to serve as an intromittent organ. A longitudinal groove on the surface of the penis directs the flow of sperm. When the spongy bodies are no longer filled with blood, the retractor muscle returns the penis to the cloacal floor. Snakes and lizards have hemipenes, paired elongated outpocketings of the caudal wall of the cloaca that extend under the skin at the base of the tail. Each hemipenis is held in place by a retractor muscle. During copulation the muscle relaxes, the pocket turns inside out and protrudes through the vent in an erect condition. Semen passes along grooves on its surface. Except in pythons, erectile tissue is lacking in hemipenes. Hemipenes protrude independently of each other and are often covered with spines. Very small hemipenes of unknown function are usually present in females.

All birds have internal fertilization, although they are not viviparous; most lack intromittent organs. Male swans, ducks, geese, tinamous, ostriches, and some other ratites (flightless birds), however, have an erectile median penis like that of crocodiles and turtles. Chickens have an organ consisting of a small amount of erectile tissue, but lymph vessels, rather than blood vessels, become engorged. Some birds have a vestigial penis.

All mammals have internal fertilization and an erectile penis. That of monotremes is of the reptilian type, nonprotrusible and in the cloacal floor. In higher mammals the penis has been modified. The groove on the surface of the embryonic penis becomes enclosed in a tube along with the corpus spongiosum and two additional erectile masses, the corpora cavernosa. The proximal ends (crura) of the corpora cavernosa are anchored laterally to the pubic and ischial bones by various muscles and constitute the root of the penis. The crura converge in the midline to enter the body of the penis, which also contains the urethra, surrounded by the corpus spongiosum. The latter begins on the pelvic floor as the bulb of the penis and contains a dilation of the urethra (urethral bulb). The body of the penis extends a variable distance beyond the body of the mammal, in contrast to the short genital tubercle of reptiles. Except in ruminants (i.e., cud-chewing animals, such as cattle and deer), cetaceans, and some rodents, the penis terminates in a glans penis, a swelling of the corpus spongiosum that caps the ends of the corpora cavernosa and contains the urinogenital aperture. The glans is supplied with nerve endings and is partly or wholly sheathed, except during erection, by a circular fold of skin, the prepuce. The inner surface of the prepuce is moistened by preputial glands, and the external surface is sometimes covered with spines or hard scales, as in the cat, guinea pig, and wombat. The glans penis of the male Virginia opossum (Didelphis virginiana), the bandicoot, and some other species is bifid (i.e., with two equal tips), correlated with the paired vaginas of females. In boars, the glans penis is corkscrew-shaped, and in goats, rams, and many antelopes a urethral (vermiform) process of much smaller diameter extends three or four centimetres (about an inch to an inch and a half) beyond the glans. In some cattle, a sigmoid, or S-shaped, flexure bends the penis, which otherwise would be too long to fit into the preputial sac. The penis of marsupials is directed backward, and that of cats and rodents is directed backward, except during copulation. In some mammals (e.g., bats) it is pendulous; and in armadillos it may extend one third the length of the body during copulation.

Erection of the mammalian penis is initiated typically by an increase in the volume of blood reaching the cavernous and spongy bodies, engorgement of the vessels, and consequent compression of the veins leaving the organ. When a retractor muscle is present (wolf, fox, dog), it relaxes as erection occurs. The amount of erectile tissue in bovines (cattle) is small, and the penis has much fibroelastic tissue. Erection in such species results primarily from relaxation of the retractor muscle, and vascular engorgement provides only rigidity. Among mechanisms that reverse the erectile state are disgorgement of blood from the cavernous spaces, elasticity of the walls of the spaces, and action of a retractor muscle. A penis bone (baculum, os priapi) is present in various degrees of development in many mammals.

Female mammals have an erectile penile organ known as the clitoris in the floor of the urinogenital sinus or vagina. In the young spider monkey Ateles, the clitoris is six or seven centimetres (2.4 to 2.8 inches) long. In a few mammals (some rodents, insectivores, lemurs, and hyenas) the urethral canal becomes enclosed within the clitoris, as in males. In hyenas, the clitoris is large and often mistaken for a penis, and female scrotal pouches, lacking gonads, are present. So much do the male and female external genitalia resemble each other that the ancients regarded the hyena as a hermaphrodite. The clitoris of female mammals often contains cartilage or bone. A specialized clitoris is present in female turtles, crocodiles, alligators, and a few species of birds in which the male has a penis.

The spermatic duct of male mammals between the seminal vesicle and the prostatic urethra has a heavy muscular coat and serves as an ejaculatory duct. In mammals in which the seminal vesicles empty directly into the urethra, the latter is ejaculatory. In birds, the terminal segments of the spermatic ducts are erectile and ejaculatory, and in fish the posterior end of whatever duct transports sperm may be ejaculatory.

Role of Gonads in Hormone Cycles

Neurosecretions formed in the brain in response to environmental stimuli regulate the synthesis and release of hormones known as gonadotropins, which, in turn, stimulate the gonads. Cyclical intervals of illumination may be the principal environmental factor regulating gonadal activity. Although cyclical temperature changes are experienced by many species, as are fluctuations in food supply, rainfall, and salinity, their precise effects and those of many other stimuli, independently or in combination, have not yet been defined for any species. Photoperiodicity, temperature, and perhaps all other cycles are attributable to the seasons, and to the 24-hour day.

As a result of rhythmic stimulation by gonadotropins secreted by the pituitary gland, the gonads grow, mature, and produce gametes and hormones. Certain of these hormones, known as androgens, are thought to be produced chiefly by interstitial cells and are more abundant in males. Hormones known as estrogens are probably produced chiefly by ovarian follicles and their thecas. Circulating progestins are produced in greatest quantities by corpora lutea. Although the gonadal hormones of different species vary somewhat in structure, their effects are essentially the same. As the quantity of pituitary gonadotropins decreases, the activity of the gonads slows and may temporarily cease.

The effects of gonadal hormones may be summarized as follows:

Gonadal hormones induce growth of and maintain the cyclical function of the reproductive tracts, accessory sex glands, and copulatory or ovipository organs. They thereby provide for the storage, nutrition, and transport of gametes; the secretion of necessary substances onto the surface of gametes; and the ultimate extrusion of sperm, eggs, or the products of conception. In mammals, therefore, they prepare the vagina for copulation and the uterus for implantation of eggs; in addition, gonadal hormones maintain pregnancy until birth or until placental hormones can take over their function. The hormonal basis for the maintenance of viviparity in vertebrates below mammals is almost unknown.

Gonadal hormones participate in the maturation of gametes still in the gonads by augmenting the metabolic effects of other hormones.

Gonadal hormones are essential for the differentiation of many secondary sex characters—the physical differences between the sexes—facilitate amplexus (copulatory embrace) and provide for the protection or nutrition of young. Secondary sex characters include scent glands; sexually linked pigmentation of the skin or its appendages; the nature of any vocal apparatus; hardened areas on the appendages that facilitate amplexus; distribution of hair; body size; mammary gland development; and other features.

Gonadal hormones participate in the induction of behaviour necessary for the union of sperm and eggs; this includes migratory phenomena, heat (estrus) in mammals, courtship, territorial defense, mating, and care of eggs or young.

Gonadal hormones participate in a mechanism that affects the pituitary, thereby imposing certain restraints on the secretion of gonadotropins.

The effects of a cyclical environment on gonads is illustrated in mammals that ovulate spontaneously. Ovulation is induced by ovulatory hormones released rhythmically from the pituitary gland. Newborn mice maintained during the first week of life in regular, natural photoperiods will, on reaching maturity, ovulate regularly. Newborn mice kept in continuous light during this interval will not ovulate regularly. The photoperiods in which these animals live as neonates, or newborn, establish an intrinsic brain rhythm that subsequently results in cyclical reproductive activity. If mature female mice that have been ovulating regularly are subjected to continuous light, ovulation ultimately becomes arrhythmical. This suggests that the rhythmical environment is the ultimate regulator of the gonads. Because of the effects of cyclical photoperiods, spontaneous ovulation occurs about the same time of day or night in all members of species intensively studied thus far. Golden hamsters ovulate shortly after midnight; chickens and Japanese rice fish ovulate in the morning. Not all mammals ovulate spontaneously, however. In those that do not (e.g., reflex ovulators), including some cats, rodents, weasels, shrews, rabbits, the act of mating substitutes for the environmental effects on the pituitary gland in releasing ovulatory hormones.

Provisions for the Developing Embryo

Among the requirements of developing embryos are nutrients, oxygen, a site in which to discharge metabolic wastes, and protection from the environment. These needs exist whether the embryo is developing outside the body of the female parent (oviparity), or within, so that she delivers living young (viviparity). Combinations of yolk, albumen, jellies, and shells contributed by the female parent, as well as membranes constructed from the tissues of the embryo meet the embryo's needs.

Oviparous eggs are usually supplied with enough nutrients to last until the new individual is able to obtain food from the environment. The alternative, postnatal parental feeding is uncommon. Oviparous animals that develop from yolk-laden eggs are not hatched until they resemble adults. Those that develop from eggs with moderate amounts of yolk hatch sooner, usually into free-living larvae; in this case the larvae transform, or undergo metamorphosis, into adults. The eggs of amphioxus, an oviparous protochordate, contain almost no nutrients; the embryos hatch in an extremely undeveloped but self-sustaining state as few as eight hours after fertilization. The yolk mass is large in some animals and becomes surrounded by a membrane called the yolk sac, the vessels of which convey yolk to the embryo. In some species, yolk also passes from the yolk sac directly into the fetal intestine.

Oviparous fishes and amphibians develop in an aquatic environment, and exchange of oxygen and carbon dioxide and elimination of metabolic wastes occur through the egg membranes. Oviparous reptiles, birds, and monotremes develop on land, and gaseous exchange is accomplished by two membranes (allantois, chorion) applied closely to the shell. The allantois also receives some wastes. Drying out or mechanical injury of embryos of reptiles, birds, and mammals is prevented by still another membrane, the amnion, which is a fluid-filled sac immediately surrounding the embryo.

Viviparity has evolved in some members of all vertebrate classes except birds. When eggs heavily laden with yolk and surrounded by a well-formed shell develop within the female, the parent may provide the developing young only with shelter and oxygen (ovoviviparity). At the opposite extreme, if eggs contain only enough nutrients to supply energy for a few cell divisions after fertilization, the female provides shelter, oxygen, and nourishment, and, in addition, excretes all metabolic wastes produced by the developing organism (euviviparity). Between these extremes are numerous intermediate degrees of dependence on the parent.

Teleosts have evolved many unusual adaptations for viviparity. In some viviparous teleosts the eggs are fertilized in the ovarian follicle, where development occurs. The granulosa cells either form a membrane that secretes nutrients and assists in respiratory and excretory functions or they may be ingested along with follicular fluid, nearby eggs, and other ovarian tissue. A common site for development is the ovarian cavity, which may become distended with as many as nine series of embryos of different ages. Embryos in this location are bathed with nutritive fluids secreted by the epithelium of the cavity. In some species, mortality rates of intraovarian young are high, and surviving individuals ingest those that die. In still other species, extensions of villi in the ovarian lining invade the mouth and opercular (gill) openings of the embryo, filling the opercular chamber, mouth, and pharynx with surfaces that secrete nutrients. The embryos also develop specialized surfaces for nutrition, respiration, and excretion. An enlarged pericardial (heart) sac or an expansion of the hindgut of the embryo may occur next to the blood-vessel containing (vascular) follicular wall. Vascular extensions may grow out of the anus, urinogenital pore, or gills of the embryo. Other embryonic surfaces—including ventral body wall, fins, and tail—may participate in the support of viviparity. These embryonic surfaces may lie in contact with the follicular or ovarian epithelium, or they may simply be bathed by ovarian fluids. One or more combinations of the maternal and embryonic specializations described above, as well as many others, make viviparity possible among teleost fishes. In a number of teleosts the eggs are incubated, or brooded, in the mouth of the male for periods as long as 80 days. The oral epithelium becomes vascular and highly glandular. In sea horses and pipefish the female deposits her eggs in a ventral brood pouch of the male, and the embryos develop there.

In viviparous elasmobranchs development takes place in the uterus, the lining of which develops parallel ridges or folds covered with villi or papillae (trophonemata) that constitute a simple placenta (site of fetal–maternal contact). In contact with this region is the yolk sac of the embryo, which serves as a respiratory and nutritive membrane. Trophonemata secrete uterine fluids that supplement the yolk as a source of energy. In one shark (Pteroplatea micrura), trophonemata extend into the spiracular chamber (an opening for the passage of respiratory water) of the young and secrete nutrients into the fetal gut. In another (Mustelus antarcticus), the uterine folds form fluid-filled compartments for each embryo. The yolk sac may lie in contact with the uterine lining, or projections of the sac may extend into uterine pits. When the stored yolk is used up before birth, the yolk sac may serve for the absorption of nutrients; i.e., as a placenta. In a few species, immature eggs that enter the oviduct are eaten by the developing young.

Very few amphibians bear living young. In the viviparous frog Nectophrynoides, all development, including larval stages, occurs in the uteri and the young are born fully metamorphosed; i.e., except for size they resemble adults. N. occidentalis, an African species, has a nine-month gestation period. There is almost no yolk in the egg and no placenta, so it is probable that uterine fluids provide nourishment and oxygen. In N. vivipara there are as many as 100 larvae in the uteri, each with long vascular tails that may function as respiratory membranes. Gastrotheca marsupiata is an ovoviviparous anuran with a gestation period of three to four months. In certain viviparous salamanders the extent of the nutritional dependence on the mother varies. After depleting their own yolk supply, the larvae of some forms eat other embryos and blood that escapes from the uterine lining. Conventional viviparity is rare among amphibians; however, they have evolved unusual alternatives. In some anurans the young develop in such places as around the legs of the male (Alytes), or in pouches in the skin of the back (some females of the genera Nototrema, Protopipa, and Pipa). In Pipa, vascular partitions in the skin pouch separate developing young, and the larvae have vascular tails that absorb substances. In Nototrema larval gills have vascular extensions with a similar function. The male Chilean toad (Rhinoderma darwinii) carries developing eggs in the vocal sac until the young frogs emerge.

Some snakes and lizards and all mammals except monotremes exhibit viviparity to some degree. The same extra-embryonic membranes found in oviparous reptiles and mammals (yolk sac, chorioallantoic membrane, and amnion) function in viviparous ones. Here, the extra-embryonic membranes lie against the uterine lining instead of against an egg shell. At special sites of fetal–maternal contact (placentas), viviparous young receive oxygen and give up carbon dioxide; metabolic wastes are transferred to maternal fluids and tissues; and, in euviviparous species, the young receive all their nutrients. Yolk-sac placentas are common in marsupials with short gestation periods (opossum, kangaroo) and in lizards. Chorioallantoic placentas (i.e., a large chorion fused with a large allantois) occur in certain lizards, in marsupials with long gestation periods, and in mammals above marsupials. The yolk-sac placenta does not invade maternal tissues, but intimate interlocking folds may occur between the two. The chorioallantoic membranes of reptiles and mammals exhibit many degrees of intimacy with maternal tissues, from simple contact to a deeply rooted condition (deciduate placentas). Chorioallantoic or chorionic placentas represent specializations in a chorionic sac surrounding the embryo. The entire surface of the sac may serve as a placenta (diffuse placenta, as in pigs); numerous separate patches of placental thickenings may develop (cotyledonary placenta, as in sheep); a thickened placental band may develop at the equator of the chorionic sac (zonary placenta, as in cats); or there may be a single oval patch of placental tissue (discoidal placenta, as in higher primates).

Canine Anatomy

Dog anatomy is as complex as human anatomy. Anatomy is the study of the structures which reside within an animal's body. Anatomy will vary from species to species. Dog anatomy simply the study of the anatomical and visible features that is encompassed within our canine companions. Anatomy does not just look at the physical characteristics of a system; instead, dog anatomy tells veterinarians how the various body systems work together to produce life.

Without a proficient foundation in dog anatomy, a veterinarian could not be a vet, a surgeon, or even a pharmacologist. This is because dog anatomy does not just about know and memorizing structures, it is also about understanding the physiology and the biochemistry of the body.

Parts of the Canine Skull

The skull of a dog can be broken down into two parts—facial and cranial. The facial region of a dog skull is made up of several bones, and these are the:

- Lacrimal bone
- Zygomatic bone
- Nasal bone
- Maxilla
- Palatine bone
- Incisive bone
- Vomer bone

As we further back towards the dog skull, we come to the cranium. Now the cranium is too made up of multiple bones, however, let us keep things simple by focusing on the neuro (cranium). The cranium is a term used to describe the bones that surround the brain. It is composed of:

- Occipital bone
- Temporal bone

- Parietal bone
- Frontal bone
- Ethmoid bone
- Sphenoid bone

Through years of selective breeding, dogs are considered the only species of animal that have three different types of skull shape.

Mesaticephalic is the term given to dogs with a normal skull conformation. Examples of dogs that fall into this category are your Golden Retrievers and Beagles. Dolicephalic refers to dogs that have a more extended and more substantial facial conformation.

Many dog breeds have a dolichocephalic facial component; some of these breeds include the Afghan hound, Doberman Pinscher, Great Dane, and Rough Collie.

Finally, Brachiocephalic refers to dogs with a shorter facial conformation. The most notorious Brachiocephalic dog breeds include the Boston Terrier, Pug, Bulldog, and Boxer.

Canine Cardiovascular System

The cardiovascular system is part of the circulatory system. It consists of the heart, blood vessels (veins and arteries), and lymphatics. Just like in human beings, a dogs heart will have four chambers—two atria and two ventricles. Within the heart are also four major blood vessels and these are a cranial and caudal vena cava, a pulmonary trunk, and a pulmonary vein.

So, on the left side of the heart, oxygenated blood (think of this as blood which has a lot of oxygen to give) enters the left atrium of the heart through the pulmonary veins. From there it enters the second chamber of the heart—the left ventricle—and it is then forcefully expelled through the aorta. In veterinary medicine, this is referred to as the system circulation. In other words, the left side of the heart is responsible for taking in oxygen-rich blood and sending it through to the heart and the rest of the body.

Now, on the right side of the heart, deoxygenated blood aka blood with little to no oxygen enters the left atrium of the heart. It enters the left atrium through two blood vessels a caudal and cranial vena cava.

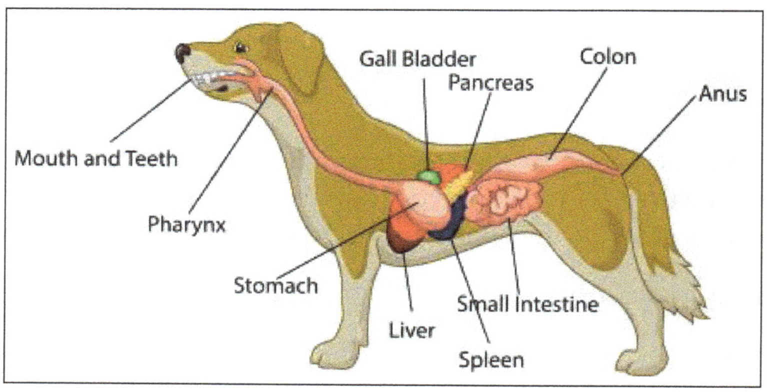

The caudal vena cava brings oxygen-poor blood from the lower half of an animal's body. And, the cranial vena cava brings oxygen-poor blood from the upper half of the body. After entering the right atrium, the oxygen-poor blood flows into the right atrium and will then be pumped out through the pulmonary trunk.

Canine Digestive System

The dog digestive system is a complex pathway that not only involves the mechanical breakdown of food, but it also consists of the absorption of nutrients. The digestive system begins at the mouth, where food is mechanically and chemically broken down into particles. Saliva is an essential component in the process of digestion. In human beings, saliva contains an enzyme called amylase.

This enzyme is responsible for the breakdown of carbohydrates. However, the saliva of our dogs and cats don't don't produce any enzymes. Instead, the function of their saliva is to naturally lubricate food, making it easier to travel down the esophagus. As the food leaves the mouth, it enters the esophagus. The esophagus is a long muscular tube that propels food down to the stomach. Now, these contractions that move food into the stomach are called peristaltic waves, and the central nervous system controls it.

Once the food enters the stomach, it undergoes further chemical and mechanical digestion. The stomach of a dog contains small folds which help with the process of grinding and breaking food down. During the churning process, gastric enzymes such as pepsin, rennin, and hydrochloric acid are secreted for the chemical breakdown of the food.

Finally, at the end of this entire process, the churned up food will enter the small intestine. There are three parts to the small intestine—the duodenum, jejunum, and ileum. The first part of the small intestine is the duodenum, and it has a close relationship with the pancreas.

The pancreas of a dog has two functions—an endocrine and exocrine function. The exocrine pancreas is responsible for secreting pancreatic juices and other enzymes into the duodenum. The purpose of the pancreatic juice is to neutralize any stomach acid that may have entered the duodenum. While the purpose of enzyme secretion is to begin the breakdown of proteins, carbohydrates, and fats.

The food then slowly beings to flow through the various other parts of the small intestine—the jejunum and ileum. If you were to look at a photomicrograph of the surface of the small intestine, you would see tiny little crypts and hair like structures.

These crypts are known as the crypts of liberkühn, and overtop of them lie villi (aka the hair-like structures). The purpose of these structures is to provide a greater surface area, so that food and nutrients can be absorbed more efficiently.

Finally, as food exits the small intestine, it enters the large intestine. Now, the large intestine is where all the water from the food bolus is absorbed back into the body.

The large intestine consists of few parts—a colon, caecum, and rectum. No digestion occurs in the colon of a dog; instead, the primary function of the colon is to store the digested food and collect any electrolytes, vitamins, and fatty acids that may be present.

This is essentially the final stage of digestion as eventually when the time is right; your pupper will release their colon contents out through their rectum.

Taste Buds in Dogs

Yes, even our canine companions have taste buds, but they don't have as many compared to us humans. It is estimated that dogs have about 1,700 tastebuds; of these they can determine sweetness, sour, salty, and bitter foods. In addition to this, dogs also have a unique tastebud for water. Now, we humans don't have a tastebud for water, but at least we have over 9,000 tastebuds.

Respiratory System of the Dog

The respiratory system of a dog is quite a complex system. The respiratory system is composed of the nose, mouth, trachea, bronchi, and alveoli. This system is crucial as it is what helps us breathe, without a proper functioning respiratory system an animal will experience shock, hypoxia, and death.

When a dog inhales, they take in oxygen through the nose and mouth. The gaseous oxygen is then transported through the nasal cavity down through to the trachea.

The trachea is known as the windpipe, and it is merely a long cylindrical tube that is composed of cartilage, muscle, and ligaments. As air flows down the trachea, it reaches the bronchi. Now the bronchi split into two halves—which are known as a bifurcation. The first half of the bronchi will branch into the right side of the lung and the second half of the bronchi will branch to the left.

As the respiratory bronchi get smaller and smaller, they begin to form a network of sacs. These sacs are referred to as the alveolar sacs, and it is where gas exchange will occur.

So, what is gas exchange? And what are alveoli? Don't worry it's a pretty simple process. Remember, how the heart sends deoxygenated blood back to the lungs?

A meshwork of capillaries will surround every alveolus. So, when a dog breathes in air, the oxygen travels into the alveoli sac and diffuses into the blood capillaries. This is how an animal receives oxygenated blood.

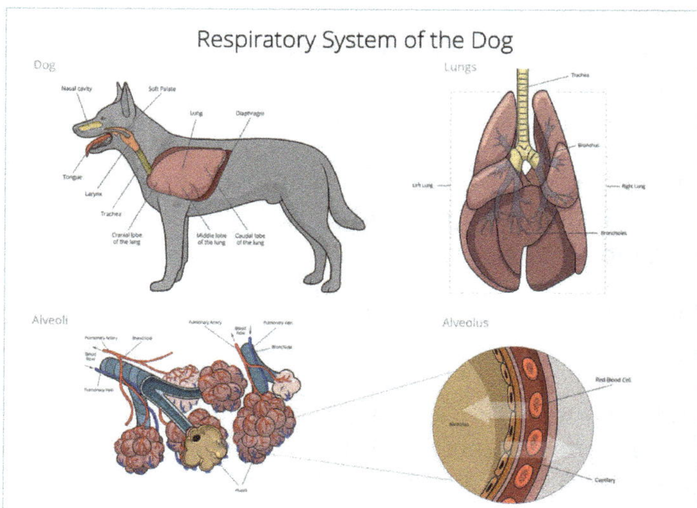

The oxygenated blood is now part of the circulatory system, where it will eventually reach the heart. The heart then pumps the deoxygenated blood back to the lungs through the veins. The deoxygenated blood contains carbon dioxide which readily diffuses across the capillary walls and to the alveoli.

So, when an animal exhales, then they are merely getting rid of that carbon dioxide.

Sweating in Dogs

Sweating is the physiological response a body has when it wants to cool down. For a mammal to sweat, they require specialized sweat glands. However, dogs don't have any sweat glands under their body, on their back, etc.

However, dogs do have sweat glands in areas where there is no fur. For example, dogs do have sweat glands on their paw pads. So although they do have sweat glands in certain regions, sweating is not the primary way dogs cool down. Instead, dogs use another mechanism to cool themselves down on a hot summer's day, and this is called panting.

The process of panting is a form of thermoregulation. Panting is an evaporative mechanism which allows a dog to cool down by increasing their breath per minute and taking shallow breaths.

Dog Muscle Anatomy

In dog anatomy, the muscular-skeletal system is composed of bone (the skeleton), cartilage, tendons, ligaments, and muscles. When working together in complete synchrony theses apparatus produce the ability to walk, run, and jump.

In canine anatomy, there are three types of muscle groups. Smooth muscles line the internal organs, such as the bladder, the esophagus, and stomach. Cardiac muscles are nonstriated muscle fibers specific to the heart. And, finally, skeletal muscles are those that are attached to the extremities of a dog.

The next part of the musculoskeletal system is ligaments. Ligaments simply hold bones together, in other words, they form bone to bone attachments. In dog anatomy, or in fact, human anatomy as well—the main function of ligaments is to stabilize joints during movement.

Tendons are often confused with ligaments, but they are distinctively different. Tendons are fibrous tissue that attaches the bone to the muscle. These tissues are highly flexible and when placed under pressure, tendons are able to initiate movement through muscle contraction.

Urogenital System of Dogs

The urogenital system of a dog comprises of the urinary tract and the sex organs. Starting at the urinary tract, the kidney is the first organ of the urogenital system. The kidney is a bean-shaped organ whose main function is to regulate electrolyte balance, produce hormones, and eliminate waste.

Attached to each of the kidneys are tube-like structures called ureter and each ureter directs the pre-formed urine into the bladder. So, when a dog needs to urinate, then the urine leaves the bladder via the urethra.

So, how is female dog anatomy different from that of male dog anatomy?

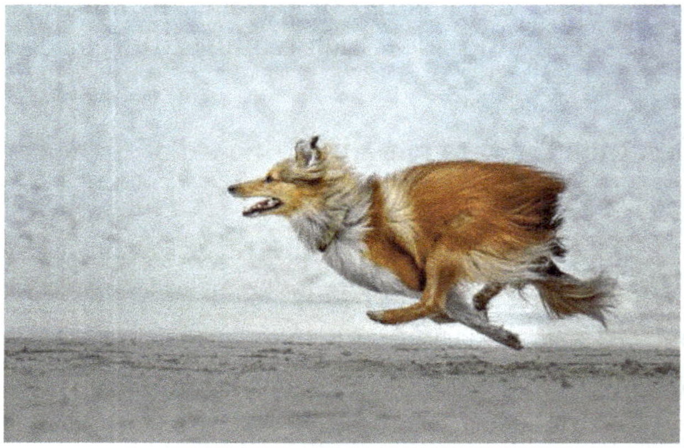

Apart from their reproductive organs, the urinary tract system is essentially the same for both genders. The female dog anatomy will consist of ovaries, a uterine horn, a uterus, uterine body, cervix, and vagina.

The male dog anatomy on the other hand simply consists of the testis which is where sperm production occurs. A spermatic cord and various sex glands such as the prostate and vesicular glands.

Equine Anatomy

Points of the Horse and Pony

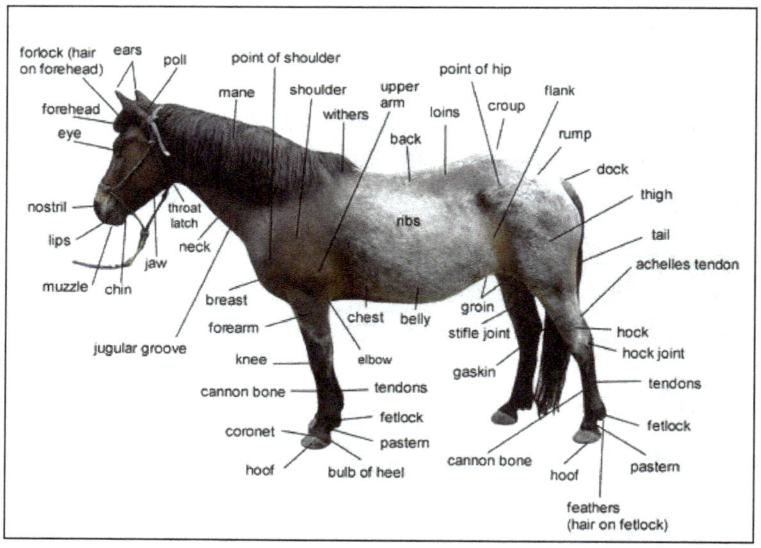

Horse Body Parts in Action

The hoofs do more than just support the horse. They act as a sort of pump as well. The bottom of the hoof is hard to the touch yet flexible enough to 'give' when the horse walks. With each step the horse takes, the blood that has been forced down the leg is now forced back upward toward the heart.

The front legs of the horse bear most of the horse's weight, while the powerful back legs act as the motor that drives the animal forward. Horses carry the weight of a rider on their backs just behind the withers. A saddle helps distribute the weight evenly over the weight bearing ribs. If the saddle is improperly set too far back toward the horse's loins, the horse will get sore and not perform well.

The tail of a horse is used quite effectively as a fly swatter, but did you know that horses use their tails to communicate as well? Much like white tail deer, horses will raise their tails when they are very alert. They also hold their tails high during mating season to help attract the attention of a mate.

Take a look at this drawing of a horse skeleton. You are looking at about 205 bones that make up the equine skeletal anatomy. The more you study this picture the better understanding you will have of how a horse is built and how he moves.

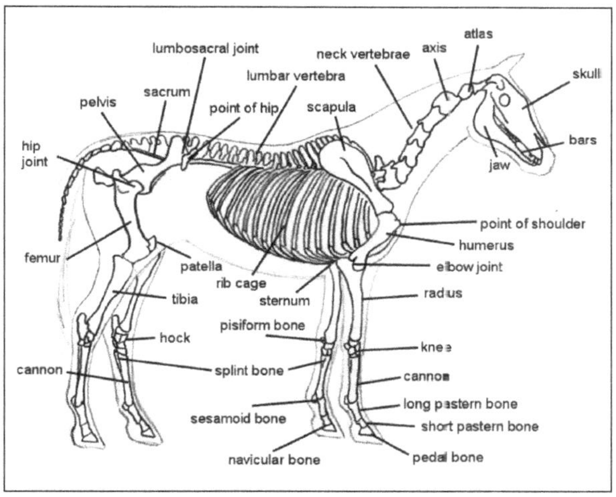

Proper nutrition during pregnancy and the early formative years of a horse will ensure a healthy bone structure. Inadequate nutrition during these times will stunt the bone growth in a foal, while an overabundance of certain nutrients will cause the bone to grow too rapidly, causing joint damage.

Good conformation in a horse starts with the bones. A horse with poor conformation will not have the endurance or hardiness of an animal born with a well formed horse skeleton. They will be more prone to injury of the joints and ligaments, and when used hard, usually do not have the longevity of usefulness over their lifetime.

The neck is the most flexible portion of the horse's spine. A quick glance at this skeleton horse will show you where the vertebrae of the neck are placed. When giving vaccines you will avoid this area of the neck. Horses with longer necks have a slight speed advantage over horses with shorter necks.

In viewing the skull, you can clearly see the bars of the horse's mouth. This is the section of the jaw that has no teeth, where the bit lies on the horse's gums. When you are fitting a bridle to a horse, you'll want to ensure the bit does not interfere or bump the teeth, causing pain.

You can see by looking at the horse skeleton that weight is best carried directly behind the withers. This area has the support of the rib cage and the sturdy shock absorbing structure of the knee bones in the front legs. Did you know that the front legs are not attached to the rest of the skeleton? The shoulders of the horse are held close to the body by layers of muscle. Kind of like a giant sling.

A Balanced Horse Skeleton is the Key to Soundness

Horses have limited flexibility of the lower spine. Poor conformation of the back legs forces the lower back to absorb more shock than it is designed for. Over time this can cause the vertebra to fuse together. Placing weight over the loin area puts undue stress on the lower back causing bone damage and stress to the kidneys.

An unhindered lower back allows the horse to reach further forward with his back legs when running, thus gaining more speed. This flexibility also allows a horse to place more weight on their back legs when maneuvering fast turns.

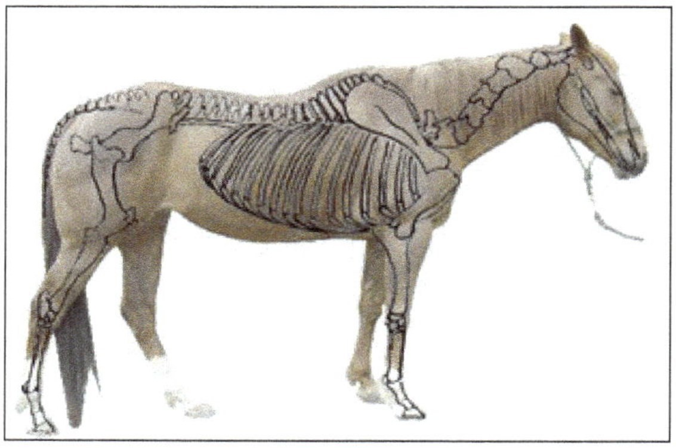

The bones of the horse skeleton are held together with ligaments, tendons and muscles. When the skeletal structure is properly proportioned the joints work smoothly. One bone works in relation to another. If the angle at witch these bones are working is compromised, the joint becomes unevenly stressed and injury to the tendons and ligaments become more likely.

Stressful angles to the joints can come from poor conformation, poor hoof trimming practices or repetitive strenuous hard work. In combination, these three factors add up to an increased likelihood of leg injury in the horse.

The better proportioned the skeleton, the better athlete the horse will be. Understanding how a particular horse is put together lets you know if that horse is capable of living up to your expectations.

In fact, not every horse has perfect conformation. Many horses with conformation faults make wonderful pleasure horses. Not every horse is expected to perform in high physically demanding athletic competitions and working conditions. With proper nutrition and exercise, horses with an imperfect equine skeletal structure can lead a very long and productive life, so long as they are not exposed to overly demanding stresses on the skeleton.

Equine forelimb anatomy is key to the performance ability of every horse. The front legs support nearly two thirds of the weight of a horse. Any conformation faults here will contribute greatly to lameness and injury of these weight bearing forelimbs.

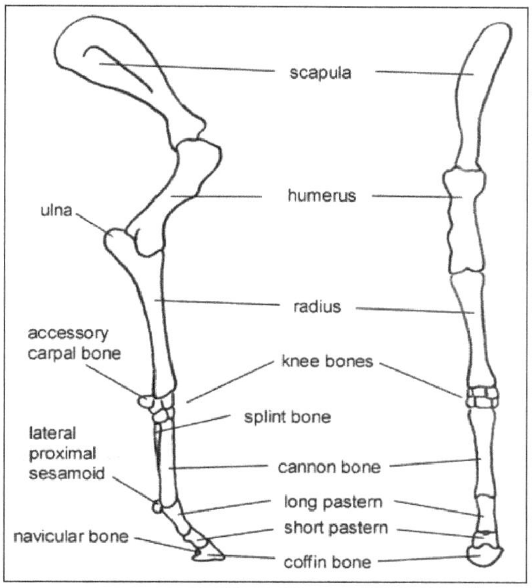

Common Forelimb Injuries

- Splints
- Navicular disease
- Bowed tendons
- Knee injuries
- Laminitis
- Windpuffs
- Ringbone
- Arthritis
- Fractures

Many of these forelimb injuries have to do with the high level of weight and concussion that the leg is subject too. All conformation flaws reduce the ability of the joints to absorb shock, thus over stressing the bones and ligaments.

Over time, repeated stresses of heavy weight and impact take their toll on the joints and surrounding tissues. A horse with flawed conformation will break down much faster.

Equine Forelimb Anatomy – the Upper Leg

The uppermost bone in the foreleg is the scapula, or shoulder blade. The point of the shoulder and the shoulder blade make up the angle of the shoulder, which should be about a 45° angle. The scapula connects to the humorous with a ball and socket type joint. The humorous connects to the radius. Neither of them connects to the spine.

The front legs of a horse are not attached to the spine, but rather held in place by a 'girdle' or sling of muscles.

The radius is the bone that makes up the forearm of the horse. It should be longer in comparison to the cannon bone. A strong front leg will have a long forearm and a short cannon bone.

The tip of the radius is called the ulna, or the elbow of the horse. The elbow should sit directly below the front of the withers. An elbow that is turned in or out puts extra strain on the fetlock joint. A turned in elbow is called 'tied in', and tends to shorten the stride; while a turned out elbow makes a horse 'paddle' (throw his feet to the side).

Equine Forelimb Anatomy – the Lower Leg

The knee is made up of 8 small bones that sit between the radius and the cannon bone. A well-shaped knee should be large and flat from the front and wide from the side. The carpal bone that is visible at the back if the knee should be well defined. The knee should sit directly over the cannon bone. Knees should not be bowed or knocked, nor set too far forward or back when viewed from the side.

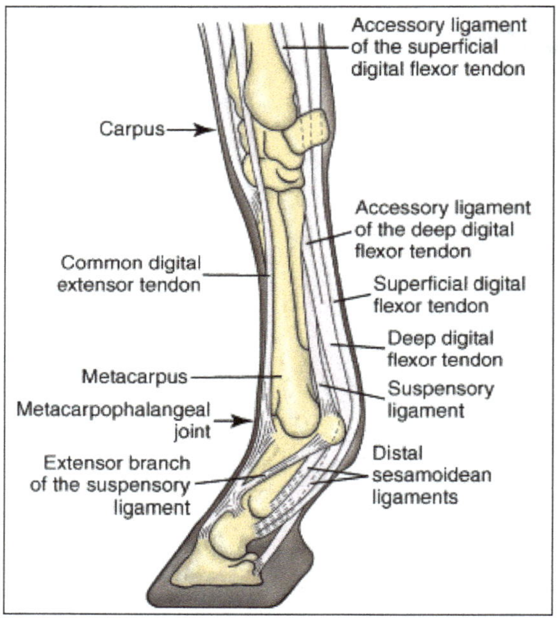

The knee is made up of 8 small carpus bones in two rows of four. The cannon bone should be relatively short in length and straight up and down. The small splint bone runs partially down the side of the cannon bone. When viewed from the side the cannon bone is wider than when seen from the front. A long cannon bone puts undue stress on the knee joint and tendons. The cannon bone in the front legs will be shorter than the cannon bones in the back legs.

The long pastern bone and the cannon bone come together to form the fetlock joint. The fetlock joint is hugely important as a shock absorber. It takes a vast amount of stress. This joint should be relatively large, but not so large as to show any signs of damage.

A horse has no muscles below the knee, only ligaments and tendons. The long pastern bone and short pastern bones come together to form the pastern, the area between the fetlock joint and the top of the hoof. This joint should be sloped at a 47°- 55° angle. Excessive sloped pastern puts too much strain on ligaments and the horse is prone to bowed tendons and navicular disease. Too upright a pastern gives a horse a choppy gait. Pasterns that are too short make a horse prone to navicular disease, windpuffs, splints, knee injuries, splints, ringbone and arthritis.

Lastly the petal or coffin bone and the tiny navicular bone make up the portion of the horse leg bones inside the horse's hoof. Equine forelimb anatomy sets the tone for the agility, endurance and speed of a horse. The closer you can get to an ideal front leg conformation the less prone your horse will be to injury.

Horse teeth continue to grow for the life of the horse. Because of this continual growth it is necessary that horses receive regular dental care with a procedure called floating. Floating teeth keeps the grinding surfaces even, ensuring proper food digestion.

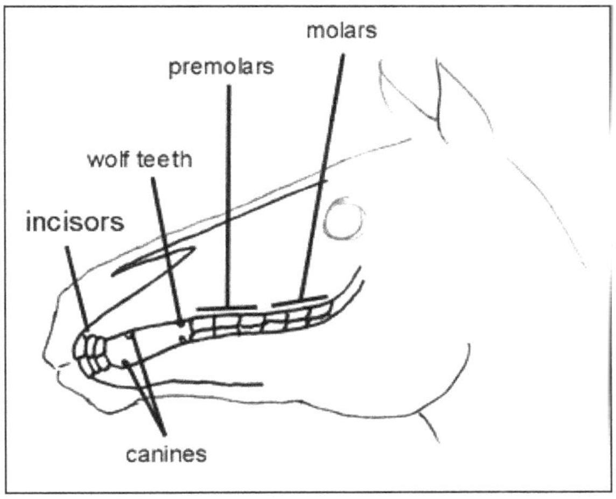

The changes that take place to the horse's teeth over time help determine the age of a horse. Aging a horse by its teeth is very accurate in young horses and during specific time periods in a horse's life. As the horse grows older, this tooth aging process becomes less accurate.

The teeth are made up of materials that vary in hardness. This variation causes portions of the teeth to wear at different rates. The combination of wear marks, the presence or absence of baby teeth, tooth shape, and identifying grooves all help in aging a horse by its teeth.

Horse Teeth and Age

- 1 yr: have 24 baby teeth;
- 2- 2½ yrs: will have second set of permanent molars;
- 3 yrs: 2 permanent central incisors erupted;
- 4 yrs: canine teeth erupted (males and some mares);
- 5 yrs: all permanent teeth are in, grinding surfaces are oval from side to side;
- 6 yrs: permanent incisors showing wear;

- 7 and 8 yrs: cups of the middle, lower incisors disappear;
- 8 and 9 yrs: cups of the corner, lower incisors disappear;
- 10 yrs: Galvayne's groove appears at gum line;
- 11 yrs: cups in corner, upper incisors disappear;
- 12 yrs: chewing surfaces on central incisors become round instead of oval;
- 14-16 yrs: corner incisors develop ridges;
- 17 yrs: all incisors have round surface
- 18 yrs: central incisors become triangular;
- 20 yrs: Galvayne's groove runs the length off the corner incisors;
- 23 yrs: all incisors become triangular;
- 24 to 29 yrs: The grinding surfaces become oval again, but this time from front to back;
- 30 yrs: Galvayne's groove gone;
- Over 30+ yrs: short teeth, small tooth nubs, loss of teeth.

An adult horse has 36 teeth: 12 incisors, 12 premolars and 12 molars.

A foal will have 24 teeth: 12 incisors and 12 premolars.

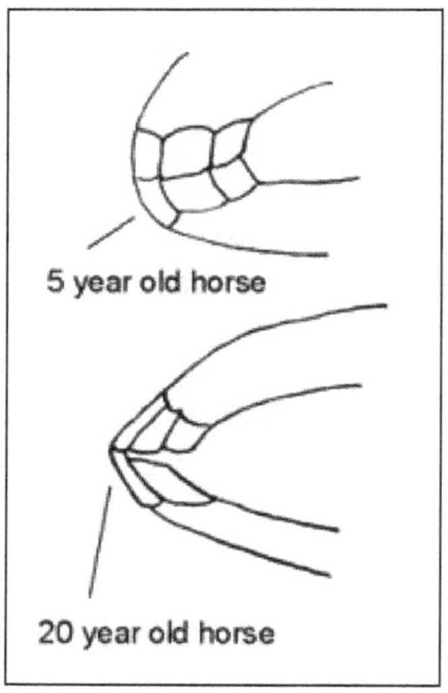

He may also have up to 4 wolf teeth and a set of 4 canine teeth. The wolf teeth come in at about 5 to 6 months of age. These are the small pointed teeth that grow in just in front of the premolars. Wolf teeth are often shed along with the baby teeth, but not always. If the wolf teeth are retained and interfere with the bit they can be removed. The horse does not need them for chewing.

Most male horses will have canine teeth and some mares will too. If a horse grows canine teeth they will erupt at about 4 years of age. These small pointed teeth grow just a little bit behind the incisors on the bars of the horse's mouth. They generally do not interfere with the bit.

A foal will have grown his first 24 baby teeth, deciduous teeth, by nine months. By 12 months he will grow his first set of permanent molars. It will take four to five years for a young horse to lose all his baby teeth and replace them with the permanent adult horse teeth.

Anatomy of Horse Teeth

A horse's tooth has a very long root that resides deep into the jaw bone. Very slowly over time tooth grows (pushes out). A very young horse will have a small bit of tooth exposed with a long root. A very old horse will have a small bit of tooth exposed with hardly any root left; as they have 'used their tooth up' over time.

The permanent teeth change shape as the horse grows older, because what you are seeing is the 'root' portion of the tooth that is slowly emerging from the jaw.

The front teeth, or incisors, are used for biting grass. The back teeth, molars and premolars, are used for grinding the grass. The horse has a large inter-dental space between the incisors and the molars. That's a fancy term for what we call the bars, the space in the horses gums that have no teeth at all.

A young horse's teeth will be shorter and straight up and down. The older a horse gets, the longer the tooth becomes, giving rise to the term "Long in the tooth." The incisors become longer and more and more slanted at a forward angle as the horse ages.

Horse Teeth and the Galvayne's Groove

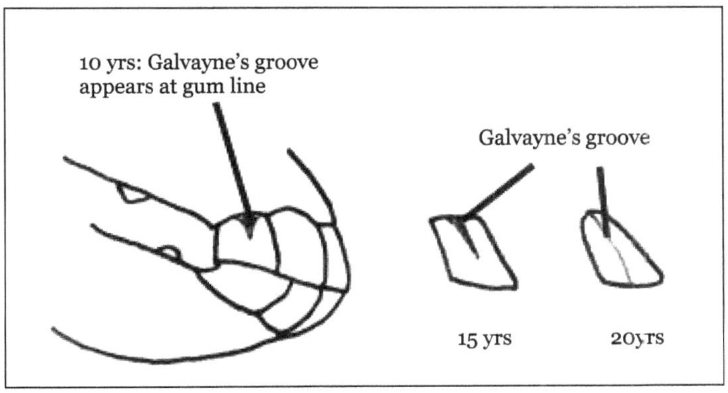

At about the age of 10, the upper corner incisors begin to show a groove at the gum line. This is the Galvayne's groove. Over the next 10 years the groove will grow all the way down the length of the tooth. A 20 year old horse will have a Galvayne's groove all the way down the upper corner incisors.

Then the groove begins to disappear, starting from the top. By the time the horse is 30 the groove will be completely gone. Eventually those long incisors will grow very short as the old horse has very little tooth left.

The hoof wall is made up of horny tissue. The hoof continues to grow throughout the life of the horse, much like fingernails in humans. Just like fingernails, the horny shell has no nerves or blood vessels. The horny hoof wall grows out from the coronary band that sits just at the hair line above the hoof.

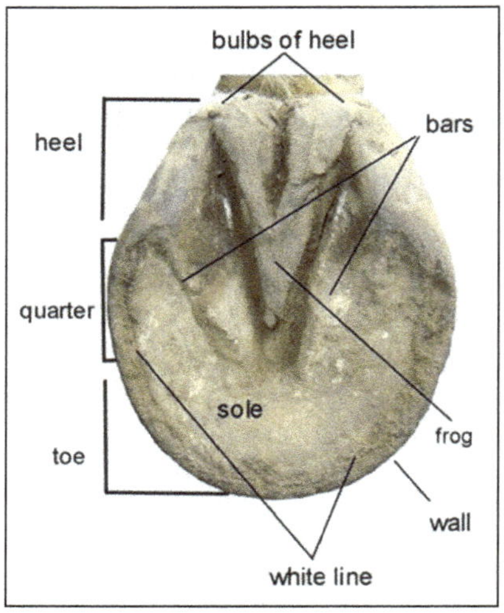

The hoof itself is thick and hard, yet pliable. The hoof wall is thickest at the toe and thinner at the heel. The ideal horse hoof anatomy should have a nice rounded toe and a wide heel base. A narrow heel suggests the presence of navicular disease or the tendency toward contracting navicular.

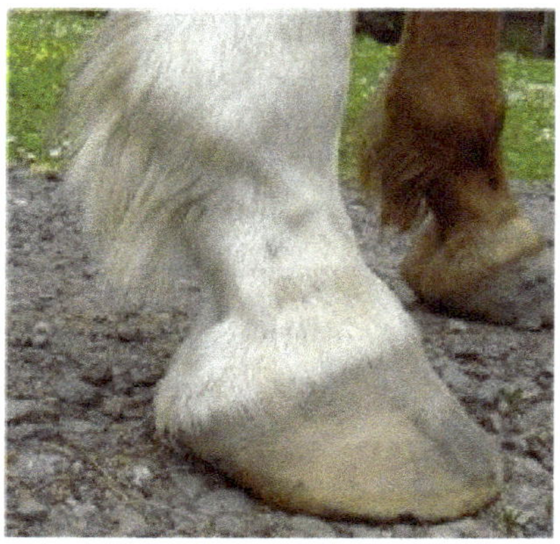

The hoof will soften in wet conditions and dry out in dry conditions. Adding a bit of vegetable oil to your horse's diet will help keep the hooves strong and moisturized from the inside out. Just like human nails and hair, the horses hoof and coat will respond to oils in the diet.

Horse Hoof Anatomy – the Bottom Side

Looking at the illustration you can clearly see the structure of the bottom of the hoof. The most pronounced feature is the triangular shaped frog. The frog acts as a shock absorber. It is the softest part of the horses hoof and expands with each step, as does the flexible heel of the hoof. Horse shoes should be slightly wider than the heel of the hoof to allow for this expansion.

The white line is the transitional tissue between the tough horny outer wall of the hoof, and the sensitive inner tissues of the hoof. When a farrier is shoeing a horse, he places the nails into the horny wall that has no nerve or blood vessels. A white line that is pierced by a farriers nail causes pain, lameness and possible infection.

The bars of the hoof serve in several ways. They help to take up some of the weight that is placed on the hoof wall and they keep the hoof from over and under expanding. The bars also spread out slightly with each step to help drive the 'heart pump' action of the hoof.

Horse Hoof Anatomy – the Inner Structure

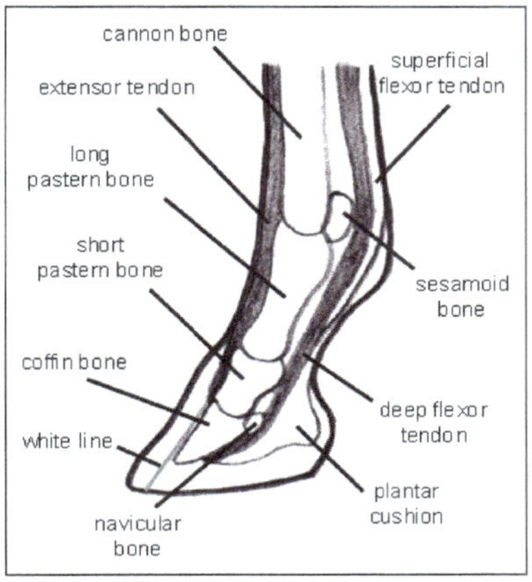

The coffin bone is the 'toe' bone of the horse's foot. This bone is shaped like a small hoof with flared sides. This is the bone that rotates downward to pierce the sole of the foot in a horse with founder. The coffin bone meets the short pastern bone while the tiny navicular bone just behind them both inside the horses hoofs.

Horse Hoof - the Second Heart

Did you know that a horse has no muscles in their lower leg? The lower leg is made up of bone, ligament and tendons, and of course the all-important hoof. The horse hoof anatomy allows the hoof to act as a second heart. With each step the horse takes, the flexible hoof expands and contracts, forcing blood back up the horses leg toward the heart.

This is why keeping a horse in a stall with little activity is so unhealthy. The lack of exercise and movement cuts down on circulation. This can cause a horse to "stock up", a condition where the lower legs are swollen from lack of circulation.

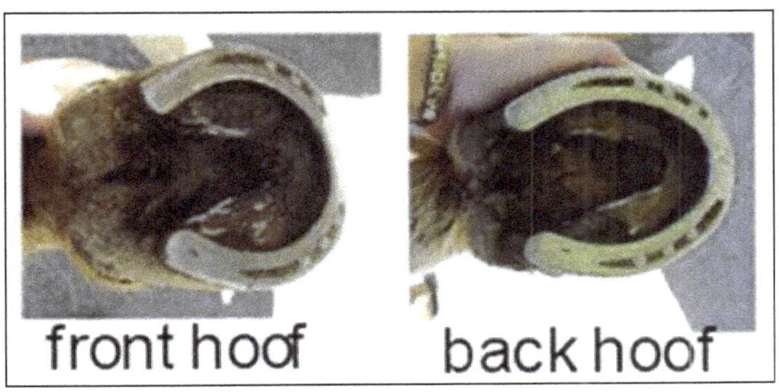

The sole of the hoof is harder than the frog and softer than the outer hoof wall. It is flexible and acts at the 'heart pump'. The sole in the front hoof is round shaped, while the sole of the back hoof is more oval shaped. A concave sole is preferable to a flat sole.

A concave sole reduces concussion to the joints in the horse's leg, offers better footing in rough terrain, is less apt to stone bruise and is less prone to navicular disease. The back hoof is usually more concave than the front hoof on a horse.

Cow Anatomy

Cows vary in all different colours, some are brown, tanned, white, black, and brown-white patched or black-white patched. In a female cow, milk is produced in the udders and extracted from the teats. A Cows udder has four compartments with one teat hanging from each.

Tiny Cells remove water and nutrients from the blood and convert it into milk. The milk forms into droplets and drips into a cistern which holds the milk. If the cow's teat is squeezed, it produces a squirt of milk and is either saved in tanks or feeds a suckling calf.

A cow's mouth is adapted for grazing; the top part of the mouth is a hard pad and the bottom part a row of flat-topped teeth. Cows have 32 teeth in all, 8 incisors on the bottom part and 6 molars on the top and bottom parts on each side.

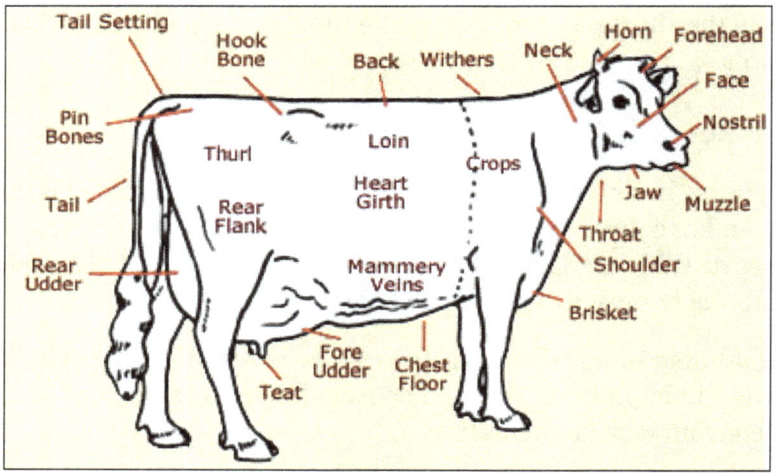

The cow tears grass from the field and grinds it between the two mouth parts. A cow's ear is very flexible and can turn in any direction. They are especially used to hear any signs of danger from many directions. Cows have long tails which they use to waft insects of them.

Bulls have horns, although some female cows have small horns too. Bull's horns are made out of similar material to our fingernails called 'Keratin'. Bull's horns can be removed without causing the cow any discomfort.

Diet: Cows are herbivores which mean they do not eat meat, only plants, grass and cereal. Cows are ruminant animals which mean they have more than one stomach.

Cows have a four part stomach, each part used for a different process. Cows swallow their food without chewing it too much at first. Cows later regurgitate a 'cud' which is then chewed well and swallowed.

Anatomy of a Cow's Stomach

Inside a cow's stomach region, there are 4 digestive departments:

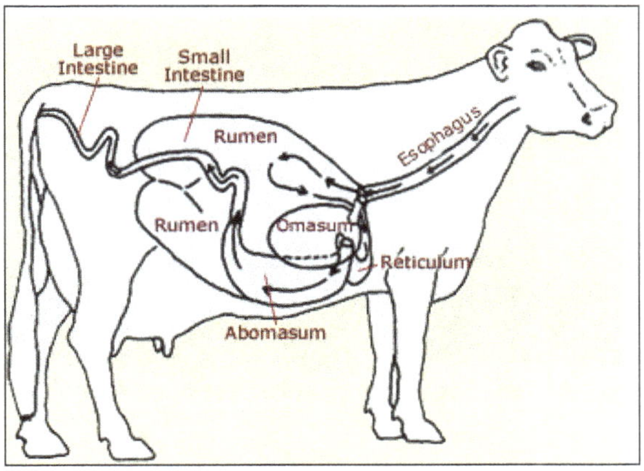

- The Rumen: This is the largest part and holds upto 50 gallons of partially digested food. This is where the 'cud' comes from. Good bacteria in the Rumen help soften and digest the cow's food and provide protein for the cow.
- The Recticulum: This part of the stomach is called the 'hardware' stomach. This is because if the cow eats something it should not have like a peice of fencing, it lodges here in the Recticulum. However, the contractions of the reticulum can force the object into the peritoneal cavity where it initiates inflammation. Nails and screws can even peroferate the heart. The grass that has been eaten is also softened further in this stomach section and is formed into small wads of cud. Each cud returns to the cow's mouth and is chewed 40 – 60 times and then swallowed properly.
- The Omasum: This part of the stomach is a 'filter'. It filters through all the food the cow eats. The cud is also pressed and broken down further.
- The Abomasum: This part of the stomach is like a human's stomach and is connected to the intestines. Here, the food is finally digested by the cow's stomach juices and essential nutrients that the cow needs are passed through the bloodstream. The rest is passed through to the intestines and produces a 'cow pat'.

Avian Anatomy

Anatomy of the Wing

- Mantle: The whole back, combined with the top surface of the wings.
- Remiges: Large flight feathers on the wings - responsible for supporting the bird during flight. The outer remiges are referred to as the primaries (longest wing feathers). These are the largest, thinnest and stiffest of the flight feathers. The inner remiges - called the secondaries (shorter, upper "arm" feathers) - are attached to the "forearm" (ulna) of a bird.

- Rectrices: The long tail feathers - they help a bird brake and steer in flight. They are in a single horizontal row on the rear margin of the tail.

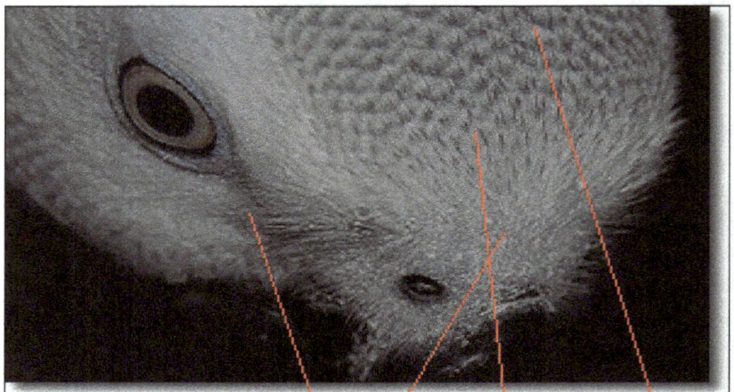

Congo African Grey lores, cere, forehead & sinciput

- Coverts or Covert Feathers: Sets of feathers covering other feathers. For example, the wing-coverts are the feathers right above the wing feathers. They cover the base of the flight feathers to provide a smoother surface for the air to flow over.
- Undertail Coverts: Feathers around the vent.
- Head Anatomy:
    - Forehead;
    - Sinciput;
    - Septum (= a partition of bone and cartilage between the nasal cavities/nostrils);
    - Crown;
    - Malar Stripe: A line angling back from the bird's chin, separating the cheek from the throat;
    - Occiput;
    - Supercilium;
    - Eye Stripe/Eye Streak;
    - Supraloral Line or supraloral feathers of a bird;
    - Loral area/Lores - The area between beak and eyes;
    - Cere - an area of soft skin surrounding the nostrils; it may be bare or covered with small, soft feathers;
    - Epaulets (shoulder patches).
- Oil Gland is also known as Uropygial Gland or Preen Gland: Located just above the tail.

Bird anatomy, or the physiological structure of birds' bodies, shows many unique adaptations, mostly aiding flight. Birds have evolved a light skeletal system and light but powerful musculature which, along with circulatory and respiratory systems capable of very high metabolic rates and oxygen supply, permit the bird to fly. The development of a beak has led to evolution of a specially adapted digestive system. These anatomical specializations have earned birds their own class in the vertebrate phylum.

Respiratory System

Due to the high metabolic rate required for flight, birds have a high oxygen demand. Development of an efficient respiratory system enabled the evolution of flight in birds. Birds ventilate their lungs by means of air sacs, structures unique to birds (and hence, perhaps dinosaurs, too). These sacs do not play a direct role in gas exchange, but to store air and act like bellows, allowing the lungs to maintain a fixed volume with fresh air constantly flowing through them.

Air always flows from right (posterior) to left (anterior) through a bird's lungs during both inhalation and exhalation. Key to a Common Kestrel's circulatory lung system: 1 cervical air sac, 2 clavicular air sac, 3 cranial thoracal air sac, 4 caudal thoracal air sac, 5 abdominal air sac (5' diverticulus into pelvic girdle), 6 lung, 7 trachea.

Three distinct sets of organs perform respiration—the anterior air sacs (interclavicular, cervicals, and anterior thoracics), the lungs, and the posterior air sacs (posterior thoracics and abdominals). The posterior and anterior air sacs, typically nine, expand during inhalation. Air enters the bird via the trachea. Half of the inhaled air enters the posterior air sacs, the other half passes through the lungs and into the anterior air sacs. The sacs contract during exhalation. Air from the anterior air sacs empties directly into the trachea and out the bird's mouth or nares. The posterior air sacs empty their air into the lungs. Air passing through the lungs as the bird exhales is expelled via the trachea. Because fresh air flows through the lungs in only one direction, there is no mixing of oxygen-rich air and oxygen-poor, carbon dioxide-rich, air as in mammalian lungs. Thus, the partial pressure of oxygen in a bird's lungs is the same as the environment, and so birds have more efficient gas-exchange of both oxygen and carbon dioxide than do mammals.

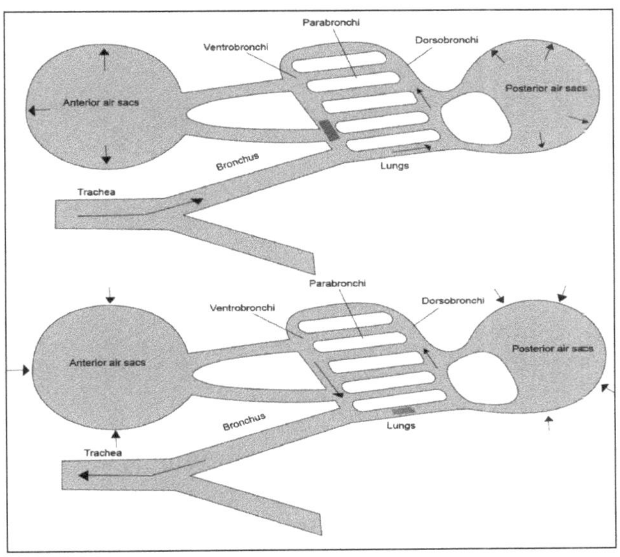

Birds lungs obtain fresh air during bothe exhalation and inhalation.

Avian lungs do not have alveoli, as mammalian lungs do, but instead contain millions of tiny passages known as parabronchi, connected at either ends by the dorsobronchi and ventrobronchi. Air flows through the honeycombed walls of the parabronchi into air vesicles, called atria, which project radially from the parabronchi. These atria give rise to air capillaries, where oxygen and carbon dioxide are traded with cross-flowing blood capillaries by diffusion.

Birds also lack a diaphragm. The entire body cavity acts as a bellows to move air through the lungs. The active phase of respiration in birds is exhalation, requiring muscular contraction.

The syrinx is the sound-producing vocal organ of birds, located at the base of a bird's trachea. As with the mammalian larynx, sound is produced by the vibration of air flowing through the organ. The syrinx enables some species of birds to produce extremely complex vocalizations, even mimicking human speech. In some songbirds, the syrinx can produce more than one sound at a time.

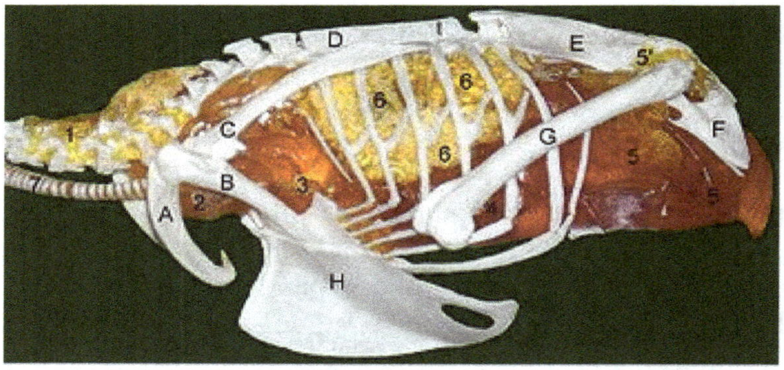

Air always flows from right (posterior) to left (anterior) through a bird's lungs during both inhalation and exhalation.

Key to a Common Kestrel's circulatory lung system:

1. Cervical air sac
2. Clavicular air sac
3. Cranial thoracal air sac
4. Caudal thoracal air sac
5. Abdominal air sac (5' diverticulus into pelvic girdle)
6. Lung
7. Trachea

Circulatory System

Birds have four-chambered heart, in common with humans, most mammals, and some reptiles (namely the crocodilia). This adaptation allows for efficient nutrient and oxygen transport throughout the body, providing birds with energy to fly and maintain high levels of activity. A Ruby-throated Hummingbird's heart beats up to 1200 times per minute (about 20 beats per second).

Digestive System

Many birds possess a muscular pouch along the oesophagus called a crop. The crop functions to both soften food and regulate its flow through the system by storing it temporarily. The size and shape of the crop is quite variable among the birds. Members of the order Columbiformes, such as pigeons, produce nutritious crop milk which is fed to their young by regurgitation. Birds possess a ventriculus, or gizzard, composed of four muscular bands that rotate and crush food by shifting the food from one area to the next within the gizzard. The gizzard of some species contains small pieces of grit or stone swallowed by the bird to aid in the grinding process of digestion, serving the function of mammalian or reptilian teeth. The use of gizzard stones is a similarity between birds and dinosaurs, which left gizzard stones called gastroliths as trace fossils.

Drinking Behavior

There are four general ways in which birds drink. Most birds are unable to swallow by the "sucking" or "pumping" action of peristalsis in their oesophagus (as humans do), and drink by repeatedly raising their heads after filling their mouths to allow the liquid to flow by gravity, a method usually described as "sipping" or "tipping up". The notable exception is the Columbiformes; in fact, according to Konrad Lorenz in 1939, "one recognizes the order by the single behavioral characteristic, namely that in drinking the water is pumped up by peristalsis of the esophagus which occurs without exception within the order. The only other group, however, which shows the same behavior, the Pteroclidae, is placed near the doves just by this doubtlessly very old characteristic."

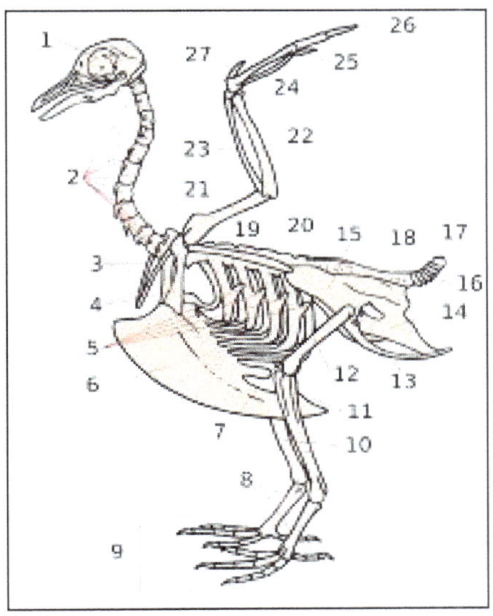

A Stylised Bird Skeleton.

1. Skull
2. Cervical Vertebrae
3. Furcula
4. Coracoid

5. Uncinate Process
6. Keel
7. Patella
8. Tarsometatarsus
9. Digits
10. Tibiotarsus (long leg bone)
11. Tibiotarsus
12. Femur
13. Ischium (innominate bone)
14. Pubi (innominate bone)
15. Illium (innominate bone)
16. Caudal Vertebrae
17. Pygostyle
18. Synsacrum
19. Scapula
20. Lumbar Vertebrae
21. Humerus
22. Ulna
23. Radius
24. Carpus
25. Metacarpus
26. Digits
27. Alula

Although this general rule still stands, since that time, observations have been made of a few exceptions in both directions.

In addition, specialized nectar feeders like sunbirds (Nectariniidae) and hummingbirds (Trochilidae) drink by using protrusible grooved or trough-like tongues, and parrots (Psittacidae) lap up water.

Skeletal System

The bird skeleton is highly adapted for flight. It is extremely lightweight but strong enough to withstand the stresses of taking off, flying, and landing. One key adaptation is the fusing of bones into single ossifications, such as the pygostyle. Because of this, birds usually have a smaller number of bones than other terrestrial vertebrates. Birds also lack teeth or even a true jaw, instead having evolved a beak, which is far more lightweight. The beaks of many baby birds have a projection called an egg tooth, which facilitates their exit from the amniotic egg.

Birds have many bones that are hollow with criss-crossing struts or trusses for structural strength. The number of hollow bones varies among species, though large gliding and soaring birds tend to have the most. Respiratory air sacs often form air pockets within the semi-hollow bones of the bird's skeleton. Some flightless birds like penguins and ostriches have only solid bones, further evidencing the link between flight and the adaptation of hollow bones.

Birds also have more cervical (neck) vertebrae than many other animals; most have a highly flexible neck consisting of 13-25 vertebrae. Birds are the only vertebrate animals to have a fused collarbone (the furcula or wishbone) or a keeled sternum or breastbone. The keel of the sternum serves as an attachment site for the muscles used for flight, or similarly for swimming in penguins. Again, flightless birds, such as ostriches, which do not have highly developed pectoral muscles, lack a pronounced keel on the sternum. It is noted that swimming birds have a wide sternum, while walking birds had a long or high sternum while flying birds have the width and height nearly equal.

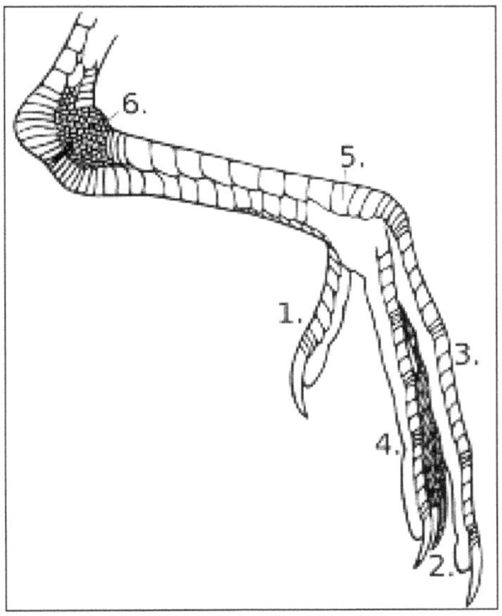

Birds have uncinate processes on the ribs. These are hooked extensions of bone which help to strengthen the rib cage by overlapping with the rib behind them. This feature is also found in the tuatara Sphenodon. They also have a greatly elongate tetradiate pelvis as in some reptiles. The hindlimb has an intra-tarsal joint found also in some reptiles. There is extensive fusion of the trunk vertebrea as well as fusion with the pectoral girdle. They have a diapsid skull as in reptiles with a pre-lachrymal fossa (present in some reptiles). The skull has a single occipital condyle.

Skeletal Composition

The skull consists of five major bones: the frontal (top of head), parietal (back of head), premaxillary and nasal (top beak), and the mandible (bottom beak). The skull of a normal bird usually weighs about 1% of the birds total bodyweight.

The vertebral column consists of vertebrae, and is divided into three sections: cervical (13-16) (neck), Synsacrum (fused vertebrae of the back, also fused to the hips (pelvis), and pygostyle (tail).

The chest consists of the furcula (wishbone) and coracoid (collar bone), which two bones, together with the scapula, form the pectoral girdle. The side of the chest is formed by the ribs, which meet at the sternum (mid-line of the chest).

The shoulder consists of the scapula (shoulder blade), coracoid, and humerus (upper arm). The humerus joins the radius and ulna (forearm) to form the elbow. The carpus and metacarpus form the "wrist" and "hand" of the bird and the digits (fingers) are fused together. The bones in the wing are extremely light so that the bird can fly more easily.

The hips consist of the pelvis which includes three major bones: Illium (top of the hip), Ischium (sides of hip), and Pubis (front of the hip). These are fused into one (the innominate bone). Innominate bones are evolutionary significant in that they allow birds to lay eggs. They meet at the acetabulum (the hip socket) and articulate with the femur, which is the first bone of the hind limb.

The upper leg consists of the femur. At the knee joint, the femur connects to the tibiotarsus (long leg bone - shin) and fibula (side of lower leg). The tarsometatarsus forms the upper part of the foot, digits make up the toes. The leg bones of birds are the heaviest, contributing to a low center of gravity. This aids in flight. A bird's skeleton comprises only about 5% of its total body weight

Birds feet are classificated as anisodactyl, zygodactyl, heterodactyl, syndactyl or pamprodactyl.

Muscular System

Most birds have approximately 175 different muscles, mainly controlling the wings, skin, and legs. The largest muscles in the bird are the pectorals, or the breast muscles, which control the wings and make up about 15 - 25% of a flighted bird's body weight. They provide the powerful wing stroke essential for flight. The muscle ventral (underneath) to the pectorals is the supracoracoideus. It raises the wing between wingbeats. The supracoracoideus and the pectorals together make up about 25 – 35% of the bird's full body weight.

The skin muscles help a bird in its flight by adjusting the feathers, which are attached to the skin muscle and help the bird in its flight maneuvers.

There are only a few muscles in the trunk and the tail, but they are very strong and are essential for the bird. The pygostyle controls all the movement in the tail and controls the feathers in the tail. This gives the tail a larger surface area which helps keep the bird in the air.

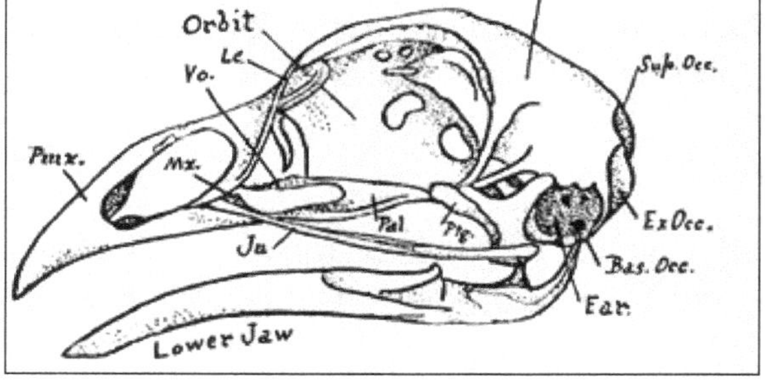

Head

Birds have acute eyesight - raptors have vision eight times sharper than humans - thanks to higher densities of photoreceptors in the retina (up to 1,000,000 per square mm in Buteos, compared to 200,000 for humans), a high number of optic nerves, a second set of eye muscles not found in other animals, and in some cases, an indented fovea which magnifies the central part of the visual field. Many species, including hummingbirds and albatrosses, have two foveas in each eye. Many birds can detect polarised light. The eye occupies a considerable part of the skull and is surrounded by a sclerotic eye-ring, a ring of tiny bones that surround the eye. This character is also seen in the reptiles.

The bills of many waders have Herbst corpuscles which help them detect prey hidden under wet sand using minute pressure differences in the water. All extant birds can move the parts of the upper jaw relative to the brain case. However this is more prominent in some birds and can be readily detected in parrots.

Birds have a large brain to body mass ratio. This is reflected in the advanced and complex bird intelligence. The region between the eye and bill on the side of a bird's head is called the lore. This region is sometimes featherless, and the skin may be tinted, as in many species of the cormorant family.

Reproduction

Although most male birds have no external sex organs, the male does have two testes which become hundreds of times larger during the breeding season to produce sperm. The female's ovaries also become larger, although only the left ovary usually functions. However, if the left ovary is damaged by infection or other problems, the right ovary will try to function.

In the males of species without a phallus, sperm is stored in the seminal glomera within the cloacal protuberance prior to copulation. During copulation, the female moves her tail to the side and the male either mounts the female from behind or in front (in the stitchbird), or moves very close to her. The cloacae then touch, so that the sperm can enter the female's reproductive tract. This can happen very fast, sometimes in less than half a second.

The sperm is stored in the female's sperm storage tubules for a week to a year, depending on the species. Then, eggs will be fertilised individually as they leave the ovaries, before being laid by the female. The eggs continue their development outside the female body.

Many waterfowl and some other birds, such as the ostrich and turkey, possess a phallus. When not copulating, it is hidden within the proctodeum compartment within the cloaca, just inside the vent.

After the eggs hatch, parents provide varying degrees of care in terms of food and protection. Precocial birds can care for themselves independently within minutes of hatching; altricial hatchlings are helpless, blind, and naked, and require extended parental care. The chicks of many ground-nesting birds such as partridges and waders are often able to run virtually immediately after hatching; such birds are referred to as nidifugous. The young of hole-nesters, on the other hand, are often totally incapable of unassisted survival. The process whereby a chick acquires feathers until it can fly is called "fledging".

Some birds, such as pigeons, geese, and Red-crowned Cranes, remain with their mates for life and may produce offspring on a regular basis.

Scales

The scales of birds are composed of the same keratin as beaks, claws, and spurs. They are found mainly on the toes and metatarsus, but may be found further up on the ankle in some birds. Most bird scales do not overlap significantly, except in the cases of kingfishers and woodpeckers. The scales of birds are thought to be homologous to those of reptiles and mammals.

Bird embryos begin development with smooth skin. On the feet, the corneum, or outermost layer, of this skin may keratinize, thicken and form scales. These scales can be organized into;

1. Cancella: Minute scales which are really just a thickening and hardening of the skin, criss-crossed with shallow grooves.
2. Reticula: Small but distinct, separate, scales. Found on the lateral and medial surfaces (sides) of the chicken metatarsus. These are made up of alpha-keratin.
3. Scutella: Scales that are not quite as large as scutes, such as those found on the caudal or hind part, of the chicken metatarsus.
4. Scutes: The largest scales, usually on the anterior surface of the metatarsus and dorsal surface of the toes. These are made up of beta-keratin as in reptilian scales.

The rows of scutes on the anterior of the metatarsus can be called an acrometatarsium or acrotarsium.

Feathers can be intermixed with scales on some birds' feet. Feather follicles can lie between scales or even directly beneath them, in the deeper dermis layer of the skin. In this last case, feathers may emerge directly through scales, and be encircled at the plane of emergence entirely by the keratin of the scale.

Feline Anatomy

The following two diagrams help you familiarize yourself with basic feline anatomy. The chart below (of a male cat) shows you were all the internal organs are located.

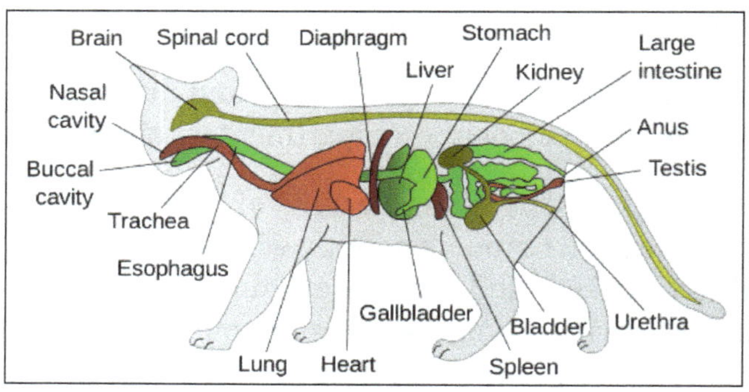

Did you know that cats have 244 bones in their body? Humans only have 206. This diagram of a feline skeleton shows you where all of your cat's bones are located.

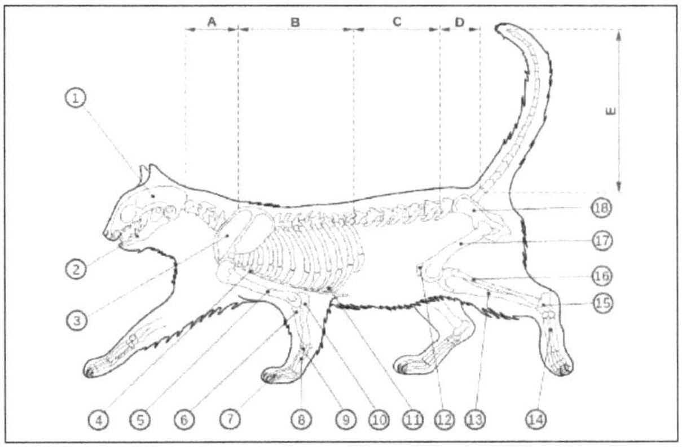

Figure shows, A – cervical bones, B – thoracic bones, C – lumbar bones, D – sacral bones, E – tail bones, 1 – cranium, 2 – mandible, 3 – scapula, 4 – sternum, 5 – humerus, 6 – radius, 7 – phalangeals, 8 – metacarpals, 9 – carpal bones, 10 – ulna, 11 – ribs, 12 – patella, 13 – tibia, 14 – metatarsals, 15 – tarsal bones, 16 – fibula, 17 – femur.

Fascinating Feline Anatomical Abilities

- Purring: The result of intermittent signaling by the diaphragmatic and laryngeal muscles.
- Whiskers: They help your cat identify and analyze everything she touches via sensitive nerve endings.
- Sandpaper tongue: To help with grooming.
- Jacobson's organ: Located in the roof of the mouth, this organ helps cats analyze scents. Your cat's mouth will be partially open when she uses this organ. This is also known as the flehmen response.
- Tail: It contains almost 10 percent of the cat's bones, and acts as a counterweight in helping him keep his balance. A cat's tail also communicates his mood. Understanding "tail speak" is an important part of reading feline body language.

Ruminant Animal Digestive System

Ruminant livestock include cattle, sheep, and goats. Ruminants are hoofed mammals that have a unique digestive system that allows them to better use energy from fibrous plant material than other herbivores. Unlike monogastrics such as swine and poultry, ruminants have a digestive system designed to ferment feedstuffs and provide precursors for energy for the animal to use. By better understanding how the digestive system of the ruminant works, livestock producers can better understand how to care for and feed ruminant animals.

Ruminant Digestive Anatomy and Function

The ruminant digestive system uniquely qualifies ruminant animals such as cattle to efficiently use high roughage feedstuffs, including forages. Anatomy of the ruminant digestive system includes the mouth, tongue, salivary glands (producing saliva for buffering rumen pH), esophagus, four-compartment stomach (rumen, reticulum, omasum, and abomasum), pancreas, gall bladder, small intestine (duodenum, jejunum, and ileum), and large intestine (cecum, colon, and rectum).

A ruminant uses its mouth (oral cavity) and tongue to harvest forages during grazing or to consume harvested feedstuffs. Cattle harvest forages during grazing by wrapping their tongues around the plants and then pulling to tear the forage for consumption. On average, cattle take from 25,000 to more than 40,000 prehensile bites to harvest forage while grazing each day. They typically spend more than one-third of their time grazing, one-third of their time ruminating (cud chewing), and slightly less than one-third of their time idling where they are, neither grazing nor ruminating.

The roof of the ruminant mouth is a hard/soft palate without incisors. The lower jaw incisors work against this hard dental pad. The incisors of grass/roughage selectors are wide with a shovel-shaped crown, while those of concentrate selectors are narrower and chisel-shaped. Premolars and molars match between upper and lower jaws. These teeth crush and grind plant material during initial chewing and rumination.

Saliva aids in chewing and swallowing, contains enzymes for breakdown of fat (salivary lipase) and starch (salivary amylase), and is involved in nitrogen recycling to the rumen. Saliva's most important function is to buffer pH levels in the reticulum and rumen. A mature cow produces up to 50 quarts of saliva per day, but this varies, depending on the amount of time spent chewing feed, because that stimulates saliva production.

Forage and feed mixes with saliva containing sodium, potassium, phosphate, bicarbonate, and urea when consumed, to form a bolus. Those bolus then moves from the mouth to the reticulum through a tube-like passage called the esophagus. Muscle contractions and pressure differences carry these substances down the esophagus to the reticulum.

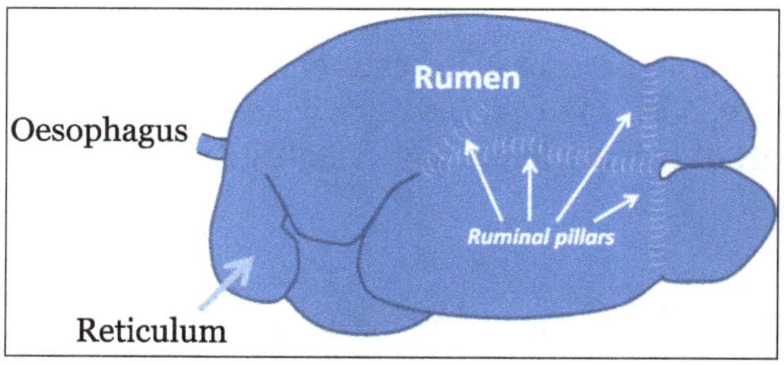

Left-sided view of ruminant digestive tract.

Ruminants eat rapidly, swallowing much of their feedstuffs without chewing it sufficiently (< 1.5 inches). The esophagus functions bidirectionally in ruminants, allowing them to regurgitate their cud for further chewing, if necessary. The process of rumination or "chewing the cud" is where forage and other feedstuffs are forced back to the mouth for further chewing and mixing with saliva. This cud is then swallowed again and passed into the reticulum. Then the solid portion slowly moves into the rumen for fermentation, while most of the liquid portion rapidly moves from the reticulorumen into the omasum and then abomasum. The solid portion left behind in the rumen typically remains for up to 48 hours and forms a dense mat in the rumen, where microbes can use the fibrous feedstuffs to make precursors for energy.

True ruminants, such as cattle, sheep, goats, deer, and antelope, have one stomach with four compartments: the rumen, reticulum, omasum, and abomasums. The ruminant stomach occupies almost 75 percent of the abdominal cavity, filling nearly all of the left side and extending significantly into the right side. The relative size of the four compartments is as follows: the rumen and reticulum comprise 84 percent of the volume of the total stomach, the omasum 12 percent, and the abomasum 4 percent. The rumen is the largest stomach compartment, holding up to 40 gallons in a mature cow.

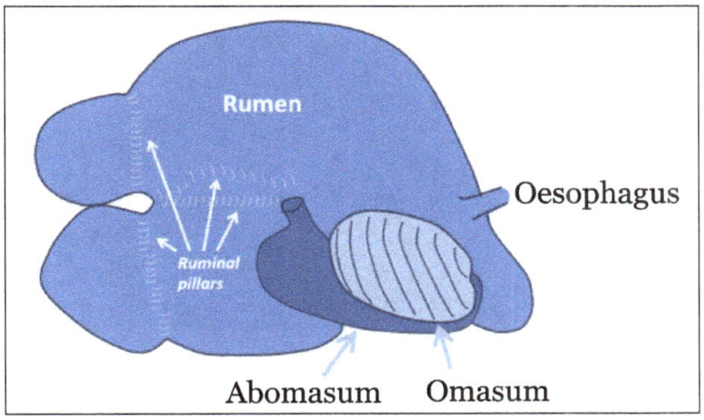

Right-sided view of ruminant digestive tract.

The reticulum holds approximately 5 gallons in the mature cow. Typically, the rumen and reticulum are considered one organ because they have similar functions and are separated only by a small muscular fold of tissue. They are collectively referred to as the reticulorumen. The omasum and abomasum hold up to 15 and 7 gallons, respectively, in the mature cow.

The reticulorumen is home to a population of microorganisms (microbes or "rumen bugs") that include bacteria, protozoa, and fungi. These microbes ferment and break down plant cell walls into their carbohydrate fractions and produce volatile fatty acids (VFAs), such as acetate (used for fat synthesis), priopionate (used for glucose synthesis), and butyrate from these carbohydrates. The animal later uses these VFAs for energy.

The reticulum is called the "honeycomb" because of the honeycomb appearance of its lining. It sits underneath and toward the front of the rumen, lying against the diaphragm. Ingesta flow freely between the reticulum and rumen. The main function of the reticulum is to collect smaller digesta particles and move them into the omasum, while the larger particles remain in the rumen for further digestion.

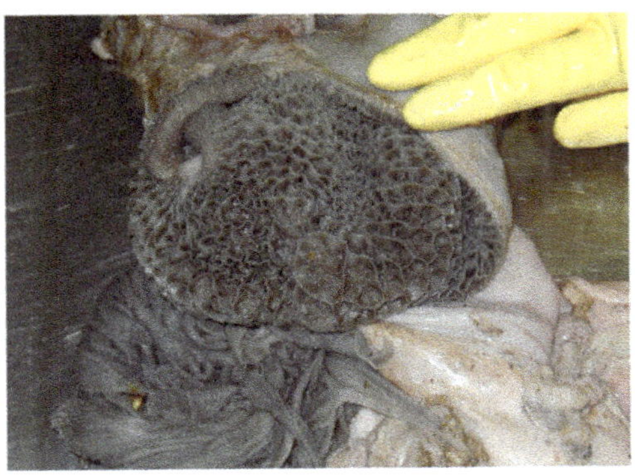

"Honeycomb" interior lining of the reticulum in an 8-week-old calf.

The reticulum also traps and collects heavy/dense objects the animal consumes. When a ruminant consumes a nail, wire, or other sharp heavy object, it is very likely the object will be caught in the reticulum. During normal digestive tract contractions, this object can penetrate the reticulum wall and make its way to the heart, where it can lead to hardware disease. The reticulum is sometimes referred to as the "hardware stomach".

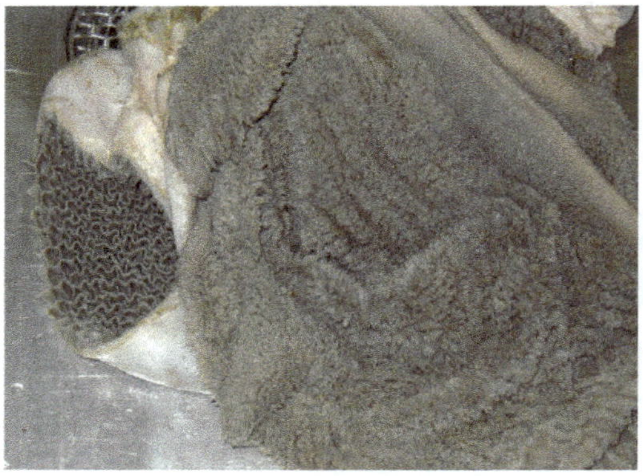

Interior lining of the rumen, revealing papilloe in an 8-week-old calft.

The rumen is sometimes called the "paunch." It is lined with papillae for nutrient absorption and divided by muscular pillars into the dorsal, ventral, caudodorsal, and caudoventral sacs. The rumen acts as a fermentation vat by hosting microbial fermentation. About 50 to 65 percent of starch and soluble sugar consumed is digested in the rumen. Rumen microorganisms (primarily bacteria) digest cellulose from plant cell walls, digest complex starch, synthesize protein from nonprotein nitrogen, and synthesize B vitamins and vitamin K. Rumen pH typically ranges from 6.5 to 6.8. The rumen environment is anaerobic (without oxygen). Gases produced in the rumen include carbon dioxide, methane, and hydrogen sulfide. The gas fraction rises to the top of the rumen above the liquid fraction.

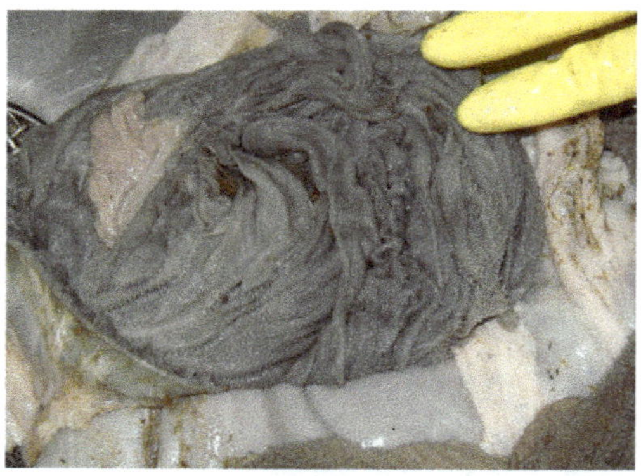

Interior lining of the omasum, revealing the "many piles" tissue folds in an 8-week-calf.

The omasum is spherical and connected to the reticulum by a short tunnel. It is called the "many piles" in reference to the many folds or leaves that resemble pages of a book. These folds increase the surface area, which increases the area that absorbs nutrients from feed and water. Water absorption occurs in the omasum. Cattle have a highly developed, large omasum.

The abomasum is the "true stomach" of a ruminant. It is the compartment that is most similar to a stomach in a nonruminant. The abomasum produces hydrochloric acid and digestive enzymes, such as pepsin (breaks down proteins), and receives digestive enzymes secreted from the pancreas, such as pancreatic lipase (breaks down fats). These secretions help prepare proteins for absorption in the intestines. The pH in the abomasum generally ranges from 3.5 to 4.0. The chief cells in the abomasum secrete mucous to protect the abomasal wall from acid damage.

The small and large intestines follow the abomasum as further sites of nutrient absorption. The small intestine is a tube up to 150 feet long with a 20-gallon capacity in a mature cow. Digesta entering the small intestine mix with secretions from the pancreas and liver, which elevate the pH from 2.5 to between 7 and 8. This higher pH is needed for enzymes in the small intestine to work properly. Bile from the gall bladder is secreted into the first section of the small intestine, the duodenum, to aid in digestion. Active nutrient absorption occurs throughout the small intestine, including rumen bypass protein absorption. The intestinal wall contains numerous "finger-like" projections called villi that increase intestinal surface area to aid in nutrient absorption. Muscular contractions aid in mixing digesta and moving it to the next section.

The large intestine absorbs water from material passing through it and then excretes the remaining material as feces from the rectum. The cecum is a large blind pouch at the beginning of the large intestine, approximately 3 feet long with a 2-gallon capacity in the mature cow. The cecum serves little function in a ruminant, unlike its role in horses. The colon is the site of most of the water absorption in the large intestine.

Ruminant Digestive Development

Immature ruminants, such as young, growing calves from birth to about 2 to 3 months of age, are functionally nonruminants. The reticular groove (sometimes referred to as esophageal groove) in these young animals is formed by muscular folds of the reticulum. It shunts milk directly to the omasum and then abomasum, bypassing the reticulorumen. The rumen in these animals must be inoculated with rumen microorganisms, including bacteria, fungi, and protozoa. This is thought to be accomplished through mature ruminants licking calves and environmental contact with these microorganisms.

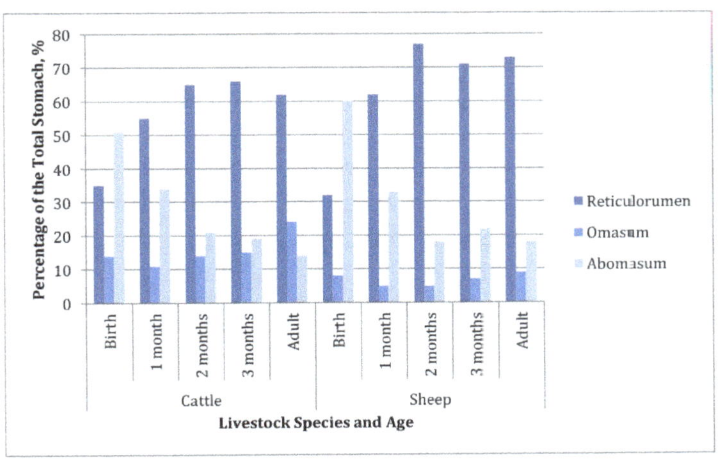

Relative proportions of stomach compartments in cattle and sheep at various ages.

Immature ruminants must undergo reticulorumen-omasal growth, including increases in volume and muscle. In a calf at birth, the abomasum is the largest compartment of the stomach, making up more than 50 percent of the total stomach area. The reticulorumen and omasum account for 35 percent and 14 percent of the total stomach area in the newborn calf. As ruminants develop, the reticulorumen and omasum grow rapidly and account for increasing proportions of the total stomach area. In mature cattle, the abomasum encompasses only 21 percent of the total stomach capacity, whereas the reticulorumen and omasum make up 62 and 24 percent, respectively, of the total stomach area. Rumen papillae (sites of nutrient absorption) lengthen and decrease in numbers as part of rumen development.

Because immature ruminants do not have a functional rumen, feeding recommendations differ for developing ruminants compared with adult ruminants. For instance, it is recommended immature ruminants are not allowed access to feeds containing non-protein nitrogen such as urea. Developing ruminants are also more sensitive to gossypol and dietary fat levels than mature ruminants. Design nutritional programs for ruminants considering animal age.

Ruminant Feeding Types

Based on the diets they prefer, ruminants can be classified into distinct feeding types: concentrate selectors, grass/roughage eaters, and intermediate types. The relative sizes of various digestive system organs differ by ruminant feeding type, creating differences in feeding adaptations. Knowledge of grazing preferences and adaptations amongst ruminant livestock species helps in planning grazing systems for each individual species and also for multiple species grazed together or on the same acreage.

Concentrate selectors have a small reticulorumen in relation to body size and selectively browse trees and shrubs. Deer and giraffes are examples of concentrate selectors. Animals in this group of ruminants select plants and plant parts high in easily digestible, nutrient dense substances such as plant starch, protein, and fat. For example, deer prefer legumes over grasses. Concentrate selectors are very limited in their ability to digest the fibers and cellulose in plant cell walls.

Grass/roughage eaters (bulk and roughage eaters) include cattle and sheep. These ruminants depend on diets of grasses and other fibrous plant material. They prefer diets of fresh grasses over legumes but can adequately manage rapidly fermenting feedstuffs. Grass/roughage eaters have much longer intestines relative to body length and a shorter proportion of large intestine to small intestine as compared with concentrate selectors.

Goats are classified as intermediate types and prefer forbs and browse such as woody, shrubby type plants. This group of ruminants has adaptations of both concentrate selectors and grass/roughage eaters. They have a fair though limited capacity to digest cellulose in plant cell walls.

Carbohydrate Digestion

Forages

On high-forage diets ruminants often ruminate or regurgitate ingested forage. This allows them to "chew their cud" to reduce particle size and improve digestibility. As ruminants are transitioned to higher concentrate (grain-based) diets, they ruminate less.

Once inside the reticulorumen, forage is exposed to a unique population of microbes that begin to ferment and digest the plant cell wall components and break these components down into carbohydrates and sugars. Rumen microbes use carbohydrates along with ammonia and amino acids to grow. The microbes ferment sugars to produce VFAs (acetate, propionate, and butyrate), methane, hydrogen sulfide, and carbon dioxide. The VFAs are then absorbed across the rumen wall, where they go to the liver.

Once at the liver, the VFAs are converted to glucose via gluconeogenesis. Because plant cell walls are slow to digest, this acid production is very slow. Coupled with routine rumination (chewing and rechewing of the cud) that increases salivary flow, this makes for a rather stable pH environment (around 6).

High-concentrate Feedstuffs

When ruminants are fed high-grain or concentrate rations, the digestion process is similar to forage digestion, with a few exceptions. Typically, on a high-grain diet, there is less chewing and ruminating, which leads to less salivary production and buffering agents' being, produced. Additionally, most grains have a high concentration of readily digestible carbohydrates, unlike the more structural carbohydrates found in plant cell walls. This readily digestible carbohydrate is rapidly digested, resulting in an increase in VFA production.

The relative concentrations of the VFAs are also changed, with propionate being produced in the greatest quantity, followed by acetate and butyrate. Less methane and heat are produced as well. The increase in VFA production leads to a more acidic environment (pH 5.5). It also causes a shift in the microbial population by decreasing the forage using microbial population and potentially leading to a decrease in digestibility of forages.

Lactic acid, a strong acid, is a byproduct of starch fermentation. Lactic acid production, coupled with the increased VFA production, can overwhelm the ruminant's ability to buffer and absorb these acids and lead to metabolic acidosis. The acidic environment leads to tissue damage within the rumen and can lead to ulcerations of the rumen wall. Take care to provide adequate forage and avoid situations that might lead to acidosis when feeding ruminants high-concentrate diets.

Protein Digestion

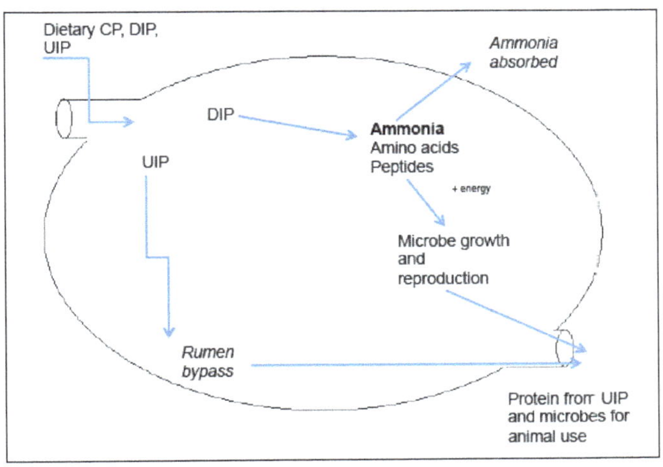

Protein digestion in the ruminant.

Two sources of protein are available for the ruminant to use: protein from feed and microbial protein from the microbes that inhabit its rumen. A ruminant is unique in that it has a symbiotic relationship with these microbes. Like other living creatures, these microbes have requirements for protein and energy to facilitate growth and reproduction. During digestive contractions, some of these microorganisms are "washed" out of the rumen into the abomasum where they are digested like other proteins, thereby creating a source of protein for the animal.

All crude protein (CP) the animal ingests is divided into two fractions, degradable intake protein (DIP) and undegradable intake protein (UIP, also called "rumen bypass protein"). Each feedstuff (such as cottonseed meal, soybean hulls, and annual ryegrass forage) has different proportions of each protein type. Rumen microbes break down the DIP into ammonia (NH3) amino acids, and peptides, which are used by the microbes along with energy from carbohydrate digestion for growth and reproduction.

Excess ammonia is absorbed via the rumen wall and converted into urea in the liver, where it returns in the blood to the saliva or is excreted by the body. Urea toxicity comes from overfeeding urea to ruminants. Ingested urea is immediately degraded to ammonia in the rumen.

When more ammonia than energy is available for building protein from the nitrogen supplied by urea, the excess ammonia is absorbed through the rumen wall. Toxicity occurs when the excess ammonia overwhelms the liver's ability to detoxify it into urea. This can kill the animal. However, with sufficient energy, microbes use ammonia and amino acids to grow and reproduce.

The rumen does not degrade the UIP component of feedstuffs. The UIP "bypasses" the rumen and makes its way from the omasum to the abomasum. In the abomasum, the ruminant uses UIP along with microorganisms washed out of the rumen as a protein source.

References

- Veterinary-anatomy-and-physiology: intechopen.com, Retrieved 2 March, 2019
- Animalcel: magnet.fsu.edu, Retrieved 5 June, 2019
- Types-of-Circulatory-Systems-in-Animals, The-Circulatory-System, General-Biology: libretexts.org, Retrieved 11 January, 2019
- Animal-reproductive-system, animal: britannica.com, Retrieved 18 July, 2019
- Dog-anatomy: certapet.com, Retrieved 20 January, 2019
- Horse-anatomy: equinespot.com, Retrieved 17 May, 2019
- Cow-anatomy: animalcorner.co.uk, Retrieved 7 August, 2019
- Anatomy: beautyofbirds.com, Retrieved 13 February, 2019
- Understanding-the-ruminant-animal-digestive-system: msstate.edu, Retrieved 10 April, 2019

Chapter 3

Animal Diseases

There are a wide variety of diseases which can affect animals such as viral diseases, fungal diseases and bacterial diseases. Apart from these, diseases can also be caused by parasites such as helminths. This chapter closely examines these types of animal diseases to provide an extensive understanding of the subject.

Animal disease is an impairment of the normal state of an animal that interrupts or modifies its vital functions.

Concern with diseases that afflict animals dates from the earliest human contacts with animals and is reflected in early views of religion and magic. Diseases of animals remain a concern principally because of the economic losses they cause and the possible transmission of the causative agents to humans. The branch of medicine called veterinary medicine deals with the study, prevention, and treatment of diseases not only in domesticated animals but also in wild animals and in animals used in scientific research. The prevention, control, and eradication of diseases of economically important animals are agricultural concerns. Programs for the control of diseases communicable from animals to man, called zoonoses, especially those in pets and in wildlife, are closely related to human health. Further, the diseases of animals are of increasing importance, for a primary public-health problem throughout the world is animal-protein deficiency in the diet of humans. Indeed, both the United Nations Food and Agricultural Organization (FAO) and the World Health Organization (WHO) have been attempting to solve the problem of protein deficits in a world whose human population is rapidly expanding.

Economic Importance

About 50 percent of the world's population suffers from chronic malnutrition and hunger. Inadequate diet claims many thousands of lives each day. When the lack of adequate food to meet present needs for an estimated world population of more than 4,600,000,000 in the 1980s is coupled with the prediction that the population may increase to 7,000,000,000 by the year 2000, it becomes obvious that animal-food supplies must be increased. One way in which this might be accomplished is by learning to control the diseases that afflict animals throughout the world, especially in the developing nations of Asia and Africa, where the population is expanding most rapidly. Most of the information concerning animal diseases, however, applies to domesticated animals such as pigs, cattle, and sheep, which are relatively unimportant as food sources in these nations. Remarkably little is known of the diseases of the goat, the water buffalo, the camel, the elephant, the yak, the llama, or the alpaca; all are domesticated animals upon which the economies of many developing countries depend. It is in these countries that increased animal production resulting from the development of methods for the control and eradication of diseases affecting these animals is most urgently needed.

Despite the development of various effective methods of disease control, substantial quantities of meat and milk are lost each year throughout the world. In countries in which animal-disease control is not yet adequately developed, the loss of animal protein from disease is about 30 to 40 percent of the quantity available in certain underdeveloped areas. In addition, such countries also suffer losses resulting from poor husbandry practices.

Role in Human Disease

Animals have long been recognized as agents of human disease. Man has probably been bitten, stung, kicked, and gored by animals for as long as he has been on earth; in addition, early man sometimes became ill or died after eating the flesh of dead animals. In more recent times, man has discovered that many invertebrate animals are capable of transmitting causative agents of disease from man to man or from other vertebrates to man. Such animals, which act as hosts, agents, and carriers of disease, are important in causing and perpetuating human illness. Because about three-fourths of the important known zoonoses are associated with domesticated animals, including pets, the term zoonosis was originally defined as a group of diseases that man is able to acquire from domesticated animals. But this definition has been modified to include all human diseases (whether or not they manifest themselves in all hosts as apparent diseases) that are acquired from or transmitted to any other vertebrate animal. Thus, zoonoses are naturally occurring infections and infestations shared by man and other vertebrates.

Although the role of domesticated animals in many zoonoses is understood, the role of the numerous species of wild animals with which man is less intimately associated is not well understood. The discovery that diseases such as yellow fever, viral brain infections, plague, and numerous other important diseases involving man or his domesticated animals are fundamentally diseases of wildlife and exist independently of man and his civilization, however, has increased the significance of studying the nature of wildlife diseases.

Animals in Research

Although in modern times the practice of veterinary medicine has been separated from that of human medicine, the observations of the physician and the veterinarian continue to add to the common body of medical knowledge. Of the more than 1,200,000 species of animals thus far identified, only a few have been utilized in research, even though it is likely that, for every known human disease, an identical or similar disease exists in at least one other animal species. Veterinary medicine plays an ever-increasing role in the health of man through the use of animals as biomedical models with similar disease counterparts in man. This use of animals as models is important because research on many genetic and chronic diseases of man cannot be carried out using humans.

Hundreds of thousands of mice and monkeys are utilized each year in research laboratories in the U.S. alone. Animal studies are used in the development of new surgical techniques (e.g., organ transplantations), in the testing of new drugs for safety, and in nutritional research. Animals are especially valuable in research involving chronic degenerative diseases, because such diseases can be induced in animals experimentally with relative ease. The importance of chronic degenerative diseases, such as cancer and cardiovascular diseases has increased in parallel with the growing number of communicable diseases that have been brought under control.

Examples of animal diseases that are quite similar to commonly occurring human diseases include chronic emphysema in the horse; leukemia in cats and cattle; muscular dystrophies in chickens and mice; atherosclerosis in pigs and pigeons; blood-coagulation disorders and nephritis in dogs; gastric ulcers in swine; vascular aneurysms (permanent and abnormal blood-filled area of a blood vessel) in turkeys; diabetes mellitus in Chinese hamsters; milk allergy and gallstones in rabbits; hepatitis in dogs and horses; hydrocephalus (fluid in the head) and skin allergies in many species; epilepsy in dogs and gerbils; hereditary deafness in many small animals; cataracts in the eyes of dogs and mice; and urinary stones in dogs and cattle.

The study of animals with diseases similar to those that affect man has increased knowledge of the diseases in man; knowledge of nutrition, for example, based largely on the results of animal studies, has improved the health of animals, including man. Animal investigations have been used extensively in the treatment of shock, in open-heart surgery, in organ transplantations, and in the testing of new drugs. Other important contributions to human health undoubtedly will result from new research discoveries involving the study of animal diseases.

Role of Ecology

Epidemiology, the study of epidemics, is sometimes defined as the medical aspect of ecology, for it is the study of diseases in animal populations. Hence the epidemiologist is concerned with the interactions of organisms and their environments as related to the presence of disease. The multiple-causality concept of disease embraced by epidemiology involves combinations of environmental factors and host factors, in addition to the determination of the specific causative agent of a given disease. Environmental factors include geographical features, climate, and concentration of certain elements in soil and water. Host factors include age, breed, sex, and the physiological state of an animal as well as the general immunity of a herd resulting from previous contact with a disease. Epidemiology, therefore, is concerned with the determination of the individual animals that are affected by a disease, the environmental circumstances under which it may occur, the causative agents, and the ways in which transmission occurs in nature. The epidemiologist, who utilizes many scientific disciplines (e.g., medicine, zoology, mathematics, anthropology), attempts to determine the types of diseases that exist in a specific geographical area and to control them by modifying the environment.

Diseases in animal populations are characterized by certain features. Some outbreaks are termed sporadic diseases because they appear only occasionally in individuals within an animal population. Diseases normally present in an area are referred to as endemic, or enzootic, diseases, and they usually reflect a relatively stable relationship between the causative agent and the animals affected by it. Diseases that occasionally occur at higher than normal rates in animal populations are referred to as epidemic, or epizootic, diseases, and they generally represent an unstable relationship between the causative agent and affected animals.

The effect of diseases on a stable ecological system, which is the result of the dominance of some plants and animals and the subordination or extinction of others, depends on the degree to which the causative agents of diseases and their hosts are part of the system. Epidemic diseases result from an ecological imbalance; endemic diseases often represent a balanced state. Ecological imbalance and, hence, epidemic disease may be either naturally caused or induced by man. A breakdown in sanitation in a city, for example, offers conditions favourable for an increase in the rodent population, with the possibility that diseases such as plague may be introduced into and spread among the human population. In this case, an epidemic would result as much from an alteration in the environment as from the presence of the causative agent Pasteurella pestis, since, in relatively balanced ecological systems, the causative agent exists enzootically in the rodents (i.e., they serve as reservoirs for the disease) and seldom involves man. In a similar manner, an increase in the number of epidemics of viral encephalitis, a brain disease, in man has resulted from the ecological imbalance of mosquitoes and wild birds caused by man's exploitation of lowland for farming. Driven from their natural habitat of reeds and rushes, the wild birds, important natural hosts for the virus that causes the disease, are forced to feed near farms; mosquitoes transmit the virus from birds to cattle and man.

Detection and Diagnosis

Reactions of Tissue to Disease

As previously noted, disease may be defined as an injurious deviation from a normal physiological state of an organism sufficient to produce overt signs, or symptoms. The deviation may be either an obvious organic change in the tissue composing an organ or a functional disturbance whose organic changes are not obvious. The severity of the changes that occur in cells and tissues subjected to injurious agents is dependent upon both the sensitivity of the tissue concerned and the nature and time course of the agent. A mildly injurious agent that is present for short periods of time may either have little effect or stimulate cells to increased activity. Strongly injurious agents in prolonged contact with cells cause characteristic changes in them by interfering with normal cell processes. Most causative agents of disease fall into the latter category.

Characteristics of Cell and Tissue Changes

Changes in cells and tissues as a result of disease include degenerative and infiltrative changes. Degenerative changes are characterized by the deterioration of cells or a tissue from a higher to a lower form, especially to a less functionally active form. When chemical changes occur in the tissue, the process is one of degeneration. When the changes involve the accumulation of materials within the cells comprising tissues, the process is called infiltration. Diseases such as pneumonia, metal poisoning, or septicemia (the persistence of disease-causing bacteria in the bloodstream) may cause the mildest type of degeneration—parenchymatous changes, or cloudy swelling of the cells; the cells first affected are the specialized cells of the liver and the kidney. Serious cellular damage may cause the uptake of water by cells (hydropic degeneration), which lose their structural features as they fill with water. The causes for the accumulation in cells of abnormal amounts of fats (fatty infiltration and degeneration) have not yet been established with certainty but probably involve fat metabolism. Poisons such as phosphorus may cause sudden increases in the accumulation of fats in the liver. An abnormal protein material may accumulate in connective-tissue components of small arteries as a result of chronic pneumonia, chronic bacterial infections, and prolonged antitoxin production (in horses); the condition is known as amyloid degeneration and infiltration. Hyaline degeneration, characterized by tissues that become clear and appear glasslike, usually occurs in connective-tissue components of small blood vessels as a result of conditions that may occur in kidney structures (glomeruli) of animals with nephritis or in lymph glands of animals with tuberculosis. Certain structures (glomeruli) of animals with nephritis result in degeneration.

The condition in which mucus, a secretion of mucous membranes lining the inside surfaces of organs, is produced in excess and accumulates in greater than normal amounts is referred to as mucoid degeneration. Major causes of this condition include chronic irritation of mucous membranes and certain mucus-producing tumours. Abnormal amounts of glycogen, which is the principal storage carbohydrate of animals, may occur in the liver as a result of certain inherited diseases of animals; the condition is known as glycogen infiltration. The abnormal deposition of calcium salts, which is known as hypercalcification, may occur as a result of several diseases involving the blood vessels and the heart, the urinary system, the gallbladder, and the bonelike tissue called cartilage. Pigments (coloured molecules) from coal dust or asbestos dust may infiltrate the lungs of certain dogs in two types of lung disease: anthracosis and asbestosis. Abnormal amounts of iron-containing coloured molecules (hemosiderin) resulting from the breakdown of hemoglobin, the oxygen-carrying protein of red blood cells, are often deposited in the liver and the spleen after diseases that involve excessive breakdown of red blood cells. A dark-coloured molecule (melanin) occurs abnormally in the livers of certain sheep suffering from Dubin–Johnson syndrome and in certain tumours called melanomas. Uric acid infiltration, which occurs in poultry, is characterized by the deposition of uric acid salts.

Necrosis, the death of cells or tissues, takes place if the blood supply to tissues is restricted; poisons produced by microbes, chemical poisons, and extreme heat or electricity also may cause necrosis. The rotting of the dead tissue is known as gangrene.

Atrophy of animal tissue involves a process of tissue wasting, in which a decrease occurs in the size or number of functional cells—e.g., in inherited muscular dystrophy of chickens. Hypertrophy—an increase in the size of the cells in a tissue or an organ—occurs in heart muscle during diseases involving the heart valves, in certain pneumonias, and in some diseases of the endocrine glands. Aplasia is the term used when an entire organ is missing from an animal; hypoplasia indicates arrested or incomplete development of an organ, and hyperplasia an increase in the production of the number of cells—e.g., the persistent callus that forms on the elbows of some dogs. Metaplasia is used to describe the change of one cell type into another; it may occur in chronic irritation of tissues and in certain cancerous tumours.

Characteristics of Inflammatory Reactions

When tissues are injured, they become inflamed. The inflammation may be acute, in which case the inflammatory processes are active, or chronic, in which case the processes occur slowly and new connective tissue is formed. The reaction of inflamed tissues is a combination of defensive and repair mechanisms. Acute inflammation is characterized by redness, heat, swelling, sensitivity, and impaired function. Several types of acute inflammation are known. Mild acute inflammations of mucous membranes resulting in the production of thin watery material (exudate) are called catarrhal inflammations; parenchymatous inflammations occur in organs undergoing degeneration. If the exudate formed in response to an injury is of a serious nature—that is, resembling blood plasma—the process is called serous inflammation. In fibrinous inflammation, a protein (fibrin) forms on membranes, including those in the lungs. In suppurative inflammation, dead tissue is replaced with pus composed of colourless blood cells (leucocytes) and tissue juices.

During the inflammatory reaction, the injured tissue is surrounded by an area of rapidly dividing cells. Specialized cells called macrophages enter the tissue and remove blood and tissue debris. Other cells, called neutrophils, ingest disease-causing bacteria and other foreign material. In chronic inflammations, the connective tissue contains fibroblasts, cells that divide and form new connective, or scar, tissue.

Characteristics of Circulatory Disturbances

An increase in the rate of blood flow to a body part, which is referred to by the term congestion, or hyperemia, occurs during inflammation; a diminished blood flow to tissues is referred to by the term ischemia, or a local anemia. Examples of hemorrhage, the escape of blood from vessels, include epistaxis, or nosebleeds, in racehorses; hematemesis, or regurgitation of blood, in dogs with uremia; hemoptysis, or blood loss from lungs; hematuria, or blood in urine, of cattle with inflammation of the urinary bladder. Edema, a condition that is characterized by abnormal accumulations of fluid in tissues, occurs not only in a tissue during inflammation but also over the entire body if the concentration of blood-serum proteins, especially albumin, is low. A thrombosis, which is a blood clot in a blood vessel, may block or slow circulation of blood to tissues; if blood vessels become blocked, the condition is known as an embolism. The term infarction describes the necrosis that occurs in tissues whose blood supply is blocked by an embolism.

Methods of Examination

Before an unhealthy animal receives treatment, an attempt is made to diagnose the disease. Both clinical findings, which include symptoms that are obvious to a nonspecialist and clinical signs that can be appreciated only by a veterinarian, and laboratory test results, may be necessary to establish the cause of a disease. A clinical examination should indicate if the animal is in good physical condition, is eating adequately, is bright and alert, and is functioning in an apparently normal manner. Many disease processes are either inflammatory or result from tumours. Malignant tumours (e.g., melanomas in horses, squamous cell carcinomas in small animals) tend to spread rapidly and usually cause death. Other diseases cause the circulatory disturbances or the degenerative and infiltrative changes. If a specific diagnosis is not possible, the symptoms of the animal are treated.

A case record of the information pertaining to an animal (or to a herd of animals) that is suspected of having a disease is begun at the time the animal is taken to a veterinarian (or the veterinarian visits the animal) and is continued through treatment. It includes a description of the animal (age, species, sex, breed); the owner's report; the animal's history; a description of the preliminary examination; clinical findings resulting from an examination of body systems; results of specific laboratory tests; diagnosis regarding a specific cause for the disease (etiology); outlook (prognosis); treatment; case progress; termination; autopsy, if performed; and the utilization of scientific references, if applicable.

The veterinarian must diagnose a disease on the basis of a variety of examinations and tests, since he obviously cannot interrogate the animal. Methods used in the preparation of a diagnosis include inspection—a visual examination of the animal; palpation—the application of firm pressure with the fingers to tissues to determine characteristics such as abnormal shapes and possible tumours, the presence of pain, and tissue consistency; percussion—the application of a short, sharp blow to a tissue to provoke an audible response from body parts directly beneath; auscultation—the act of listening to sounds that are produced by the body during the performance of functions (e.g., breathing, intestinal movements); smells—the recognition of characteristic odours associated with certain diseases; and miscellaneous diagnostic procedures, such as eye examinations, the collection of urine, and heart, esophageal, and stomach studies.

General Inspection

Deviation of various characteristics from the normal, observation of which constitutes the general inspection of an animal, is a useful aid in diagnosing disease. The general inspection includes examination of appearance; behaviour; body condition; respiratory movements; state of skin, coat, and abdomen; and various common actions.

The appearance of an animal may be of diagnostic significance; small size in a pig may result from retardation of growth, which is caused by hog-cholera virus. Observation of the behaviour of an animal is of value in diagnosing neurological diseases; e.g., muscle spasms occur in lockjaw (tetanus) in dogs, nervousness and convulsions in dogs with distemper, dullness in horses with equine viral encephalitis, and excitement in animals suffering from lead poisoning. Subtle behavioral changes may not be noticeable. The general condition of the body is of value in diagnosing diseases that cause excessive leanness (emaciation), including certain cancers, or other chronic diseases, such as a deficiency in the output of the adrenal glands or tuberculosis. Defective teeth also may point to malnutrition and result in emaciation.

The respiratory movements of an animal are important diagnostic criteria; breathing is rapid in young animals, in small animals, and in animals whose body temperature is higher than normal. Specific respiratory movements are characteristic of certain diseases—e.g., certain movements in horses with heaves (emphysema) or the abdominal breathing of animals suffering from painful lung diseases. The appearance of the skin and hair may indicate dehydration by lack of pliability and lustre; or the presence of parasites such as lice, mites, or fleas; or the presence of ringworm infections and allergic reactions by the skin changes they cause. The poisoning of sheep by molybdenum in their hay may be diagnosed by the loss of colour in the wool of black sheep. Distension of the abdomen may indicate bloat in cattle or colic in horses.

Abnormal activities may have special diagnostic meaning to the veterinarian. Straining during urination is associated with bladder stones; increased frequency of urination is associated with kidney disease (nephritis), bladder infections, and a disease of the pituitary gland (diabetes insipidus). Excessive salivation and grinding of teeth may be caused by an abnormality in the mouth. Coughing is associated with pneumonia. Some diseases cause postural changes: for example, a horse with tetanus may stand in a stiff manner. An abnormal gait in an animal made to move may furnish evidence as to the cause of a disease, as louping ill in sheep.

Clinical Examination

Following the general inspection of an animal thought to have contracted a disease, a more thorough clinical examination is necessary, during which various features of the animal are studied. These include the visible mucous membranes (conjunctiva of the eye, nasal mucosa, inside surface of the mouth, and tongue); the eye itself; and such body surfaces as the ears, horns (if present), and limbs. In addition, the pulse rate and the temperature are measured.

The veterinarian examines the visible mucous membranes of the eye, nose, and mouth to determine if jaundice, hemorrhages, or anemia are present. The conjunctiva, or lining of the eye, may exhibit pus in pinkeye infections, have a yellow appearance in jaundice, or exhibit small hemorrhages in certain systemic diseases. Examination of the nose may reveal ulcers and vesicles (small sacs containing liquid), as in foot-and-mouth disease, a viral disease of cattle, or vesicular exanthema, a viral disease of swine. Ulceration of the tongue may be apparent in animals suffering from actinobacillosis, a disease of bacterial origin.

A detailed examination of the eye may show abnormalities of the cornea resulting from such diseases as infectious hepatitis in dogs, bovine catarrhal fever, and equine influenza. Cataract, a condition in which the passage of light through the lens of the eye is obstructed, may result from a disorder of carbohydrate metabolism (diabetes mellitus), infections, or a hereditary defect.

An elevated temperature, or fever, resulting from the multiplication of disease-causing organisms may be the earliest sign of disease. The increase in temperature activates the body mechanisms that are necessary to fight off foreign substances. Measuring the pulse rate is useful in determining the character of the heartbeat and of the circulatory system.

Tests as Diagnostic Aids

In many cases, the final diagnosis of an animal disease is dependent upon a laboratory test. Some involve measuring the amount of certain chemical constituents of the blood or body fluids, determining the presence of toxins (poisons), or examining the urine and feces. Other tests are designed to identify the causative agents of the disease. The removal and examination of tissue or other material from the body (biopsy) is used to diagnose the nature of abnormalities such as tumours. Specific skin tests are used to confirm the diagnoses of various diseases—e.g., tuberculosis and Johne's disease in cattle and glanders in horses.

Confirmation of the presence in the blood of abnormal quantities of certain constituents aids in diagnosing certain diseases. Abnormal levels of protein in the blood are associated with some cancers of the bone, such as multiple myeloma in horses and dogs. Animals with diabetes mellitus have a high level of the carbohydrate glucose and the steroid cholesterol in the blood. The combination of an increase in the blood level of cholesterol and a decrease in the level of iodine bound to protein indicates hypothyroidism (underactive thyroid gland). A low level of calcium in the serum component of blood confirms milk fever in lactating dairy cattle. An increase in the activities of certain enzymes (biological catalysts) in the blood indicates liver damage. An increase in the blood level of the bile constituent bilirubin is used as a diagnostic test for hemolytic crisis, a disease in which red blood cells are rapidly destroyed by organisms such as *Babesia* species in dogs and in cattle and Anaplasma species in cattle.

The examination of the formed elements of blood, including the oxygen-carrying red blood cells (erythrocytes), the white blood cells (neutrophils, eosinophils, basophils, lymphocytes, and monocytes), and the platelets, which function in blood coagulation, is helpful in diagnosing certain diseases. Examination of the blood cells of cattle may reveal abnormal lymphocytic cells characteristic of leukemia. Low numbers of leucocytes indicate the presence of viral diseases, such as hog cholera and infectious hepatitis in dogs. Neutrophil levels increase in chronic bacterial diseases, such as canine pneumonia and uterine infections in female animals. Elevated monocyte levels occur in chronic granulomatous diseases; e.g., histoplasmosis and tuberculosis. Canine parasitism and allergic skin disorders are characterized by elevated eosinophil levels. Prolonged clotting time may be associated with a deficiency of platelets.

Anemia has many causes. They include hemorrhages from blood loss after injuries; the destruction of red blood cells by the rickettsia Haemobartonella felis in cats; incompatible blood transfusions in dogs; the inadequate production of normal red blood cells, which occurs in iron or cobalt deficiency after exposure to radioactive substances; general malnutrition; and contact with substances that depress the activity of bone marrow.

Poisonings occur commonly in animals. Some species are more sensitive to certain poisons than others. Swine develop mercury poisoning if they eat too much grain that has been treated with mercury compounds to retard spoilage. Dogs may be poisoned by the arsenic found in pesticides or by strychnine, which is found in rat poison. Many plants are poisonous if eaten, such as bracken fern, which poisons cattle and horses, and ragwort, which contains a substance poisonous to the liver of cattle.

Examination of an animal's urine may reveal evidence of kidney diseases or diseases of the entire urinary system or a generalized systemic disease. The presence of protein in the urine of dogs indicates acute kidney disease (nephritis). Although constituents of bile normally are found in the urine of dogs, the quantity increases in dogs with the presence of infectious hepatitis, a disease of the liver. The presence of abnormal amounts of the simple carbohydrate glucose and of ketone bodies (organic compounds involved in metabolism) in an animal's urine is used to diagnose diabetes mellitus, a disease in which the pancreas cannot form adequate quantities of a substance (insulin) important in regulating carbohydrate metabolism. The urine of horses with azoturia (excessive quantities of nitrogen-containing compounds in the urine) or muscle breakdown may contain a dark-coloured molecule called myoglobin.

The presence of eggs or parts of worms in the excrement of animals suspected of suffering from intestinal parasites, such as roundworms, tapeworms, or flatworms, aids in diagnosis. Feces that are light in colour, have a rancid odour, contain fat, and are poorly formed may indicate the existence of a chronic disease of the pancreas. Clay-coloured fatty feces suggest obstruction of the bile duct, which conveys bile to the intestine during digestion.

The identification of a disease-causing microorganism within an animal enables the veterinarian to choose the best drug for therapy. Agglutination tests, which utilize serum samples of animals and microorganisms suspected of causing a disease, many times confirm the presence of the following bacterial diseases: brucellosis in cattle and swine, salmonellosis in swine, leptospirosis in cattle, and actinobacillosis in swine and cattle. Other tests measure the antibodies (specific proteins formed in response to a foreign substance in the body) formed against a disease-causing agent, such as those that cause brucellosis, foot-and-mouth disease, infectious hepatitis in dogs, and fowl pest.

The modern veterinary diagnostic laboratory performs, in addition to the tests mentioned, tests of cells in the bone marrow; specific-organ-function tests (liver, kidney, pancreas, thyroid, adrenal, and pituitary glands); radioisotope tests, tissue biopsies, and histochemical analyses; and tests concerning blood coagulation and body fluids.

Survey of Animal Diseases

Infectious and Noninfectious Diseases

Diseases may be either infectious or noninfectious. The term infection, as observed earlier, implies an interaction between two living organisms, called the host and the parasite. Infection is a type of parasitism, which may be defined as the state of existence of one organism (the parasite) at the expense of another (the host). Agents (e.g., certain viruses, bacteria, fungi, protozoans, worms, and arthropods) capable of producing disease are pathogens. The term pathogenicity refers to the ability of a parasite to enter a host and produce disease; the degree of pathogenicity—that is, the ability of an organism to cause infection—is known as virulence. The capacity of a virulent organism to cause infection is influenced both by the characteristics of the organism and by the ability of the host to repel the invasion and to prevent injury. A pathogen may be virulent for one host but not for another. Pneumococcal bacteria, for example, have a low virulence for mice and are not found in them in nature; if introduced experimentally into a mouse, however, the bacteria overwhelm its body defenses and cause death.

Many pathogens (e.g., the bacterium that causes anthrax) are able to live outside the animal's body until conditions occur that are favourable for entering and infecting it. Pathogens enter the body in various ways—by penetrating the skin or an eye, by being eaten with food, or by being breathed into the lungs. After their entry into a host, pathogens actively multiply and produce disease by interfering with the functions of specific organs or tissues of the host.

Before a disease becomes established in a host, the barrier known as immunity must be overcome. Defense against infection is provided by a number of chemical and mechanical barriers, such as the skin, mucous membranes and secretions, and components of the blood and other body fluids. Antibodies, which are proteins formed in response to a specific substance (called an antigen) recognized by the body as foreign, are another important factor in preventing infection. Immunity among animals varies with species, general health, heredity, environment, and previous contact with a specific pathogen.

As certain bacterial species multiply, they may produce and liberate poisons, called exotoxins, into the tissues; other bacterial pathogens contain toxins, called endotoxins, which produce disease only when liberated at the time of death of the bacterial cell. Some bacteria, such as certain species of Clostridium and Bacillus, have inactive forms called spores, which may remain viable (i.e., capable of developing into active organisms) for many years; spores are highly resistant to environmental conditions such as heat, cold, and chemical compounds called disinfectants, which are able to kill many active bacteria.

The term infestation indicates that animals, including spiny-headed worms (Acanthocephala), roundworms (Nematoda), flatworms (Platyhelminthes), and arthropods such as lice, fleas, mites, and ticks, are present in or on the body of a host. An infestation is not necessarily parasitic.

Noninfectious diseases are not caused by virulent pathogens and are not communicable from one animal to another. They may be caused by hereditary factors or by the environment in which an animal lives. Many metabolic diseases are caused by an unsuitable alteration, sometimes brought about by man, in an animal's genetic constitution or in its environment. Metabolic diseases usually result from a disturbance in the normal balance of the physiological mechanisms that maintain stability, or homeostasis. Examples of metabolic diseases include overproduction or underproduction of hormones, which control specific body processes; nutritional deficiencies; poisoning from such agents as insecticides, fungicides, herbicides, fluorine, and poisonous plants; and inherited deficiencies in the ability to synthesize active forms of specific enzymes, which are the proteins that control the rates of chemical reactions in the body.

Excessive inbreeding (i.e., the mating of related animals) among all domesticated animal species has resulted in an increase in the number of metabolic diseases and an increase in the susceptibility of certain animals to infectious diseases.

Zoonoses

As stated previously, zoonoses are human diseases acquired from or transmitted to any other vertebrate animal. Zoonotic diseases are common in currently developing countries throughout the world and constitute, with starvation, the major threat to human health. More than 150 such diseases are known.

Zoonoses may be separated into four principal types, depending on the mechanisms of transmission and epidemiology. One type includes the direct zoonoses, such as rabies and brucellosis, which are maintained in nature by one vertebrate species. The transmission cycle of the cyclozoonoses, of which tapeworm infections are an example, requires at least two different vertebrate species. Both vertebrate and invertebrate animals are required as intermediate hosts in the transmission to humans of metazoonoses; arboviral and trypanosomal diseases are good examples of metazoonoses. The cycles of saprozoonoses (for example, histoplasmosis) may require, in addition to vertebrate hosts, specific environmental locations or reservoirs.

Most animals that serve as reservoirs for zoonoses are domesticated and wild animals with which man commonly associates. People in occupations such as veterinary medicine and public health, therefore, have a greater exposure to zoonoses than do those in occupations less closely concerned with animals.

In addition to the numerous human diseases spread by contact with the parasitic worm helminth and by contact with arthropods, many diseases are transmitted by the bites and venom of certain animals; poisonous or diseased food animals also transmit diseases. Dog bites may seriously injure tissues and also can transmit bacterial infections and rabies, a disease of viral origin. The bite of a diseased rat may transmit any of several diseases to man, including plague, salmonellosis, leptospirosis, and rat-bite fevers. Cat scratch disease may be transmitted through cat bites, and the deadly herpes B virus can spread by monkey bites. The bites of venomous snakes and fish account for considerable human discomfort and death. About 200 of the 2,500 known species of snakes can cause human disease. One estimate for snakebite deaths worldwide is 30,000 to 40,000 per year, the vast majority of them in Asia. Poisonous wild animals inadvertently used for food include animals harbouring the anthrax bacillus and those containing the causative agents of salmonellosis, trichinosis, and fish-tapeworm infection. The flesh of various types of fish is toxic to man. Japanese puffers, for example, contain the poisonous chemical compound tetrodotoxin; scombroid fish harbour Proteus morganii, which causes gastrointestinal diseases; and mullet and surmullet can cause nervous disturbances.

Approaches to the control of zoonoses differ according to the type under consideration. Because the majority of direct zoonoses and cyclozoonoses and some saprozoonoses are most effectively controlled by techniques involving the animal host, methods used to combat these diseases are almost entirely the responsibility of veterinary medicine. A good example is the elimination of stray dogs, for they are an important factor in the control of zoonoses such as rabies, hydatid disease, and visceral larva migrans. In addition, the control of diseases such as brucellosis and tuberculosis in cattle involves a combination of methods—mass immunization, diagnosis, slaughter of infected animals, environmental disinfection, and quarantine. Several supportive measures for the control of disease are useful in some cases. Air-sanitation measures are helpful in direct zoonoses in which human illness is spread by droplets or dust, and zoonotic infections that are spread through a fluid medium, such as water or milk, sometimes can be controlled. Heat, cold, and irradiation are effective in killing the immature forms of Trichinella spiralis, the causative agent of trichinosis, in meat; and certain antibiotic drugs help to prevent deterioration of food.

The control of metazoonoses may be directed at the infected vertebrate hosts, at the infected invertebrate host, or at both. Particularly effective in this instance has been the use of chemical insecticides to attack the invertebrate carriers of specific infections, even though several difficulties have been encountered—for example, the inaccessibility of the invertebrate to the chemicals, which occurs with organisms that breed in swiftly flowing waters or in dense vegetation, and the development of insecticide resistance by the organisms. Insecticides are used to destroy the mosquitoes that spread malaria (Anopheles). Mechanical filters placed across irrigation ditches help to prevent the dissemination of the snails that transmit Schistosoma mansoni, a parasitic flatworm.

Disease Prevention, Control and Eradication

Prevention is the first line of defense against disease. At least four preventive techniques are available for use in the prevention of disease in an animal population. One is the exclusion of causative agents of disease from specific geographic areas, or quarantine. A second preventive tool utilizes control methods such as immunization, environmental control, and chemical agents to protect specific animal populations from endemic diseases, diseases normally present in an area. The third preventive measure concerns the mass education of people about disease prevention. Finally, early diagnosis of illness among members of an animal population is important so that disease manifestations do not become too severe and so that affected animals can be more easily managed and treated.

Quarantine—the restriction of movement of animals suffering from or exposed to infections such as bluetongue and scrapie (in sheep), foot-and-mouth disease (in cattle), and rabies (in dogs)—is one of the oldest tools of preventive medicine. It was applied to domesticated animals as early as Roman times. The establishment of international livestock quarantine in the United States in 1890 provided for the holding of all imported cattle, sheep, and swine at the port of entry for 90, 15, and 15 days, respectively. In this way, such diseases as Nairobi sheep disease, surra, and infections caused by Brucella melitensis were eliminated or excluded from the United States, but international quarantine barriers did not prevent the entry of bluetongue, scrapie, and the tick Rhipicephalus evertsi, which is a carrier for several animal diseases. On the other hand, long-term quarantine of all dogs entering Great Britain has been effective since its initiation in 1919 (the quarantine also includes cats). It is possible that aircraft may pose new problems regarding livestock-disease quarantine since many disease carriers (e.g., insects and viruses) may be accidentally brought by plane into a country.

Mass immunization as a preventive technique has the advantage of allowing the resistant animal freedom of movement, unlike environmental control, in which the animal is confined to the controlled area; immunization may, however, provide only short-lived and partial protection. Mass-inoculation techniques against diseases such as Newcastle disease in chickens and distemper in mink and dogs have been successful. Animal diseases have been prevented by methods involving environmental control, including the maintenance of safe water supplies, the hygienic disposal of animal excrement, air sanitation, pest control, and the improvement of animal housing. One specific environmental program, called the portable-calf-pen system, involves routine movement of the pens to avoid a concentration of specific pathogens in them. Other programs involve the utilization of automatic and sanitary watering and feeding equipment and buildings with environmental controls. The use of chemical compounds to prevent illness (chemoprophylaxis) includes a variety of pesticides, which are used to kill insects that transmit diseases, and substances either used internally or applied to the animal's body to prevent the transmission or the development of a disease. An example is the use of sulfonamide drugs in the drinking water of poultry to prevent coccidiosis. Environmental-control methods in the poultry industry have resulted in the most efficient means of poultry production developed thus far.

The early detection of a disease in a population of animals—a herd of cattle, for example—is particularly useful in controlling certain chronic infectious diseases, such as mastitis, brucellosis, and tuberculosis, as well as certain noninfectious diseases such as bloat. Laboratory tests—the agglutination test in pullorum disease, the tuberculin skin test for tuberculosis, the examination of feces for eggs of specific parasites, the physical and chemical tests performed on milk to diagnose bovine mastitis—are used for the early detection of diseases in an animal population.

Methods of disease control and eradication have been successful in various countries. In the United States, for example, the test-and-slaughter technique, in which simple tests are used to confirm the existence of diseased animals that are then slaughtered, has been of great value in controlling infectious and hereditary diseases, including dourine, a venereal disease in horses, fowl plague, and foot-and-mouth disease in cattle and deer. Bovine tuberculosis has been eliminated from Denmark, Finland, and The Netherlands and reduced to a low level in various other countries, including Great Britain, Japan, the United States, and Canada, by the test-and-slaughter method. Many infectious diseases have been eradicated from Great Britain—sheep pox, rinderpest, pleuropneumonia, glanders, and rabies. Diseases eliminated from Australia by a combination of methods—control of agents that carry disease, the test-and-slaughter technique, the use of chemical agents, and, more recently, biological control—include hog cholera, rinderpest, scrapie, glanders, surra, rabies, and foot-and-mouth disease.

In biological control, enemies of the agents that transmit the disease, enemies of the reservoir host, or a specific parasite are introduced into the environment. If a natural enemy of the tsetse fly could be found, for example, African sleeping sickness in man and trypanosomiasis in cattle could be controlled in West Africa. Successful biological control of the European-rabbit population in Australia has been accomplished through the use of the myxomatosis virus, which is transmitted by mosquitoes and causes the formation of malignant tumours. Although the Brazilian white rabbit is relatively unaffected by the virus, it causes rapid death in the European rabbit. The elimination of the European rabbit in France by the virus was accompanied by a decrease in tick-borne typhus in people, suggesting that the rabbit may be a significant intermediate host for the causative agent, Rickettsia conorii. Screwworms, an immature form of the fly Cochliomyia hominivorax, have been eradicated in the United States by the release of more than 3,000,000,000 sterilized males.

Disease control and elimination programs require many sophisticated techniques in addition to diagnosis and the slaughter of affected animals. They include: the control of insects known to transmit diseases; the cooperation of animal owners; the development through research of new diagnostic tests for use on large populations; the eradication of animal species from areas in which they are known to transmit disease; sterilization of strains of animals known to carry inheritable metabolic diseases; and effective meat inspection.

Viral Diseases in Farm Animals

Swamp Fever

Equine Infectious Anaemia (EIA), also known as swamp fever is a horse disease caused by a retrovirus and transmitted by bloodsucking insects. The EIA virus is mechanically transmitted from one horse to another by the bloodsucking horse flies, deer flies (Tabanus), stable flies (Stomoxys spp.), mosquitoes and possibly midges. Symptoms include recurrent fever, weight loss, an enlarged spleen, anemia, and swelling of the lower chest, abdominal wall, penile sheath, scrotum, and legs. Horse tires easily due to a recurrent fever and anemia, may relapse to acute form even several years after the original attack.

The EIA virus is a slow acting virus of the lenti-retrovirus group. Retroviruses cause leukemia in cats, mice and cattle, arthritis, pneumonia and neurological diseases in small ruminants and acquired immune deficiency syndrome (AIDS) in humans. These viruses localize and multiply in macrophages of many organs, especially in the spleen, liver, kidney, and lymph nodes, where they take over the cell and sit and wait to become activated. Upon activation, the cell reproduces more viruses, which bursts free from the cell to infect other cells. This causes recurring cycles, in which the horse seems normal and then ill.

There is no known treatment that can eliminate the virus from the body. To date there are no satisfactory vaccines for EIA. The Coggins' test is agar gel diffusion (AGID) test, which is a practical diagnostic test for identifying horses infected with EIA. This test is used to detect the EIA antibody.

Equine Encephalomyelitis

Equine encephalomyelitis is an inflammation of the brain and spinal cord that affects horses but is also deadly for humans. The virus was isolated, characterized, and vaccines were produced in the 1930s. The viruses responsible for causing these diseases are members of a family of viruses called the alphavirus. The mosquito transmits the virus from small infected animals such as birds and rodents to horses.

The warm, humid weather of the summer is good for mosquito breeding and this is when outbreaks are more common. Transmission of EEE is not horse to human, but bird or rodent to human via the mosquito.

Approximately two days after equine infection with encephalomyelitis, there is an infection and low-grade fever. The first apparent signs are at four to five days. At that time, the animal generally has a fever and rapid heart rate, is showing signs of anorexia, depression, and variable other neurological signs. As the illness progresses the brain stem and spinal cord are affected. Muscle weakness becomes apparent and there are behavioural changes and dementia. Notable symptoms include aggression, head pressing, wall leaning, compulsive circling, and blindness. Other signs might include uncontrolled twitching of the eyeball, and facial muscle paralysis. As the disease progresses, a semi-comatose and convulsive state occurs. Death usually follows two or three days later. If the animal survives, residual nervous system problems result.

Encephalomyelitis vaccines are available for horses from several different companies. They are packaged as single or combination vaccines.

African Horse Sickness

African horse sickness (AHS) is a highly infectious non-contagious, vector born viral disease affecting all species of Equidae. It is classified as an Orbivirus of family Reoviridae, of which there are 9 serotypes. All serotypes are distributed throughout Africa, although there is a variation in their temporal distribution. It is endemic to the African continent, and is characterised by respiratory and circulatory damage, accompanied by fever and loss of appetite. The disease manifests in three ways, namely the lung form, the heart form and the mixed form.

The lung (dunkop) form is characterised in the following manner:

- Very high fever (up to 41 degrees).
- Difficulty in breathing, with mouth open and head hanging down.
- Frothy discharge may pour from the nose.
- Sudden onset of death.
- Very high death rate (90%).

The heart (dikkop) form is characterised in the following manner:

- Fever, followed by swelling of the head and eyes.
- In severe cases, the entire head swells.
- Loss of ability to swallow and possible colic symptoms may occur.
- Terminal signs include bleeding in the membranes of the mouth and eyes.

- Slower onset of death, occurring 4 to 8 days after the fever has started.
- Lower death rate (50%).

This disease is spread by insect vectors such as midges but can also be transmitted by species of mosquitoes including Culex, Anopheles and Aedes, and species of ticks such as Hyalomma and Rhipicephalus.

There is currently no treatment for AHS. Control of outbreak in an endemic region involves quarantine, vector control and vaccination.

Japanese B-encephalitis

This is a fatal disease of pigs, horses, sheep, birds and man. The infection is caused by a flavivirus, a single stranded RNA virus. It is transmitted by the bite of the Culex tritaeniorhynchus mosquito. The virus multiplies at the site of the bite and in regional lymph nodes before viraemia develops that can lead to inflammatory changes in the heart, lungs, liver, and reticulo-endothelial system. The endemic area for Japanese encephalitis spreads across Asia from Pakistan to the coast of Siberia and includes Japan.

The incubation period is 6 to 16 days. There is fever, headache, nausea, diarrhea, vomiting, and myalgia, which may last for several days. This may be followed by a spectrum of neurological disease ranging from mild confusion, to agitation, to overt coma. It is more common in children, while headache and meningism are more common in adults. Tremor or other involuntary movements are common.

Japanese Encephalitis-VAX was a formalin-inactivated vaccine derived from mouse brain against Japanese B Encephalitis, produced since 1992 by BIKEN (Japan). The new vaccine available in the UK is the Japanese Encephalitis Green Cross vaccine (GC vaccine).

Swine Pox

Swinepox is a worldwide disease of pigs caused by a virus of the family Poxviridae and the genus Suipoxvirus, which can survive outside the pig for long periods of time and is resistant to environmental changes. Symptoms include small circular red areas 10-20mm in diameter that commence with a vesicle containing straw-coloured fluid in the centre. After two to three days the vesicle ruptures and a scab is formed which gradually turns black.

The disease is most frequently seen in young pigs but all ages may be affected. After an incubation period of 1 week, small red areas may be seen most frequently on the face, ears, inside the legs, and abdomen. These develop into papules and, within a few days, pustules develop that change into small vesicles. The centres of the pustules become dry and scabbed and are surrounded by a raised, inflamed zone. Later, dark scabs form, giving affected piglets a spotted appearance. These eventually drop or are rubbed off without leaving a scar. The early stage of the disease may be accompanied by mild fever and dullness. Virus is abundant in the lesions and can be transferred from pig to pig by the biting louse (Haematopinus suis). The disease also may be transmitted, possibly between farms, by other insects acting as mechanical carriers. Recovered pigs become immune. There is no specific treatment. Eradication of lice is important.

Fowl Pox

Fowl pox is a worldwide disease of poultry caused by viruses of the family Poxviridae and the genus Avipoxvirus. There are two forms of the disease. The first is cutaneous form (dry pox) that is spread by biting insects, especially mosquitoes that causes lesions on the comb, wattles, and beak. The second form is diphtheritic form (wet pox), which is spread by inhalation of the virus and causes a diphtheritic membrane to form in the mouth, pharynx, larynx, and sometimes the trachea. Symptoms include weight loss, reduced egg production, lesions, small whitish or yellowish areas, nodules or scabs, raised white or opaque nodules which may join to form yellow, cheesy, necrotic lesion. The virus, abundantly present in the lesions is transmitted by contact to pen mates through abrasions of the skins. Mosquitoes and other biting insects can have a mechanical role in the transmissions. Modified live fowl pox virus vaccines are available commercially.

Cow Pox

Cow pox is a disease of the skin that is caused by a virus known as the Cow pox virus. The pox is related to the vaccinia virus, and got its name from dairy maids touching the udders of infected cows. The cow pox virus is within the family Poxviridae and the genus Orthopoxvirus. The ailment manifests itself in the form of red blisters and is transmitted by touch from infected animals to humans. When it is gone, the person is immune to small pox. Cow pox virus has been found only in Europe and in adjacent parts of the former Soviet Union. Despite its name, the reservoir hosts of cow pox virus are rodents, from which it can occasionally spread to cats, cows, humans, and zoo animals, including large cats and elephants. Transmission to humans has traditionally occurred via contact with the infected teats of milking cows. However, currently, infection is seen more commonly among domestic cats, from which it can be transmitted to humans.

The pathology of the skin lesions caused by cow pox virus is similar to that of small pox. However, there is greater epithelial thickening and less rapid cell necrosis. There is also more involvement of the mesodermal tissues. The most significant pathological feature of cow pox is the presence of two types of cytoplasmic inclusion bodies: irregular B-type inclusion bodies, and numerous large, homogenous, acidophilic, A-type inclusion bodies.

Human cow pox usually responds to treatment with antivaccina immunoglobulin. However, this should be restricted to the most severe cases. Usually, the lesions regress spontaneously. Identification and isolation of animals infected with cow pox can help decrease the incidence of human infections.

Foot and Mouth Disease

Foot-and-mouth disease (FMD) or hoof-and-mouth disease is a highly contagious and sometimes fatal viral disease of domestic animals such as cattle, water buffalo, sheep, goats and pigs, as well as antelope, bison and deer. It is caused by foot-and-mouth disease virus. Seven main types of Foot and Mouth Virus are believed to exist that belong to the genus Aphthovirus of the family Picornaviridae. Picornaviruses are tiny viruses (27-30 nm across) that are not enveloped with an icosahedral capsid and contain a single strand of positive sense RNA.

The disease is characterised by high fever that declines rapidly after two or three days; blisters inside the mouth that lead to excessive secretion of stringy or foamy saliva and to drooling; and blisters on the feet that may rupture and cause lameness. Adult animals may suffer weight loss from which they do not recover for several months as well as swelling in the testicles of mature males, and in cows, milk production can decline significantly. Symptoms of the Foot and Mouth in Cattle include, Slobbering and smacking lips, Shivering, Tender and sore feet, Reduced milk yield, Sores and blisters on feet and Raised temperature.

Zoonotic Diseases

Zoonotic Diseases (also known as zoonoses) are caused by infections that spread between animals and people. Every year, tens of thousands of Americans get sick from diseases spread between animals and people. These are known as zoonotic diseases. Zoonotic means infectious diseases that are spread between animals and people. Because these diseases can cause sickness or death in people, CDC is always tracking and reporting them.

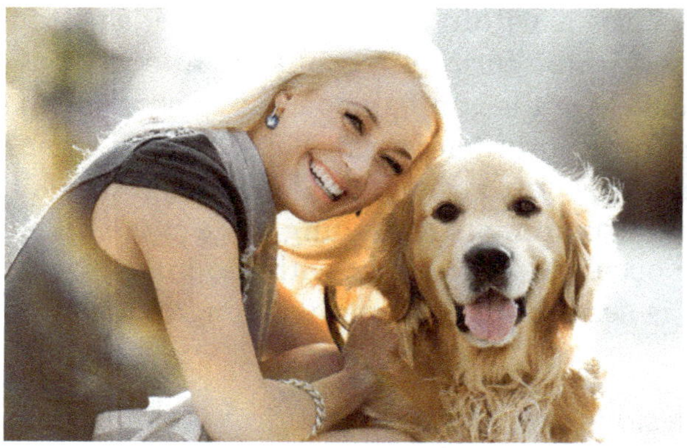

Animals provide many benefits to people. Many people interact with animals in their daily lives, both at home and away from home. Pets offer companionship and entertainment, with millions of households having one or more pets. We might come into close contact with animals at a county fair or petting zoo, or encounter wildlife while enjoying outdoor activities. Also, animals are an important food source and provide meat, dairy, and eggs.

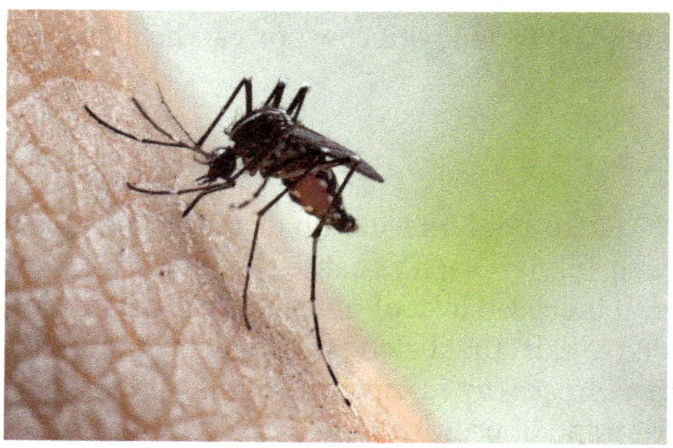

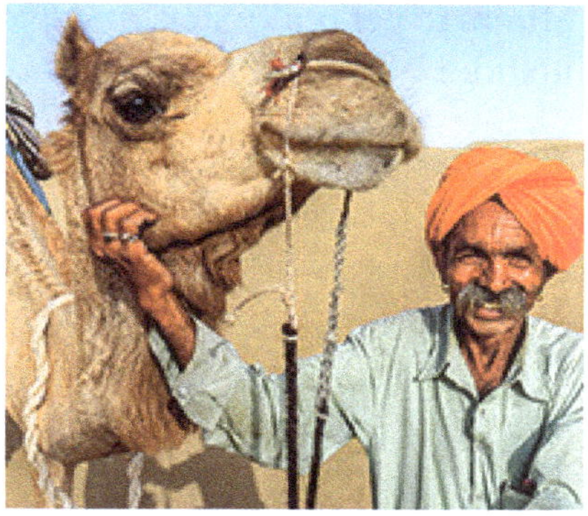

However, some animals can carry harmful germs that can be shared with people and cause illness – these are known as zoonotic diseases or zoonoses. Zoonotic diseases are caused by harmful germs like viruses, bacterial, parasites, and fungi. These germs can cause many different types of illnesses in people and animals ranging from mild to serious illness and even death. Some animals can appear healthy even when they are carrying germs that can make people sick.

Zoonotic diseases are very common, both in the United States and around the world. Scientists estimate that more than 6 out of every 10 known infectious diseases in people are spread from animals, and 3 out of every 4 new or emerging infectious diseases in people are spread from animals. Every year, tens of thousands of Americans will get sick from harmful germs spread between animals and people. Because of this, CDC works 24/7 to protect people from zoonotic diseases.

Germs Spread between Animals and People

Because of the close connection between people and animals, it's important to be aware of the common ways people can get infected with germs that can cause zoonotic diseases. These can include:

- Direct contact: Coming into contact with the saliva, blood, urine, mucous, feces, or other body fluids of an infected animal. Examples include petting or touching animals, and bites or scratches.
- Indirect contact: Coming into contact with areas where animals live and roam, or objects or surfaces that have been contaminated with germs. Examples include aquarium tank water, pet habitats, chicken coops, plants, and soil, as well as pet food and water dishes.
- Vector-borne: Being bitten by a tick, or an insect like a mosquito or a flea.
- Foodborne: Each year, 1 in 6 Americans get sick from eating contaminated food. Eating or drinking something unsafe (such as unpasteurized milk, undercooked meat or eggs, or raw fruits and vegetables that are contaminated with feces from an infected animal).

Risk of Serious Illness from Zoonotic Diseases

Anyone can become sick from a zoonotic disease, including healthy people. However, some people may be more at risk than others and should take steps to protect themselves or family members.

These people are more likely than others to get really sick, and even die, from infection with certain diseases. These groups of people include:

- Children younger than 5.
- Adults older than 65.
- People with weakened immune systems.

Bacterial Diseases of Animals

Actinobacillosis

Synonym: Wooden tongue.

Actinobacillosis is a chronic infectious disease chiefly of cattle but occasionally of sheep and is characterised by the formation of granuloma which is firm and hard like fibroma, over the tongue and, gums and, sometimes, elsewhere.

Etiology and Modes of Infection

It is due to infection of Actinobacillus lignieresi and it occurs through injuries, abrasions, specially of oral cavity and other soft tissues.

Symptoms

The seats of predilection are chiefly the tongue, gums, pharynx, palate and neighbouring lymph glands.

In the tongue, there is varying degree of enlargement and induration. The whole or only a part of the organ may be affected and sometimes may even protrude from the mouth. Partial involvement also causes distortion. Large or small superficial ulcers may be found on the surface.

Actual abscesses are not usually seen in the wooden tongue, but they may be found at the root of the organ. In the gums and palates, the lesions are characterised by the ulceration of the mucosa and diffused thickening of the submucous tissue due to formation of granulation tissue. When lymph glands in the throat are affected, the swelling and pressure caused mastication and breathing difficult.

Changes may also occur in the wall of pharynx, lungs, rumen, omasum, abomasum and reticulum. When the tongue is affected, there is constant dribbling of saliva from the mouth. Later, the saliva becomes thick, purulent and foul smelling and resembles pus. The lesions in the pharynx and stomach frequently assume a polypoid appearance and project in the lumen.

Treatment

Intravenous injection of Sodium Iodide should be given and one or two injections in many cases make recovery complete. The effect of treatment may be enhanced by painting the lesions by Tine.

Iodine and glycerine and by injection of Lugol's solution (10 ml to 15 ml) into the growth. The treatment with antibiotic, especially penicillin is very promising and should be given intramuscularly in proper dose according to body weight.

Caution

This is a zoonotic disease and can be transmitted to man. Therefore, care must be taken over washing the hands etc. after handling the animal affected with the disease.

Actinomycosis

Synonym: Lumpy jaw, Ray fungus disease.

Etiology and Mode of Infection

Actinomycosis is a specific infectious disease mainly affecting cattle, swine, man and occasionally other animals caused by Actinomycis bovis or Streptothrix bovis—commonly known as Ray fungus—an anaerobic organism and characterised by connective tissue proliferation and suppurative processes with characteristic granular bodies in the pus. It is caused by wounds. It is normally present in digestive system of cattle and becomes pathogenic by invading the tissues through wounds.

Symptoms

The lesions bear a considerable resemblance to those of Actinobacillosis and are often mistaken as Actinobacillosis. As a rule, this disease in bovine is found to affect bones particularly maxillae and bones of the skull occasionally. Sometimes, soft structures such as gums, palate and tongue may become affected as a result of direct extension.

In the maxillae the lesions appear as suppurative ostitis which is usually centered in the medullary cavity of the bone. The lesion is composed of a granulation tissue with soft purulent centre, rich in granules. The adjacent healthy bone becomes affected and rarefied and the spaces becoming filled with the proliferation of fibrous tissue which is characteristic of the disease and the appearance described as lumpy jaw.

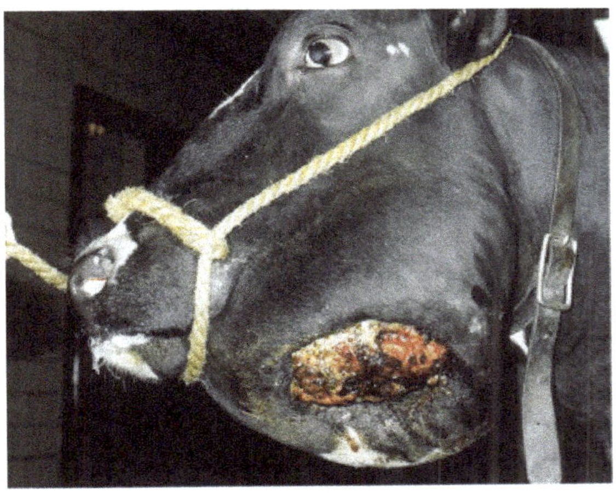

Actinomycosis

Considerable quantities of pus may be formed in such lesions which is discharged through sinuses leading to the surface. In most cases when the mouth or throat is affected, there is constant dribbling of saliva in varying amounts from the mouth.

Treatment

Same as Actinobacillosis. Penicillin or Streptomycin is quite effective. Sulpha drugs may also be used. In addition, surgical treatment should be resorted to where possible.

Anthrax

Synonym: Splenic fever, Splenic apoplexy Charbon, in vernacular—Tarka and in human "malignant pustule", "Malignant Carbuncle" and "Wool-sorter's disease".

Anthrax is an acute infectious disease of septicaemic nature caused by Bacillus anthracis and characterised clinically by an acute febrile course and anatomically by acute swelling of the spleen and Sero-haemorrhagic infiltration of the subcutaneous and subserous tissues.

Bacteriology

Bacillus anthracis is a sporulating, rod-shaped, non-motile, aerobic organism measuring 4 to 8^{μ} x 1 to 1.5^{μ}. The rods have characteristic square or slightly cupped ends and a capsule. In the blood, the bacilli are found singly or in short chains of 2 to 4 and can only be found in the blood for a short time at the earliest 16 to 18 hours before death.

As putrefaction soon destroys them, the blood should be examined as early as possible after death of the animal. The bacilli multiply in living body by fission, which is stopped after death of the animal for want of oxygen. Sporulation never occurs inside the body during life or after death; so long the body remains unopened as sporulation occurs only when there is a supply of free oxygen and a limited supply of food.

Culture

The bacillus is easily cultured on any of the common media under aerobic condition, but the capsule is not demonstrable in bacillus from culture media unless the same contain blood or serum. In culture media, long filaments composed of many individuals are formed and owing to the rapidity of the division, the segments are shorter than those seen in the body fluid.

Staining

The capsule is the most important diagnostic feature of B. anthracis and is only well seen in Bacillus from the blood. It is the last part of the bacillus to disappear under putrefactive influences.

It has special staining property which is demonstrable by staining the blood smear as under:

Mac Fadyean's Reaction

1. Make a thick film of blood on a glass slide.

2. Dry in the air.
3. Fix in the heat.
4. Stain for one minute with 1% aqueous solution of Methylene blue.
5. Wash in water, dry in air and examine under $^1/_{12}$ oil immersion objective.

The bacilli are stained blue and capsules purple. Blood smear obtained from anthrax cases and stained as above present a purple appearance even to the naked eye when the smear is seen in a reflected light, which is diagnostic. The purple colouration is also discerniable in smears even from semi-decomposed carcasses when the bacilli have completely degenerated. However, this phenomenon is lost in quite putrid blood.

Incidence

Anthrax bacilli deposited with blood, faeces etc. of infected animals may remain alive in the superficial layer of the soil for a long time and under suitable conditions of temperature and moisture may even multiply by fission or by spores. The spores can resist both desiccation and moisture and also cold and heat, and when the external conditions are favourable, the spores germinate and form bacilli, which again multiply and form spores. In this way, a soil once infected may continue for a long time, may become source of continually recurring disease.

According to Pasteur, spores may remain alive in a dry state for over 12 years. Hence, anthrax is endemic in certain localities, so called anthrax districts where the damp, marshy or periodically flooded soil favours their growth. In such areas, the disease appears nearly every year in varying degrees of severity, especially in the warm months.

Animals Susceptible

All domestic animals, birds and human beings are susceptible. Algerian sheep and the cattle of the plains show considerable resistance to artificial inoculation, but in both cases, the disease occurs naturally. The disease is most common in cattle and younger animals are more easily affected than the older ones.

Animals usually acquire prolonged immunity after recovery from anthrax if they do survive at all.

Modes of Infection

The commonest mode in animals is by ingestion of spores contained in contaminated fodder. Bacilli may infect from the mouth or throat provided there is a wound or sore, but they may even infect through intact pharyngeal mucosa.

The bacilli are destroyed by the gastric juice on reaching the stomach but the spores are unharmed by gastric juice and germinate into bacilli after passing on to the intestines.

It is also possible, though not common in animal for the bacilli or their spores to give rise either to local or general infection through injuries on the skin, or infection may be transmitted through biting flies.

Man becomes infected through wounds while handling diseased animals or animal products from diseased animals (Malignant pustule or Carbuncle) or by inhalation of anthrax spores with the dust in Wool factories (wool sorter's disease).

Pathogenesis

On reaching the surface of pharyngeal mucosa, the bacilli proliferate in the tonsillar tissue and are then carried by the lymphatic vessels to the lymphatic glands.

Ingested spores on reaching the intestine develop into bacilli which penetrate through the intestinal glands and lymphatic follicles into the lymph spaces in mucosa or submucosa and multiply there.

Bacilli which have entered through lesions in the skin or mucosa enter the connective tissue directly.

In this way, the bacilli multiply at the points of infection and enter the blood (Anthrax septicemia) the animal soon manifests severe symptoms of the disease often in a few hours and dies suddenly.

At points where large number of bacilli accumulates, as at the site of infection, the capsule substance swells from gradual absorption of fluid. This fluid absorbed by capsule substance becomes more gelatinous and thus prevent them from reentering the circulation giving rise to oedematous swellings at the affected places. As the bacilli also accumulate in the capillaries and cause injury to the walls of the vessels, effusion of blood takes place both in the centre of the oedematous swelling, as well as, in other organs with slow circulation such as spleen, liver and brain.

Postmortem Lesions

Carcasses of animal dead of anthrax undergo rapid putrefaction owing to incoaguable condition of the blood and also due to an anaerobic condition of the system created by absorption of oxygen by aerobic anthrax bacilli, which makes it ideal for rapid multiplication of the anaerobic putrefactive bacteria.

As a result of early putrefaction, the carcass becomes rapidly distended and the Rigor mortis is either absent or incomplete. Dark red blood exudes from the body opening. The visible mucosa are cyanotic and the rectum is often prolapsed which is studded with haemorrhagic spots.

In throat cases, the region is markedly swollen and firm and on incision, gelatinous oedema is to be seen. The same condition is also noticed in other regions where the bacilli penetrated.

Cattle

As a rule, the primary lesions are in the alimentary canal in the shape of gastroenteritis, which is haemorrhagic in character with severe congestion of the neighbouring blood vessels and corresponding lymphatic glands which become dark like spleen pulp.

The spleen is greatly enlarged, sometimes to five times its normal size with the capsule tense and infiltrated with blood. It may occasionally be ruptured. The spleen pulp is very dark or nearly black and is soft or even fluid.

In cattle, rare cases are sometimes seen in which the spleen remains normal. In some cases, there may be gelatinous oedema in regions where the bacilli penetrated. However, the swelling of the throat is not as common in cattle as in the horse or pig. The liver and kidneys are congested, enlarged, brittle and fragile.

Pigs

The changes are usually limited chiefly to the pharyngeal region with marked gelatinous blood stained infiltration of the peripharyngeal connective tissue which may extend to the neck and thorax. The tonsils are covered with a pale yellow, firmly adherent slough and are surrounded by greatly swollen mucous membrane. Spleen not enlarged.

Sheep

There is severe gastro-enteritis. Splenic enlargement is not characteristic and there is no throat lesion. Putrefaction is most rapid in case of sheep because the fleece keeps the carcass in a more warm state than in animals with short hairs.

Horses

The lesions usually resemble those seen in cattle except in splenic enlargement, but if the animal survives a few days as is frequently the case, then swellings appear at different parts of the body — especially in the throat region, due to a subcutaneous gelatinous oedema.

In every case of anthrax, the blood is usually thick and dark red or tarry in colour and is not coagulated or coagulated imperfectly.

The dark coloration of the blood is ascribed to anoxemia and probably excess of CO_2 and other gas in the blood. The imperfect coagulability of the blood is probably due to precipitation of the blood calcium. Some authors attribute this phenomenon to the presence of some type of haemolysin which, however, is contradicted by others.

Incubation period: 24 hours to 3 days or it may even up to 14 days.

Symptoms

Peracute Cases

Which are usually common in cattle—animals which are well nourished and appeared healthy, suddenly fall down with blood stained foam issuing from the mouth and nose and sometimes pure blood from the anus followed by signs of asphyxia, convulsions and death. This form is most frequently observed at the beginning of an outbreak than in the later stage.

Acute Cases

The disease commences with sudden rise of temperature (104 °F or 40 °C to 108° F or 42.2 °C) is characterised by restlessness and excitement during which the animal bellows, stamps its feet and butts against hard objects, or it may develop with symptoms of severe general disease, unequal distribution of body temperature, accelerated respiration due to deficient oxidation of the blood, tremors of the thighs or pelvic region or of the whole body and also acute colicky pain with severe bloody diarrhoea and haematuria. There is complete loss of appetite with cessation of rumination and secretion of milk in case of female and a moderate degree of flatulency.

In severe cases, there may be blood-stained foamy discharge or even blood from-mouth, nose and anus followed by signs of asphyxia, convulsions and death.

Duration of this form of disease is from 10 to 36 hours.

Sub-acute Cases

In this form, the common symptom is oedematous swelling of neck, chest, flank, lumbar region or external genital organs. The swellings develop rapidly, are more or less extensive, hot and firm to the touch or may pit on pressure. The overlying skin may be fissured—releasing a yellow serous fluid. The swelling of the neck is often associated with severe pharyngitis and oedema of the glottis. As a result, dyspnoea — which is more or less present is considerably aggravated.

Duration of this form of the disease is 2 to 5 days, occasionally 7 to 9 days.

Horse

The disease is manifested usually by severe continuous colic not accompanied by accumulation of faeces and gas. Usually, there is also oedema of the pharyngeal region or neck or chest, under surface of the sheath and also shoulders which are rapid in developments, hot and painful and later cold and doughy. Dyspnoea and cyanosis are also pronounced. Haemorrhagic evacuation from the intestine and bladder are common symptoms.

Duration of the disease is from 8 to 36 hours or may last 3 to 8 days.

Sheep and Goats

Due to cerebral apoplexy — which is generally the case — the animal is suddenly attacked with vertigo, staggering, grinding of the teeth and dies in a few minutes after twitching and haemorrhage from the natural body openings. In less severe cases, the symptoms are similar to acute forms seen in cattle.

Pigs

There is acute diphtheretic inflammation of the tonsils and the pharynx accompanied by swellings of the lymph glands and surrounding tissues of the throat, which may become so extensive as to suffocate the animal and the animal dies in 3 or 4 days, but more 'often it disappears after 3 weeks and the animal recovers.

Dogs and other Carnivore

There are either symptoms of severe gastroenteritis or symptoms resembling those of pigs.

Poultry

Anthrax causes sudden death with haemorrhage from the body openings. Sometimes, an affection of short duration with debility, staggering, haemorrhagic evacuations from the intestines and cyanosis of the visible mucosa of the head region is seen.

Mortality — 80% to 100%.

Diagnosis

Refer Culture

Anthrax bacilli may be isolated from admixture with other organisms by sowing the material on agar or gelatin plates, when the anthrax colonies are picked off under a low power. Anthrax spores can also be free from admixture of non-sporing organisms by heating at 80°C for 10 minutes and sowing on platelet media.

Mice, guinea pigs and rabbits (not rats as they are very resistant) are highly very susceptible. Inoculation with virulent materials kills the animals within 72 hours. Application of anthrax material by skin scarification is regarded to be better, as there is less danger of killing the animal with extraneous organisms. After the animals death, autopsy must be held and the bacilli found by microscopic examination and culture from the heart blood.

Ascoli's Reaction

Anthrax immuned serum apart from its immunising value possesses the property of producing precipitation in extracts from anthrax bacilli or organs of animals affected with anthrax. This property is due to the presence in the bacilli, especially in their capsules, a substance—precipitinogen which gives rise to specific antibodies (precipitins) in the bodies of animals treated with such bacilli. The precipitins, when they come in contact with the precipitinogen, unite with it to form an insoluble precipitate.

Precipitinogen is resistant to advance putrefaction and heat (it was present in material putrid for more than 1½ years and in dried splenic pulp after 19 years), hence a positive reaction is possible even with extracts from extremely putrefying organs in which the presence of anthrax bacilli cannot be demonstrated by other methods. The precipitate must appear immediately, as normal serum will give a precipitate in 15 minutes.

Treatment

In cases which are not too far advanced, curative treatment with anti-anthrax serum gives good result. Intravenous injection of not less than 100 ml given once reduces the- temperature within 6 hours and affects complete recovery in 12 hours. The treatment with serum should start at once and an initial dose of 250 ml of anti-anthrax serum is more effective. When no effect is produced or when the temperature again goes up, it is advisable to repeat the serum injection.

Penicillin 1,000 Iμ. to 2,000 Iμ/51b (2.25 kg.) body weight given intravenous or intramuscularly with immuned serum and repeated at intervals of 6 hours is reported to be of immense value in'-the treatment of anthrax. Sulphathiazole may also be used and is of some value. Treatment with drugs has no fixed result but this is occasionally practiced with good results, especially towards the end of an outbreak.

Cases of Swelling

Injection of 5% .to 10% phenol solution into the carbuncles or swellings and also application of the same to the swelling externally is of advantage.

Prophylaxis

- Isolation of in-contact animals;
- Disposal of carcasses;
- Disinfection of stall, byres, sick room etc.;
- Treatment of sick ones, if any.

Preventive inoculation to in-contact and other healthy animals of the locality with anthrax immuned serum in the following doses:

- Cattle (according to the size) — 10 ml to 25 ml,
- Sheep and goat — 25 ml to 30 ml Ponies, mules,
- Country bred horses — 25 ml to 50 ml,
- Imported horses — 100 ml and upwards.

A bottle of serum, once opened, must not be used after 24 hours.

The immunity conferred by a single dose of serum is of short duration (approximately 2 weeks), hence animals subjected to infection for a longer period should be reinjected—say, after 15 days of the first dose.

Active Immunity

Anthrax spore vaccine 1 ml (saponin glycerinated spore suspension) given subcutaneously confers a positive active immunity. There is practically no reaction other than a mild local or thermal reaction lasting 2 or 3 days. Vaccine from virulent uncapsulated strains of anthrax bacilli developed in the Onderstepoort Laboratory of Vety. Science, in the Union of South Africa, is superior to the other forms of spore vaccine.

Disposal of Carcasses

The animal carcass along with blood, discharges and other material should be disinfected with Bleaching powder in a hot 10% solution which kills both bacilli and spores almost instantaneously and buried at least 6 feet deep; profuse quantity of bleaching powder should be sprinkled over it and the place to be cordoned off with fencing. The milk from in contact animals must be regarded as dangerous until such time as these are considered to be out of danger.

Disease Bacillary White Diarrhoea

Synonym: Pullorum disease.

This is a highly infectious and fatal disease of septicae mic nature, chiefly affecting chicks caused by Salmonella pullorum—a bacterium of the Coli-typhoid group measuring about 1-3μ x 0.4 to 0.6μ and is non-motile and nonsporing rod-shaped organisms.

Species Susceptible

Pullorum disease is principally a disease of the newly hatched chicks. Infection is greatest during first 48 hours of life and is unusual after the 5th day. Most frequently, chicks are infected before they are hatched, that means the disease is passed on to them by their parents, as matured hens, which survive the disease. Chicks, often carry the infection as a chronic ovariam disease, and as such, remain as carriers. The only evidence of the presence of this condition in adult hens is a reaction to the agglutination test.

Pullorum disease in a few instances has also been noted in turkeys, pheasants, ducks and other wild birds.

Modes of Infection

The principal method of infection is through infected eggs laid by carrier hens, the organisms being in the yolk.

Although a small portion of chicks are born infected, the disease spreads rapidly to others by ingestion of contaminated food, particularly if the chicks are reared in incubators.

Incubation Period

2 to 10 days in natural infection.

Symptoms

The chicks may die in the shell. Deaths occur from the first day of hatching and are heaviest during the first six days. The affected chicks are weak, without appetite, drowsy, huddled up together and often chirp. The wings droop and the feathers ruffle. Diarrhoea is common, the droppings being chalky white and pasty, which usually mat the feathers around the vent and occlude it.

Postmortem Lesions

Liver enlarged and sometimes mottled and may show minute white spots. The lungs are usually congested and in about 50% of cases yellowish-white necrotic nodule are present varying from pinhead to areas involving almost a whole lobe. Similar lesions may be found in heart muscles and walls of gizzard.

There is usually catarrhal enteritis and the caeca often distended with semisolid yellow creasy casts. The presence of unabsorbed yolk-sac in chick over 4 days old is also a feature of this condition.

Carrier Hens

The lesions are principally confined to the ovary, which contains ova, both of normal and abnormal appearances, the latter being angular, flattened and reddish-green in colour, firmer in consistency and are attached by long stalks instead of short ones. It may be remembered that normal ova are round and of a golden yellow colour and attached by short stalks.

In acute cases in matured birds, which are not very common, the lesions vary. There is usually enteritis and necrotic regions may be present in the lungs, liver, spleen, heart and pancreas, besides the diseased ovary as in carriers.

Mortality

Up to 90% after an average duration of 2 to 3 days.

Treatment

Curative treatment is of no use; however, intestinal antiseptics may be tried if desired. Sulphamezathene and Sulphamerazene; have some effects as curative agents. Unaffected chicks in the affected flock should have Pot. Permanganate or corrosive sublimate or still better or any sodium salt of the two sulpha drugs. Sour milk is of some value in preventing infection. This should either the given as drink or mixed up with mash Iodised milk may also be given.

Prevention

Survivors from the disease should not be used for breeding. Breeding stocks should be periodically subjected to agglutination test and reactors eliminated and never used for breeding.

Infected runs, coops etc. to be disinfected with quick lime. Similarly, all infected incubators, brooders etc. are to be thoroughly disinfected before next use.

Black Quarter

Synonym: Black leg, Quarter-ill, Emphysematous gangrene, Quarter evil, Symptomatic anthrax.

It is an enzootic, acute febrile, infecting but non-contagious disease of toxaemic nature affecting cattle and characterised by crepitant swellings in the muscles of the various parts of the body, specially the quarters but never in the tail or below the knee or hock joint and caused by:

- Clostridium chauvoei, which is responsible for True Black quarter,
- CI. septique
- CI. oedematiens, both being responsible for a few cases of so-called Clinical Black quarter,
- CI. septique is also responsible for a disease in sheep known as Braxy.

Bacteriology

The microorganism of true Black quarter—CI. chanvoei is a gram positive, sporulating, straight or slightly curved rod found singly or in pairs and measures 3^{μ} to 5^{μ} x 0.5^{μ}. The spores are oval and are of greater diameter than the bacteria and lie centrally, terminally or sub- terminally—giving them the appearance of lemon (Clostridia form), tennis racket or pears. Sporulation occurs freely in fluids and tissues of the body and in the culture media after 24 hours.

CI. septique and CI. oedematiens resemble CI. chanvoei morphologically. All the three are non-capsulated and anaerobic and leading saprophytic life in the soil, this being in all probabilities its main habitat.

Staining

The organisms stain readily by aqueous solution of any aniline dyes, the most common of which is Methylene Blue in 1% solution.

As the organisms remain in the muscle tissue of the affected area and not in the blood, a smear made of blood is of no use. Smears are to be made from the affected muscle tissue which is to be obtained by pinching-off a small portion with a pair of forceps, preferably from the centre of the affected region after making an incision over the skin.

Incidence

As has been told earlier, the organisms live in the soil as saprophytes. They are most concentrated on permanent pastures and heavily manured lands; hence, the disease occurs in certain regions called Black Quarter districts, usually with the commencement of rains.

Animals Susceptible

The disease usually affects cattle between the ages of 6 months to 2 years. Suckling calves are seldom affected, but in severely infected areas, this may occur shortly before or directly after weaning. Cattle over 2 years, as a rule, are affected only when they are transferred from uninfected areas to infected areas.

In sheep, variations in susceptibility due to age are at present unknown.

Modes of Infection

The natural method of infection is not always easy to demonstrate, though there is some evidence that infection may occur through the alimentary canal. The precise way in which this occurs is not known.

Experimentally one cannot infect by feeding cultures. It is possible that in many cases the disease arises from wound infection, and in others, is due to bruising of muscles in which the spores are lying dormant.

Pathogenesis

After gaining entrance into the system, the spores invade the blood stream and finally become localised in tissues, specially muscles, germinate into bacilli and multiply by fission liberating a toxin which causes degeneration of the muscular tissues and decomposition of muscle sugar, forming rancid organic acids and gas. This toxin and the products of decomposition are absorbed by the circulation resulting in general infection (Toxaemia).

The most suitable muscular tissue is previously unhealthy area or where an extravasation of blood is present.

Postmortem Lesions

Putrefaction develops rapidly except in the affected muscles and extreme bloat is present shortly after death. Due to severe tympany, the legs on the upper side extend straight out. Besides, the most characteristic lesion is the crepitant swelling in some muscular part of the body, the skin over which is usually normal. Rarely the skin of the area may be dark coloured and parchment-like due to dry gangrene.

The muscles are found to be infiltrated with discoloured bloody serum and gas and often emit a peculiar rancid odour. Bloody froth often exudes from the mouth, nostrils and anus. The spleen is usually normal but may be swollen and haemorrhagic. Liver and kidneys are swollen and congested Endocarditis is frequent in calves.

Incubation Period

Usually 1 to 3 days, seldom more than 5 days.

Symptoms

The disease usually begins with sudden rise of temperature (106 °F or 41.1 °C to 107 °F or 41.7 °C) within a few hours and the animal ceases to take food or ruminate. This is soon followed by stiffness of one leg or limping. In Clinical Black Quarter—the fever is less severe or it may be absent altogether. Soon after the limping begins, swelling develops in one of the muscular parts of the body—mostly in the gluteal, sacral, femoral or lumbar regions but never in the tail or below the knee or hock.

The swellings may be circumscribed or diffused, is at first hot and painful, but later cold and painless, so much so, the animal manifests no pain on palpation or even on incision. The swelling is crepitant on palpation and tympanitic on percussion. The surrounding tissues are oedematous and the regional lymphatic glands are considerably enlarged. In some cases, there may be symptoms of colic but usually dyspnoea develops gradually, followed by death.

The duration of the disease is generally 12 hours to 48 hours but extend to 4 to 10 days.

Mortality

It is very high. Recovery, though very rare, confers high degree of immunity which is reported to be life-long.

Treatment

Owing to rapid course of the disease, the treatment is not very hopeful. Penicillin is reported to be effective, which is to be given in similar manner and doses suggested in the case of Anthrax. It may be noted that treatment with penicillin is effective only when commenced early. Intravenous injection of 60 ml 100 ml of immuned serum followed by 20 ml given subcutaneously every 2 to 4 hours gives favourable result at the onset of the disease, as well as in the lingering cases. Penicillin in the dose 1,00,000 to 2,00,000 units every 3 to 4 hours, combined with serum, has been followed by recovery.

Besides, local treatment may be adopted which consists in making several incisions in the swellings and after squeezing out the fluid and gas, as much as possible, as well as, the damaged tissue and finally treatment with strong antiseptic solution—hydrogen peroxide, 3% carbolic acid, 0.1% formalin.

Prophylaxis

Isolation, disinfection and disposal of carcasses in the similar manner as suggested under Anthrax. Subcutaneous injection of Black Quarter serum to the in-contact and healthy animals in actual outbreaks. The dose of the serum is 15 ml for cattle and 10 ml for sheep. The immunity is of short duration, hence re-inoculation should be done if the outbreak lingers, the interval of two injections being 2 weeks or less.

Active immunity lasting at least a year is produced by subcutaneous injection of polyvalent Black Quarter vaccine in doses of 5 ml to 10 ml in cattle and 1 ml to 2 ml in sheep. It is advisable that inoculation of this vaccine should be done about a month before the onset of the season when outbreaks are commonly known to occur. A second dose after 9 to 10 weeks still further enhances the degree of immunity.

Braxy

It is a disease of the digestive tract of the sheep, specially weaned lambs, and characterised by short period of illness and high mortality.

Etiology

Clostridium septique is regarded as cause of Braxy. It gains entrance to the alimentary canal by way of the mouth.

Symptoms

It develops suddenly being noticed by shepherds and often found dead when nothing unusual was seen. The affected animal shows loss of appetite, dullness, abdominal pain and diarrhoea. Temperature goes up to 107 °F (41.7 °C), respiration difficult and pulse imperceptible. A typical odour is perceptible from the breath just prior to death.

Postmortem Lesions

There is marked deep inflammation of the abomasum, sometimes with oedema. It is some sort of "gas gangrene" of the stomach. This is the primary lesion. There is excess of peritoneal fluid. Gas phlegmon may be present in the muscles.

Prevention

Vaccination at the beginning of epidemic season, especially in winter, say September, so that animals have time to develop immunity. A second vaccination after 2 weeks may be given.

Disease Botulism

Botulism is a form of food poisoning in man and animals, as well as, birds caused by the soluble exotoxin of Clostridium botulinurri from the alimentary canal characterised by symptoms of paralysis, especially of cranial nerves and great muscular weakness. Botulism is not an infection but intoxication, the toxins having been formed on the foodstuff outside the body and which is not destroyed in the digestive tract.

Bacteriology

CI. botulinum is a saprophyte, morphologically identical to other Clostridia and like all other Clostridia, it also lives a saprophytic existence in the soil, vegetation etc. and is widespread in nature.

Five types of the bacillus have so far been identified and these are known as type A, B, C, D and E. The toxin is destroyed by cooking, that is boiling.

Canned and preserved vegetable and meat, as well as, the Salter fish are the usual source of infection in man. Mouldy vegetables and grains in herbivorious birds and putrid and decaying animal products in carnivorous birds. The sources for animals are the decomposing carcasses, particularly bones with particles of decomposed flesh. Decaying vegetation, mouldy hay, mouldy ensilage etc. are also sources for animals.

Incidence

It is very common in animals that graze on a pasture land strewn with bodies of dead animals in various stages of decomposition. It is still very common in cattle fed on a phosphorus deficient diet (Aphosphorosis) and also in animals suffering from Pica.

Modes of Infection

The commonest method is by ingestion of toxin along with the food. Recent researches indicate that ingestion of bacilli as well, plays an important part by proliferation and elaboration of toxin in the intestine. Direct infection of wounds with the toxin may also set up intoxication.

Postmortem Lesions

Carcass of animal dead of Botulism does not show any lesion, discernible by naked eye.

Incubation Period

It ranges from few hours to 10 days depending upon the amount of toxin ingested.

Symptoms

In acute form, the animal is usually seen to lie down with coma developing soon. In comparatively less acute form — the symptoms seen are restlessness, hurried respiration with comparatively normal pulse, dyspnoea and death. In mild form — the symptoms observed are paralysis of the jaws, tongue and oesophagus resulting in difficulties of mastication, re-mastication and deglutition with salivation.

These are followed by great muscular weakness which compels the animal to lie prostrate with consciousness undisturbed. There is no pyrexia and the appetite unchanged but for paralysis of the organs stated above, the animal is unable to eat and drink.

A chronic form is also noticed in which the symptoms observed are loss of appetite, prostration and emaciation, often ending in death.

Treatment

Remove the food suspected to be responsible for the intoxication and give a drastic purgative. Specific and polyvalent antitoxic serum may be given but its efficacy is questionable.

Prophylaxis

Vaccination with botulinum toxoid confers a high degree of immunity that lasts for at least one year.

Botryomycosis

Synonym: Discomycosis.

This is a chronic infectious disease chiefly of horses characterised by formation of granuloma with suppurating foci and caused by Staphylococcus aureus, which is also named as Discomyces or Micrococcus ascoformans. The essential feature is the presence in the pus the large collection of cocci forming the so-called Botryomyces granules.

The granuloma is also known as Botryomycoma.

Symptoms

The common sites for the lesions in the horse are the skin and subcutaneous tissues of the shoulder and sternal region, as well as, the tail after docking and the spermatic cord after castration. The lesions are nearly always tumour like in form and may attain a large size, particularly those which occur in the neighbourhood of shoulder. On the surface of the tumour, sinuses communicating with deep seated lesions may open or superficial abscesses may break and discharge the pus and heat up at intervals.

The pus is usually golden yellow (or may be brownish) in colour, creamy or mucoid in nature and contains numerous granules called Botryomyces granules. The regional lymphatic glands are usually unaffected.

In cattle and pigs—the condition is a chronic mastitis.

Treatment

Excise the tumours wherever possible and dress with Povidone-iodine lotion or ointment. Internal administration of Sodium iodide is also recommended.

Bumble Foot

This means the appearance of small abscess like painful swellings on the pads of the poultry's feet or in between the digits caused by the entrance through some abrasion or scratch of Staphylococcus aureus.

Treatment

In the superficial form, soak the affected foot in tepid warm Sodi Bicarb solution and then apply Povidone-iodine lotion.

In case of deeper lesions, foment or poultice for reducing the pain and also to hasten suppuration. When mature, open them with cross incisions and remove the pus and core and apply as the first dressing some strong antiseptic lotion and subsequently treat them as open wounds.

In persistent cases, applications of Povidone Iodine ointment are effective and apply once or twice. Administration of sulpha drugs extent beneficial results.

Contagious Abortion of Cattle

Synonym: Brucellosis; Bang's disease; Infectious abortion.

This is a specific disease of cattle characterised by catarrhal inflammation of the gravid uterus resulting in abortion and caused by Brucella abortus bovis or Bang's bacillus.

Bacteriology

The organism is a short non-motile, non-sporulating rod-like organism measuring 1^{μ} to 2^{μ} x 0.5^{μ}. Still shorter forms are sometimes met with which have the appearance of oval cocci. It stains well with Giemsa and dilute carbol-fuchsin.

The organism does not lead a saprophytic existence but may remain alive on pasture long enough to cause infection of grazing cows. Under suitable conditions of shade and moisture, the organisms may live outside for about 3 months.

Modes of Infection

The most common method of infection is ingestion of contaminated food and water. Infection may also take place by coition, the organism either being excreted with seminal fluid or mechanically transmitted by contaminated genitals of the bull. Infection is also possible through the conjunctiva and the skin.

Course

When a herd first becomes infected, the disease spreads rapidly with high number of abortions. But in succeeding years although excessive infection may be present in the herd, abortions become fewer and fewer—provided no new animals are introduced into the herd abortion. Abortion is not a constant symptom and it has been estimated that roughly one-third of the infected herd never abort.

Despite this, they are highly dangerous spreaders of infection when they calve. 80% of cattle which abort do so only once, some abort twice in successive pregnancies, but rarely more than twice. When new and susceptible animals are introduced into the infected herd, those become infected and abort.

Sometimes, without the introduction of new stock, the disease flares up again in the herd after a period of few years. Infection may be harboured in the system for life.

Pathogenesis

On entering the body, the bacilli soon reach the regional lymphatic glands at the site of infection and from there enter the blood circulation in which they remain for 10 to 21 days setting up a sort of bacteriaemia resulting in a rise of temperature (up to 106 °F or 41.1 °C with daily variation of 1 °F). After their stay in the blood, they migrate to various organs such as liver, spleen, diaphragm etc. and, in about 48 days after the infection, they settle into the tissues of udder.

The organisms have a special prediliection for the embryonic tissues of the foetal and maternal placenta, as well as the uterus. Whereas they do not find the tissues of a non-pregnant uterus suitable for their propagation and disappear in a few days when introduced into its cavity and settle in the udder to infect the uterus when it became gravid at a later date.

In calves and young non-pregnant heifers, the infection may be eliminated from the body within a short time, the disease being one of sexual maturity only.

The organisms in the gravid uterus multiply chiefly in the epithelium of the embryonic chorionic villi and spread between the chorion and uterine mucosa. The villi then undergo fatty degeneration and autolysis and a fibrino-purulent exudate forms on their surfaces which gradually loosens their connections with the maternal cotyledons and leads to a gradual separation of foetal membranes which results in expulsion of the foetus with its membranes.

After abortion or premature birth or birth in time, major portion of the bacilli contained in the infected uterus are discharged externally and, after 3 weeks, there is usually none left in the uterine cavity as those, that may remain undischarged go back and settle in the tissues of the udder, as well as in the neighbouring lymphatic glands such as supra mammary and iliac and occasionally in the liver and spleen, where from after fresh fertilisation, they are conveyed by the blood to the developing foetal membranes to repeat the above specific processes. Thus, repeated abortion may take place in the absence of any fresh infection. A second repetition is not common and multiple abortion is exceptional, as by prolonged infection, a state of immunity is established.

During their stay in the tissues of udder after abortion, some of the bacilli are excreted by the milk, ingestion of which causes “undulant fever” in man. Excretion of bacilli through milk may continue for $2^1/_2$ to 4 months.

Postmortem Lesions

The foetal membranes are infiltrated by subchoroidal gelatinous oedema and the chorion shows leather-like wrinkling of the intercotyledonary portions. The foetal and maternal cotyledons are thickened, distorted, eroded and yellow and necrotic looking various quantities of a dirty grey mucoid or viscid exudate mixed with flakes or clumps of pus are found between the uterine mucosa and the chorion.

Incubation Period

It is extremely variable and varies between 14 to 180 days—30 to 75 days being the usual. Abortion may occur anytime during the pregnancy but in most cases occur within the last three months.

Symptoms

In some cases, there may not be any premonitory symptoms, abortion occurring without effort while, in other cases, there may be usual signs of approaching labour, in which case, besides the usual signs of parturition, a greyish white or greyish red, odourless, mucoid or muco-purulent, occasionally sanguinuous discharge appears from the vagina, which continues till after abortion and, in normal cases, ceases in a few days and, in other cases, one to two weeks at the latest.

Diagnosis

The very appearance of the foetal membranes is sufficient to establish a diagnosis (Postmortem) but to differentiate positively between a non-infections abortion and abortion by brucella, bacteriological diagnosis is essential and indispensable. The organism are found in all exudates and discharges—but is found in the stomach of the foetus in pure culture.

To detect the presence of infection in a herd, the simplest and widely used method is the agglutination test and ring test.

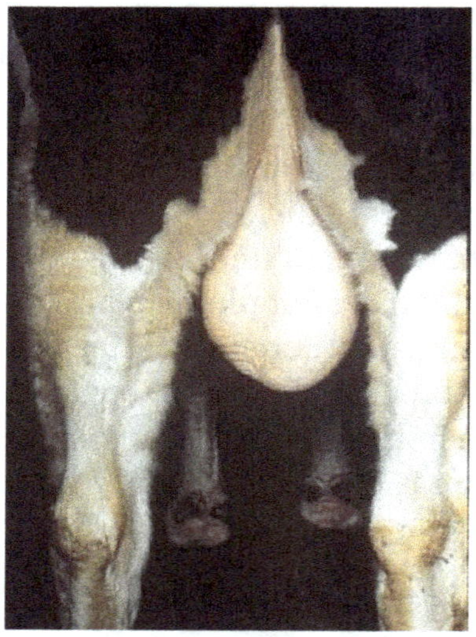

Abscess of the testicle due to B. abortus.

Treatment

There is no treatment. When the organisms have become located in the uterus, neither their multiplication can be influenced nor the death of the foetus prevented by medicinal treatment.

Immunity

Pregnant animals should not be vaccinated. Bulls should not be vaccinated because they are not naturally infected unless housed with or allowed to run with infected cows.

The best method of vaccination which has been accepted by all arid gained a great deal of attention in recent years consists in injecting calves with a vaccine of medium virulence—(Strain 19) and it produces an immunity that seemed to continue through the second gestation.

Calf-hood vaccination with Strain-19 at an age of from 4 to 8 months produces a satisfactory immunity against natural exposure to Bang's disease. It is a suspension of live organisms in 0.85% sodium chloride containing 5 billion organisms per ml bottled in single dose containers. The vaccine may deteriorate rapidly in storage or due to variations in temperature; this should be used within 3 months to ensure the use of live suspensions.

Pasteurellosis

Under collective term of Pasteurellosis are included various diseases of animals and birds, which, in their acute forms, manifest symptoms of septicaemia often accompanied with haemorrhage and are caused by Pasteurella group of bacteria which are short round-ended rods (almost oval) measuring 1.2^{μ} by 0.3^{μ} lying singly or in pairs or in group. They are Gram-negative, aerobic, non-sporing and non-motile.

When stained by Leishman's stain, they exhibit bipolar staining, i.e. the ends are deeply stained leaving a clear unstained centre with the envelope showing as delicate lateral lines linking the stained poles; hence they are termed bipolar organisms.

The names of the species under the Pasteurella group are listed below together with the diseases they produce in animals and birds noted against each:

1. P. boviseptica: The cause of H. S. in Cattle.
2. P. bubaliseptica: The cause of H. S. in Buffalo.
3. P. aviseptica: The cause of Fowl cholera.
4. P. oviseptica: The cause of Sheep pneumonia.
5. P. suiseptica: The cause of so-called swine plague.
6. P.equiseptica: Associated with Equine influenza.
7. P. leoiseptica: Associated with Snuffles in rabbits.

It is not possible to differentiate these species precisely one from another on morphological, cultural or serological grounds and are distinguished only by the conditions they set up in different species of animals and birds. As Pasteurella organisms are indistinguishable from one another, they are now called Pasteurella multocida and classified into different types.

Distribution

There seems to be little doubt that members of this genus live a saprophytic existence in the bodies of healthy animals, particularly in the upper air passages. In some cases, their presence in the body is the result of previous infection, whereas in others, there is no history of this having occurred. These 'carriers' probably constitute the chief method of spread of the organism and are the principal agents in perpetuating the infection.

The theory that Pasteurella lead a saprophytic existence outside the body in soil, mud, stagnant Water etc. has been declared as obsolete; however, excretions and secretions, as well as blood from diseased animals remain infective long enough outside the body to be a source of danger to animals.

In the carcasses of animal's dead of acute infection, the organisms are easily found microscopically in films of blood, excretions and the parenchyma of internal organs. In chronic cases, the organisms are easily confined to the regions of the body where lesions exist.

Resistance

Pasteurella species exhibit only weak power of resistance to heat, sunlight and disinfectants.

Fungal Diseases of Animals

Epizootic Lymphangitis

This is a chronic disease of horses caused by a fungus Histoplasma (Cryptococcus) farciminosus and characterised by inflammation and suppuration of the cutaneous and subcutaneous lymphatic vessels and glands.

Animals Susceptible

Chiefly horses, mules and donkeys but cases have been recorded in cattle.

Modes of Infection

It gains entry through a wound or abrasion either on the skin or of a mucous surface. The disease is spread by harness, grooming tools etc. which have come in contact with diseased animals. The parasite shows considerable vitality outside the animal body.

Incubation Period

It is usually a matter of weeks or months (average 6 to 8 weeks) and the spread of disease is slow and insidious. Even by means of experimental inoculation, incubation takes one month.

Symptoms

The first signs of the disease are often thickening or "cording" of a lymphatic vessel and adjacent gland. The lesions start from a wound or abrasion on any part of the body, the commonest site being the legs. The first sign noted are nodules up to a size of a walnut along the lymphatic vessels leading from the site of infection which, as the disease progresses, suppurate. The lymph glands into which the vessel drains swell and often develop large abscesses.

These abscesses and suppurated nodules referred to above ultimately burst—discharging creamy white or faintly yellow thick pus. Later on, these areas turn into ulcers with a red granulating base which have little tendency to heal. The forelimb—from the shoulder to the knee—is perhaps the usual site. Tumour-like masses may be seen at the shoulder and a thick cord may run down the limb. The larger masses may not burst at all if left alone.

When a limb is affected, it shows considerable thickening from chronic lymphangitis.

The characteristic feature of the disease is that the affected animal presents no constitutional disturbance even when extensive lesions are present.

Diagnosis

This disease may be confused for Farcy. In this disease, the pus is thick and creamy, on examination of which Histoplasma (Cryptococcus) farciminosus is demonstrable; whereas in Farcy, the pus is yellowish grey, viscid, occasionally reddish and is oily in appearance. Besides, there is the Mallein test to differentiate Farcy from Epizootic lymphangitis.

Treatment

Benign cases may heal spontaneously but malignant cases resist all forms of treatment. In general, exposure to direct sunlight, dry air, good feeding with much nitrogenous food and rest have a favourable influence on the disease and this explains why in tropical and subtropical regions, recovery is' more frequent than in other countries.

Treatment consists in surgical excision of all affected nodes, cords and ulcers with antiseptic dressing. An ulcer treated locally with 0.2% methylene blue solution hastens their healing.

Injection of the following is reported to have excellent results:

Rx

Bismuth Iodide	–	gr xv	16 mm
Pot. Iodide	–	3 iss	6 ml.
Aquà	–	Z iii	90 ml.

This is given intravenously once a day for 8 days and after a gap of one week for another 8 days.

Ringworm (Dermatomycosis)

This is a parasitic skin disease of man and animals of a contagious nature and is caused by the fungi belonging to the genera Microsporon and Trichophyton. The organisms belong to the two genera of fungi Imperfecti, a large group of fungi whose life history is not completely known.

Incidence

It occurs in all animals. It is commonest in cattle, occurring chiefly in calves. Then, in order of susceptibility — horses, dogs, cats, pigs and sheep. The young ones in all species are more susceptible because of their finer skin, the same applying to fine skin breeds irrespective of age.

Infection may spread from one species to another and to man by direct contacts or indirectly through infected articles.

Predisposing Causes

It must be remembered that two important contributory causes of ringworm are:

1. Over-crowding of animals into unhygienic, badly ventilated buildings and
2. General debility due to under-nourishment. There is of course seasonal variation.

Symptoms

At the commencement, rounded areas without hairs or with stumps of broken hairs are seen. The first manifestation of ringworm is that the skin becomes reddened or inflamed and a little whitish, greyish or yellow serum exudes from its surface and little nodule or vesicle form at each follicle. As a result, greyish or yellowish scales and later thick crusts or scabs form over, the areas, with subsequent development of suppurating surface under them, which, in course of time, causes these crusts to become loose and fall off.

These areas heal with new hairs growing over them. Sometimes, the lesions coalesce to form large irregular-shaped areas. New patches appear and repeat the process. Itching is most pronounced during the initial and terminal stages.

The lesion with crust formation is most common in cattle and in case of horses and other animals, the patches are usually scaly or have a scab.

Cattle

This is due to Trichophyton verrucosum infection. The lesions are nearly always on the head and neck, rarely on the body. Specially the eyelids, lips, ears and above the jaw are affected. The lesions begin as a raised ring-like patch on which the hairs stand erect. In a short time, the hairs fall off and the surface of the skin becomes covered with masses of scales heaped up into greyish-yellow crust. In calves, round the mouth and above the eyes, infection having taken place from the mother.

Horses

The infection is due to either Trichophyton or Microsporum. The lesions occur on the shoulder, back and flanks. The lesions occur in regular circles and seldom with any pruritis. The hair becomes matted in patches and this gradually extends until the whole area is denuded. The skin becomes raised and greyish white crusts are formed.

Dogs

The infection is caused by four varieties — Trichophyton, Microsporum, Oidmella or Oospora. The lesions are most on head and limbs. These occur in circular patches which become denuded of hairs and later covered with loose crusts or scabs.

Cats

Infection is due to Trichophyton, Microsporum and Achorion. The lesions are similar to what are seen in other animals.

Treatment

Oral administration of Griseofulvin is the best and simplest method. Hard crusts must be softened and removed before applying the remedy. For softening, equal parts of soft soap and lard are best which is applied with rubbing and left over for 2 to 4 days, with repetition if necessary. Addition of little quantity of Pot. Carbonate to the above expedites the softening.

Antiparasitic remedies such as Acid Salicyl, Resorcin, Coal tar, Napthalene, Creosote etc. in an ointment form is to be applied after cleaning.

The fungi are known to be sensitive to oil and fat, hence, antiparasitic remedies should have oil or fat base.

In cases in which the lesions are not extensive, good results are obtained by application of the following:

- Part of Iodine in 1 to 5 parts of alcohol or Xylol. Since this remedy is irritating, it must be used with care.
- Several antifungal ointments are now available and can be used safely without causing any irritation.

Aspergillosis

This is a disease of mammals and birds produced by the growth of the fungus Aspergillus in the tissues of the body. The most commonly affected is the respiratory tract but it has also been seen in ears, mouth, throat and liver. It runs a slow course and often mistaken for tuberculosis.

Etiology

The disease is produced by fungus Aspergillis where it causes a necrosis or death of cells and formation of small abscesses. Within the body, they grow out hyphae and produce more spores and these spread the infection further.

Symptoms

Cattle

The animal appears dull and weak and the appetite is poor. There is no rise of temperature. The disease resembles contagious pleuro pneumonia or tuberculosis but symptoms are not characteristic. The breathing is difficult and often accompanied by a dry cough. The animal does not thrive. The nasal discharge contains fungus or its spores.

Horse

The disease is not common. It is manifested by sore throat, bronchitis, pneumonia, according to the seat of fungus. It may resemble anthrax or anaemia.

Dogs

Normally the animal contracts the infection from poultry. It is manifested by epileptic-form convulsions or symptoms that are not unlike those of rabies. There is severe scratching or rubbing of the muzzle and there is discharge from nostrils which may be blood-stained. The disease runs a rapid course. Almost all the cases have occurred in the nasal cavities.

Poultry

The air passages become filled with cheesy material in which the fungus develops and breathing becomes extremely difficult. The bird gapes with its beak and gasps. Frequent sneezing and coughing are noticed. The sick bird remains isolated from the rest of the flock and there may be diarrhoea. A discharge with a repulsive odour trickles from the mouth and nostrils.

Treatment

There is no specific treatment and very unsatisfactory. Local infusions of Nystatin may be tried in case of valuable animals.

Diseases Caused by Helminth Parasites in Animals

Hepatic Fascioliasis

It is caused by members of the genera Fasciola, Fascioloides and Dicrocoelium and they are all liver flukes. The principal parasites are Fasciola hepatica, Fasciola gigantica, Fascioloides magna and Dicrocoelium dendriticum. The term hepatic fascioliasis is reserved for infestation with Fasciola hepatica.

Symptoms

In acute cases, which are rare, the animal dies suddenly; blood-stained froth appears at the nostrils and blood is discharged from anus resembling Anthrax.

Sheep

The sheep shows a temperature and is generally off colour. This is followed by an increasing anaemia/ muscular weakness, loss of appetite, pale mucosa and oedema. Skin becomes dry and doughy to the touch; the wool is dry and falling out in patches. Debility, emaciation and general depression increase and there may be occasional constipation or diarrhoea and also fever. At this stage, death may occur.

Cattle

The most characteristic symptoms are digestive disturbances. Constipation is marked and faeces are passed with difficulty, being hard and brittle. In extreme stages, diarrhoea is seen. Emaciation and weakness lead to prostration, especially in calves. Emaciation and weakness are prominent symptoms in other animals.

Pathogenesis

Very little damage is done during passage through the intestinal wall and the peritoneal cavity, although small haemorrhagic spots may be seen on the peritoneum where the worms attack themselves. The young flukes wandering in the liver parenchyma destroy the latter and, as they grow, the amount of destruction increases causing important lesions.

Massive infections may cause rupture of the liver capsule and haemorrhage into the peritoneal cavity. The adult flukes in the bile ducts feed on liver tissue and they also produce a haemolytic toxin. It may cause cholangitis and cirrhosis of liver. The worms block the ducts and may result in jaundice.

Postmortem Lesions

Anaemia, ascites, hydrothorax and hydropericardium, fatty degeneration and cirrhosis of liver. The bile ducts contain the parasites and gall stones. The liver is congested and enlarged and shows numerous small dark red foci. Haemorrhagic foci also seen in the lungs and also peritonitis.

Diagnosis

It is confirmed by finding the eggs in the faeces.

Treatment

Carbon tetrachloride is the commonly used drug. In recent years, many broad spectrum antibiotics with high efficiency are available, e.g Rafoxanide, Diamphenethide, Choxanide, Ranide 20% water dispersible powder, Hexachlorophene tablets are very effective against both adult and immature flukes.

Taeniasis in Dogs and Cats

Pathogenesis and Symptoms

The larger parasites are more pathogenic than the smaller ones but the severity of infection is of greater importance and, as well as, the age of the host.

Tapeworms may cause colic or chronic enteritis. The animals may become voracious or appetite may be diminished Unthriftiness, a shaggy coat and emaciation are frequent. Convulsions and epileptic form fits may occur in dogs only. Dogs often show symptoms of irritation in the abdomen by rubbing the abdomen on the ground. Irritation of anus is also noticed due to presence or ripe segments in the rectum.

Postmortem Lesions

Croupous or haemorrhagic enteritis are seen especially in heavy infections of Echinococcus granulosus. The worms are found in the small intestines and they may have migrated to the stomach or colon after death. Sometimes, heavy masses of worms occlude the lumen of the gut.

Treatment

Dichlorophen, Diphenthane, Dicestal are the drug of choice and to be given in suitable doses.

Taeniasis in Cattle and Swine

Taenia saginata (Beef Tapeworm) is the most common tapeworm of man. The matured parasite is harboured in the small intestine of man. It is a flat, white, jointed worm. From 12 to 25 (3.6 – 7.5 m) feet or more in length and usually only a single worm is present. Cattle become infected with the larval form (Cysticercus bovis) by swallowing eggs in food or water contaminated with infected human faeces.

The larvae penetrate the intestinal wall and develop into cysticerci in the flesh or organs. The favourite sites are in the heart and masseter muscles. The presence of these cysts in the muscles is known as "measly beef". There are no clinical symptoms in animals. Man becomes infected by eating raw or half cooked meat infected with cysticerci.

Taenia solium is quite common. The adult worm is 6 to 12 feet (1.8 – 3.6 m) in length. Swine become infected with the larval form by ingestion of food and water contaminated with egg from human sources. The larvae pass to the muscles and organs and become encysted (Cysticercus cellulosae).

The cysts are from 3 mm to 6 mm in diameter. They are oval and whitish in colour. Man gets infected by consumption of cysticerci (measly pork) infected raw or insufficiently cooked pork and its products. A clinical symptom in swine is negligible. Severe symptoms may develop in man as the larval form may also be found in human muscles.

Trichinosis

In swine, natural infection does not induce symptoms. But after a heavy artificial infection, there may be high fever, diarrhoea, stiffness, colic, difficulty in eating and swallowing, dyspnoea and oedema. Swine are infected by offals of pork containing the encysted parasites.

Trichinella spiralis occurs in two stages of development, mature intestinal trichinae and larval trichinae which are encapsulated in muscles. The adult parasite is a round worm from 1.5 to 4 mm. in length with a pointed head and a somewhat rounded tail. Its normal habitat is the small intestine of swine, rats and other mammals including man. The larval form is from 0.6 to 1 mm in length. When flesh containing the larvae is eaten by man or any animal in which development is possible, the capsule is digested and the trichinae are set free.

They become sexually mature in the small intestine about the third day and, beginning with the seventh day, the females deposit the living embryos directly into the crypts of intestinal glands. These embryos are carried in the circulation to the muscles where encapsulation takes place.

Then calcification of the encapsulated trichinae begins and continues for one and half years—this makes the cyst visible. The favourite locations of the larvae are in the muscular portions of the diaphragm, pharynx and the tongue and in the abdominal and intercostal muscles. Intensity of infestation with trichinae in garbage-fed swine is much greater than in grain-fed swine.

In man, trichinosis may be a severe and fatal disease. The usual source of infection is from ingestion of raw or insufficiently cooked trichinous pork.

Treatment

Practically, there is no treatment, once the larvae are encapsulated in the muscles.

Prevention

It consists in the thorough cooking of all pork before it is eaten by man or swine. There animals are normally fed with hotel wastes conforming pork products.

References

- Animal-disease, science: britannica.com, Retrieved 3 April, 2019
- Viral-diseases-of-animals: iaszoology.com, Retrieved 14 July, 2019
- Zoonotic-diseases: cdc.gov, Retrieved 9 May, 2019
- 10-major-diseases-caused-due-to-bacteria-in-animals: biologydiscussion.com, Retrieved 19 February, 2019
- Diseases-caused-due-to-fungi-in-animals, diseases-animals, animals: biologydiscussion.com, Retrieved 19 June, 2019
- Diseases-caused-by-helminth-parasites-in-animals, diseases-animals, animals: biologydiscussion.com, Retrieved 22 March, 2019

Chapter 4

Veterinary Ethology

The domain of veterinary science which is involved in the study of the behavior of animals in their natural habitat is termed as veterinary ethology. The topics elaborated in this chapter will help in gaining a better perspective about veterinary ethology as well as the different types of animal behavior.

Ethology is a branch of veterinary science concerned with the study of animal behavior. Ethologists take a comparative approach, studying behaviors ranging from kinship, cooperation, and parental investment, to conflict, sexual selection, and aggression across a variety of species. Today ethology as a disciplinary label has largely been replaced by behavioral ecology and evolutionary psychology. These rapidly growing fields tend to place greater emphasis on social relationships rather than on the individual animal; however, they retain ethology's tradition of fieldwork and its grounding in evolutionary theory.

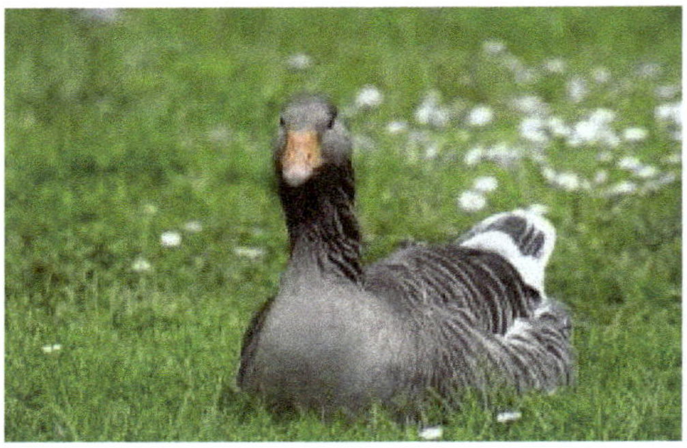

The egg-rolling behavior of the greylag goose is a widely cited example of a fixed-action pattern, one of the key concepts used by ethologists to explain animal behavior.

The study of animal behavior touches upon the fact that people receive joy from nature and also typically see themselves in a special role as stewards of creation. Behavior is one aspect of the vast diversity of nature that enhances human enjoyment. People are fascinated with the many behaviors of animals, whether the communications "dance" of honeybees, or the hunting behavior of the big cats, or the altruistic behavior of a dolphin. In addition, humans generally see themselves with the responsibility to love and care for nature.

The study of animal behavior also helps people to understand more about themselves. From an evolutionary point of view, organisms of diverse lineages are related through the process of descent with modification. From a religious point of view, human also stand as "microcosms of nature". Thus, the understanding of animals helps to better understand ourselves.

Ethologists engage in hypothesis-driven experimental investigation, often in the field. This combination of lab work with field study reflects an important conceptual underpinning of the discipline: behavior is assumed to be adaptive; i.e., something that makes it better suited in its environment and consequently improves its chances of survival and reproductive success.

Ethology emerged as a discrete discipline in the 1920s, through the efforts of Konrad Lorenz, Karl von Frisch, and Niko Tinbergen, who were jointly awarded the 1973 Nobel Prize in Physiology or Medicine for their contributions to the study of behavior. They were in turn influenced by the foundational work of, among others, ornithologists Oskar Heinroth and Julian Huxley and the American myrmecologist (study of ants) William Morton Wheeler, who popularized the term ethology in a seminal 1902 paper.

Important Concepts

One of the key ideas of classical ethology is the concept of fixed action patterns (FAPs). FAPs are stereotyped behaviors that occur in a predictable, inflexible sequence in response to an identifiable stimulus from the environment.

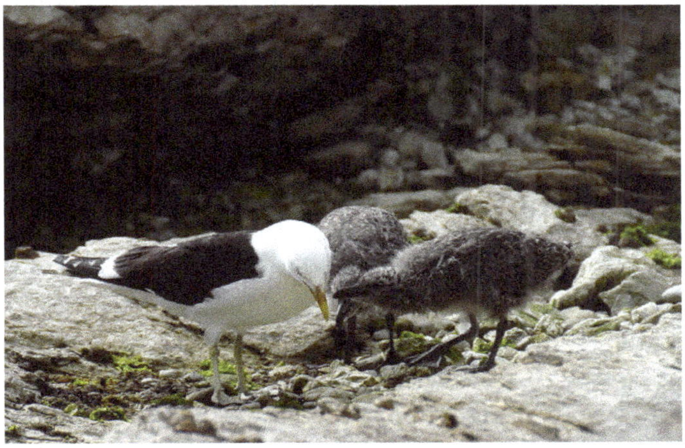

Kelp Gull chicks peck at a red spot on their mother's beak to stimulate the regurgitating reflex, another example of a fixed action pattern.

For example, at the sight of a displaced egg near the nest, the greylag goose (Anser anser) will roll the egg back to the others with its beak. If the egg is removed, the animal continues to engage in egg-rolling behavior, pulling its head back as if an imaginary egg is still being maneuvered by the underside of its beak. It will also attempt to move other egg-shaped objects, such as a golf ball, doorknob, or even an egg too large to have been laid by the goose itself.

Another important concept is filial imprinting, a form of learning that occurs in young animals, usually during a critical, formative period of their lives. During imprinting, a young animal learns to direct some of its social responses to a parent or sibling.

Despite its valuable contributions to the study of animal behavior, classical ethology also spawned problematic general theories that viewed even complex behaviors as genetically hardwired (i.e., innate or instinctive). Models of behavior have since been revised to account for more flexible decision-making processes.

Methodology

Tinbergen's Four Questions for Ethologists

The practice of ethological investigation is rooted in hypothesis-driven experimentation. Lorenz's collaborator, Niko Tinbergen, argued that ethologists should consider the following categories when attempting to formulate a hypothesis that explains any instance of behavior:

- Function: How does the behavior impact the animal's chance of survival and reproduction?
- Mechanism: What are the stimuli that elicit the response? How has the response been modified by recent learning?
- Development: How does the behavior change with age? What early experiences are necessary for the behavior to be demonstrated?
- Evolutionary history: How does the behavior compare with similar behavior in related species? How might the behavior have arisen through the evolutionary development of the species, genus, or group?

The four questions are meant to be complementary, revealing various facets of the motives underlying a given behavior.

Using Fieldwork to Test Hypotheses

As an example of how an ethologist might approach a question about animal behavior, consider the study of hearing in an echolocating bat. A species of bat may use frequency chirps to probe the environment while in flight. A traditional neuroscientific study of the auditory system of the bat would involve anesthetizing it, performing a craniotomy to insert recording electrodes in its brain, and then recording neural responses to pure tone stimuli played from loudspeakers. In contrast, an ideal ethological study would attempt to replicate the natural conditions of the animal as closely as possible. It would involve recording from the animal's brain while it is awake, producing its natural calls while performing a behavior such as insect capture.

Key Principles and Concepts

Behaviors are Adaptive Responses to Natural Selection

Because ethology is understood as a branch of biology, ethologists have been particularly concerned with the evolution of behavior and the understanding of behavior in terms of the theory of natural selection. In one sense, the first modern ethologist was Charles Darwin, whose book The Expression of the Emotions in Man and Animals has influenced many ethologists. Darwin's protégé George Romanes became one of the founders of comparative psychology, positing a similarity of cognitive processes and mechanisms between animals and humans.

Note, however, that this concept is necessarily speculative. Behaviors are not found as fossils and cannot be traced through the geological strata. And concrete evidence for the theory of modification by natural selection is limited to microevolution—that is, evolution at or below the level of species. The evidence that natural selection directs changes on the macroevolutionary level necessarily involves extrapolation from these evidences on the microevolutionary level. Thus, although scientists frequently allude to a particular behavior having evolved by natural selection in response to a particular environment, this involves speculation as opposed to concrete evidence.

Animals use Fixed Action Patterns in Communication

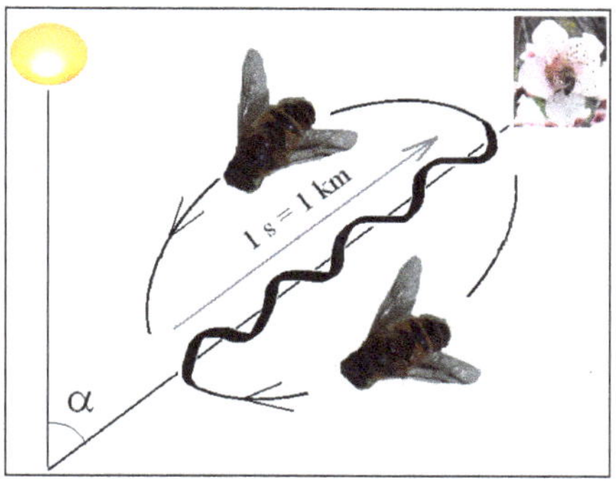

The honeybee's figure: eight dance is a fixed-action pattern that communicates information to other members of the group: the angle from the sun indicates the direction of a food source; the duration signifies its distance.

A fixed action pattern (FAP) is an instinctive behavioral sequence produced by a neural network known as the innate releasing mechanism in response to an external sensory stimulus called the sign stimulus or releaser. Once identified by ethologists, FAPs can be compared across species, allowing them to contrast similarities and differences in behavior with similarities and differences in form (morphology).

An example of how FAPs work in animal communication is the classic investigation by Austrian ethologist Karl von Frisch of the so-called "dance language" underlying bee communication. The dance is a mechanism for successful foragers to recruit members of the colony to new sources of nectar or pollen.

Imprinting is a Type of Learning Behavior

Imprinting describes any kind of phase-sensitive learning (i.e., learning that occurs at a particular age or life stage) during which an animal learns the characteristics of some stimulus, which is therefore said to be "imprinted" onto the subject.

The best known form of imprinting is filial imprinting, in which a young animal learns the characteristics of its parent. Lorenz observed that the young of waterfowl such as geese spontaneously followed their mothers from almost the first day after they were hatched. Lorenz demonstrated how incubator-hatched geese would imprint on the first suitable moving stimulus they saw within what he called a critical period of about 36 hours shortly after hatching.

Sexual imprinting, which occurs at a later stage of development, is the process by which a young animal learns the characteristics of a desirable mate. For example, male zebra finches appear to prefer mates with the appearance of the female bird that rears them, rather than mates of their own type. Reverse sexual imprinting has also observed: when two individuals live in close domestic proximity during their early years, both are desensitized to later sexual attraction. This phenomenon, known as the Westermarck effect, has probably evolved to suppress inbreeding.

Relation to Comparative Psychology

In order to summarize the defining features of ethology, it might be helpful to compare classical ethology to early work in comparative psychology, an alternative approach to the study of animal behavior that also emerged in the early 20th century. The rivalry between these two fields stemmed in part from disciplinary politics: ethology, which had developed in Europe, failed to gain a strong foothold in North America, where comparative psychology was dominant.

Broadly speaking, comparative psychology studies general processes, while ethology focuses on adaptive specialization. The two approaches are complementary rather than competitive, but they do lead to different perspectives and sometimes to conflicts of opinion about matters of substance:

- Comparative psychology construes its study as a branch of psychology rather than as an outgrowth of biology. Thus, where comparative psychology sees the study of animal behavior in the context of what is known about human psychology, ethology situates animal behavior in the context of what is known about animal anatomy, physiology, neurobiology, and phylogenetic history.
- Comparative psychologists are interested more in similarities than differences in behavior; they are seeking general laws of behavior, especially relating to development, which can then be applied to all animal species, including humans. Hence, early comparative psychologists concentrated on gaining extensive knowledge of the behavior of a few species, while ethologists were more interested in gaining knowledge of behavior in a wide range of species in order to be able to make principled comparisons across taxonomic groups.
- Comparative psychologists focused primarily on lab experiments involving a handful of species, mainly rats and pigeons, whereas ethologists concentrated on behavior in natural situations.

Since the 1970s, however, animal behavior has become an integrated discipline, with comparative psychologists and ethological animal behaviourists working on similar problems and publishing side by side in the same journals.

Veterinary ethology appears to form the common ground where animal welfare activists and veterinarians can meet. Ethological parameters seem to be adequate when evaluating animal welfare and well-being, as well as for correcting situations of animal abuse. This approach in assessing animal welfare avoids either a mechanistic or an emotional evaluation of the quality of life of an animal. The object of veterinary ethology is to teach responsible animal ownership.

Ethological parameters can be used to evaluate the welfare and well-being of animals and can often supply acceptable answers in heated debates on animal welfare issues. Ethological principles must be based on the genetic and environmental factors which contribute to the behaviour of the animal. This approach is summarised in table.

Ethological approach to animal welfare	
Genetics	Environment
Basic animal needs	Standards in the usual environment of an animal
Adaptation capabilities	The human factor

An appropriate checklist could also be established to evaluate the welfare and wellbeing of specific animals. Some factors are primarily of a qualitative nature, as welfare deals mostly with the quality of life. The main factors mentioned in table are discussed, to illustrate how these can be used in the evaluation of animal welfare.

Genetic Factors

Certain basic needs must be fulfilled for any animal to have an acceptable quality of life. Ethologists may term these needs “instincts” or “species-specific behaviour”. The term “basic” relates to primary requirements (needs), rather than secondary requirements (wants) which are not necessary for an acceptable quality of life.

Generally accepted indicators are used to establish whether the basic needs of an animal are being fulfilled. The basic behavioural needs of an animal can be determined by an ethogram, supplemented by a description of the developmental, social and specific physiological needs of the animal.

Ethogram

A few variations exist in the form which an ethogram may take, but the description given below is applicable to most animals. The ethogram is a useful tool for evaluating the basic needs of animals: the list of behavioural systems is flexible and criteria can be used as necessary. The importance of each system is related to the length of time an animal is kept, the purpose for which the animal is kept and the type of animal being kept.

Epimeletic Behaviour

Caring behaviour, as between dam and offspring, is very important in nature. However, in domestic animals, man often interferes in this process and, in some cases; the task of nurturing the young is purposefully taken away from the dam at a very early stage. In this regard, is it acceptable in animal welfare to keep female animals with poor epigenetic behaviour in breeding programmes? Or would such an approach be to the detriment of the breed in the long term? Furthermore, does the human being truly substitute the natural mother in all respects? Does the natural mother have the necessary time, privacy and space to care for her offspring?

The presence or absence of self-care (which is part of epigenetic behaviour) could also serve as an indication of the well-being of the animal.

Etepimeletic Behaviour

In domestic animals, there is a dependency on human care which goes beyond the care-seeking behaviour of the young. It is based on an inter-species epigenetic/etepimeletic situation, which lasts throughout the life of the animal. Another facet of this behaviour is that the decision to make use of veterinary services could be seen as a form of special care-seeking behaviour, which is performed by the owner on behalf of the animal in need.

Ingestion Behaviour

In domestic environments, a specific type of feed is provided in a particular place at a given time. Such intense control leaves little opportunity for variation of the ingestion behaviour of the animal.

To ensure the welfare of the animal requires knowledge of the nutritional requirements of the animal and the appropriate feeding methods. Competition for food must never be a cause of agonistic behaviour.

Excretory Behaviour

Accommodation of excretory behaviour is a very important aspect of the keeping of animals and is often insufficiently provided for. This not only comprises maintenance of hygiene and effective removal of faeces and urine, but also provision of appropriate surfaces onto which the excretions may be deposited, adequate space to ensure individual hygiene and the time necessary to carry out these behavioural patterns.

Comfort-seeking Behaviour

For domestic animals, species-specific needs should be met with regard to the provision of proper housing or shelter, to afford protection against excessive rain, snow, wind, cold, heat, sunlight (ultra-violet rays) and for some animals - to provide safety and privacy.

Surfaces on which the animals live should be considered. In certain circumstances, bedding (including regular replacement with clean, fresh material) should be evaluated as a basic need.

Investigatory Behaviour

Although inquisitiveness in animals tends to decrease with age, animals of any age kept in a confined space over a period of time may become bored with their environment. In such cases, the necessary environmental stimuli must be supplied to fulfil the investigatory needs of the animal. Some species will have a greater need to explore than others. There may also be differences between the exploratory behaviour of males and females, as well as between sterilised and non-sterilised animals.

Relaxation Behaviour

Animals need time and space to relax. Behaviour such as resting, stretching, rolling, playing, yawning, sleeping and informal exercise must be considered, especially if animals are kept on a long-term basis. Different animals will have different needs in this regard.

Allellomimetic Behaviour

Some animals have stronger needs for the social facilitation of certain kinds of behaviour. Examples of such behaviour are eating, playing or moving together. If animals with natural tendencies towards allellomimetic behaviour are kept separately for long periods, this may have a negative effect on their welfare.

Sexual Behaviour

Wherever breeding programmes are part of the keeping of animals, the necessary provision has to be made for natural breeding behaviour, including the observation of sex cycles, mattings, pregnancies and parturition. If artificial breeding procedures are used, these must also be adapted to the basic needs of the animal. These programmes should also consider effects such as inbreeding, the humane culling of surplus animals and the disposal of offspring.

Agonistic Behaviour

Agonistic behaviour of animals may be unacceptable to humans, but this behaviour can usually be explained in terms of the survival strategies of the animal. A thorough knowledge of the agonistic behaviour of an animal is necessary, either to prevent a situation which can cause aggressiveness or to manage the situations which arise when animals become aggressive. From a welfare point of view, the aim is to minimise injury to humans and animals in such situations. Preparations should include not only the required knowledge, but also suitable equipment and facilities to effectively handle aggressive animals. Serious injury can occur when no provision is made for the agonistic behaviour (e.g. belligerent) of animals. Some people simply refuse to believe that domestic animals will show such behaviour until it is too late.

Developmental Needs

One method of evaluating the welfare of animals over a lengthy period of time is to use a developmental calendar for the specific species. Such a calendar should indicate the behavioural patterns which can be expected and the provision which should be made to accommodate these patterns during various stages of development. Monitoring of behaviour could commence by recording the post-natal phases, doubling of birth mass, the change (in some animals) from mainly motor to sensory behaviour, socialisation, changing of teeth, group formation (where applicable), puberty, adult behaviour and geriatric behaviour, as well as the lifespan of the animal compared to the life-expectancy of the species. Not only species differences, but also breed differences should be incorporated into these calendars. During every developmental stage, the behaviour of an animal can then be compared to the average expected behaviour, to establish whether any deviations are taking place.

Social Needs

The social needs of animals should be known and provided for, and there may also be species or breed differences in these needs. Social needs are often underestimated and because non-fulfilment causes psychological rather than physical abuse, this is often not reported. For welfare purposes, it is thus important to use ethological knowledge of a specific animal to determine whether the social needs of an animal are met. The choice of a suitable animal for a specific environment could help to prevent problems in this regard.

Social needs usually concern the interaction of an individual animal with members of its own species, but these needs could also be fulfilled on an inter-species basis if animals are carefully mixed. With companion animals, the human is often the other species which has to provide the necessary social contact.

Social structures also involve the perception of living spaces by the individual animal. This refers to a number of different parameters, as follows:

- Physical space must allow for body movement, especially around the head. This space can be of great importance during transport.

- Social space can be defined as the distance between animals of the same species which is allowed without eliciting any special reaction. The same species could also be replaced by other accepted species and still be accepted as part of the same social system.
- Safe space determines the critical distance for the "fight or flight" decision and is defined as the area within which the intrusion of strange animals will cause an animal to react.
- Home range is applicable to free-ranging animals and is usually determined by considering the number of animals present per unit of available space, food and water.

Specific Physiological Needs

Consideration should be given to the specific physiological needs of different animals, e.g. the effect of long hair or smooth hair coats of dogs in hot and cold weather, and the lack of pigmentation in breeds which are exposed to lengthy periods of sunlight (ultraviolet rays). To evaluate welfare, such specific needs of animals must also be addressed.

Adaptation

It would be incorrect to use ethological parameters in evaluating animal welfare in a mechanistic way, because this denies the complexity of biology. Lay people with a sentimental or emotional approach to animal welfare often disagree with ethnologists on this point. If all of the above parameters are applied in a rigid manner it may appear, in certain circumstances, that the needs of the animal are not being met. However, if the animals appear to be relaxed and without any detrimental symptoms, it is possible that proper adaptation has taken place. This factor should always be considered. Adaptation to an environment may be difficult to define, but in broad terms it can be described as the absence of disease, trauma or abnormal behaviour over a period of time. Adaptive capacities of animals vary and may be influenced by genetics. The selection of animals in breeding programmes with phlegmatic temperaments, or animals which are easily trainable, could be a strategy for acquiring animals which are more adaptable. In genetic terms, this means that the animals are selected even further to fit "unnatural", human environments. Such a programme will exclude nervous animals and those which can cope less well with stress in general. However, the welfare implications of this decision should also be taken into consideration.

Lack of adaptation could also be evaluated according to stress-related parameters such as production, performance and reproduction. Furthermore, superficial measurements of stress (e.g. increased pulse rate, respiration, sweating, enlarged pupils, raised hair, anxiety or apathy) can also be considered. More sophisticated measurements could include the determination of blood levels of metabolites such as Cortisol and adrenalin; white blood cell counts could also indicate significant changes.

Environmental Factors

Environmental factors affecting domesticated animals can be controlled and can often be precisely measured. From a welfare evaluation point of view, it could thus be easier to identify any shortcomings in an environment if set standards for a specific animal are known. These standards are usually based on knowledge of the basic needs of the animal. The human (client/owner) factor will obviously play a determining role in the environment of the animal.

Environmental Factors

Three major influences which could ensure a balance between the animal and its environment are briefly discussed below.

Housing

"Housing standards" must be seen as a collective term for many measurable preconditions which could make the keeping of animals in more intensive conditions acceptable. The housing standards will depend on the period of keeping, breed, age, gender, the number of animals and also whether housing is provided for breeding purposes. Some housing facilities require a highly controlled atmosphere, and this can become very unnatural. Despite such intensive control, housing should provide an environment where the basic needs of the animal can be met. The design of housing should include specific measurements of space, proper shelter, adequate hygiene, management, the durability of the construction material and an escape-proof area. A budget for maintenance must be included from the outset. Poor maintenance may lead to trauma and unhygienic conditions (disease). Housing of animals can be expensive and must be carefully planned if this is to be cost-effective.

Nutrition

Animal nutrition is a specialised field for every species, and specific rations are available for different stages of the reproductive cycle as well as for improved production or performance. Feeding can be expensive and must also be planned in a cost-effective way, often using computer programmes. Nutrition is also affected by the preparation processes used, the source of nutrients, and the handling and storage of feeds. Furthermore, there are different methods of feeding, and both quality and quantity play a role in the welfare of the animal. Adequate provision of water may appear to be an obvious need, but water is often provided in insufficient amounts, or is left exposed to the sun, contaminated, or even placed where it is inaccessible to the animal. In proper care clean, cool water must be available at all times.

Handling Facilities

The mere provision of housing facilities is not sufficient. Special facilities should always be provided whereby animals can be handled appropriately, especially if veterinary care is required. It is the duty of the veterinarian to indicate the necessity of such facilities. The design of handling facilities is important from a welfare point of view, as proper handling facilities can prevent injuries to both animals and humans.

Human Factor

Bearing the definition of domestication in mind, the human factor is crucial to the keeping of domestic animals. Surprisingly, this fact has not been dealt with for a long time.

Selection

Man became the main selector of the genetic tendencies of animals mainly for his own benefit. On ethical grounds, therefore, the implications of this selection should be given serious consideration. Negative genetic traits can no longer be ascribed to "mother nature", but rather to "father man". Much animal suffering has been and still is caused by irresponsible genetic experimentation or by pampering the genetically weak for further breeding. It is possible that negative genetic traits are concealed or kept, in some instances, to profit from such animals. The breeder is concerned only to cover costs and has little feeling for the animal. The selection of animals for breeding must always bear in mind the health of the animal, with regard to form and function.

Conditioning

Man is clearly in charge of most of the learning and training experiences of domestic animals. Owners of animals should ensure that sensitive learning periods in the young, such as socialisation, are positive experiences. Unnecessary wants should not be created in animals, and acceptable conditioning methods should be used when animals are trained. Often it is a complete lack of training, rather than incorrect conditioning, which is detrimental to an animal. Training should provide important positive influences on the temperament and adaptative capacity of the animal. A trained animal may have increased confidence, as it knows what to expect from humans and its environment. For some animals, the establishment of a routine in their lives can be a significant type of training which develops certainty and avoids misplaced expectations. However, all training procedures should clearly take the welfare of the specific animal into account.

Care

Animal care covers many different aspects, including everything which is encompassed by the term "management". The care of the animals embraces all decisions concerning the aims of keeping animals, the control necessary to reach these goals and the evaluation of the extent to which these goals are reached. Animal management is concerned with day-to-day care as well as long-term planning, and is also linked to monetary budgets in terms of the amount which the owner is prepared to spend on the care of the animals and the output gained from such care. Decisions concerning animal care will also determine whether and to what extent veterinary care will be used. Such care is often only used if the owners of the animals are aware of the value of these services. This also underlines the importance for animal welfare of the relationship between the veterinarian and the client. A veterinarian is able to provide special care and, by giving sound advice, becomes intrinsically involved with every aspect of animal welfare, i.e. the provisional planning for keeping animals, the selection of appropriate animals, the creation of a suitable environment for such animals, the management and care of these animals, and finally achieving optimum production and performance from the animals. Other factors which should be considered in animal care are the selection of suitable personnel to work with the animals, and all relevant aspects of record keeping.

Responsible Animal Ownership

The success of the relationship between the veterinarian and the client contributes greatly to responsible animal ownership, and epitomises the importance of the human factor in animal welfare. In defining responsible animal ownership, the following points could be considered:

- The selection of healthy animals for a specific purpose and environment after consultation with a veterinarian.
- The use of acceptable conditioning processes based on species-specific behavioural traits.
- The provision of an environment where management and care (general and veterinary) is to the advantage of the animal.
- Good neighbourliness (i.e. the keeping of animals should not disturb other humans or animals in an area).

If veterinary ethology can promote responsible animal ownership, this will contribute to human society in general, and enhance the use of veterinary services. The value which the owner attaches to an animal remains a significant factor and influences the decision to use veterinary services. Responsible animal ownership will help to increase the value of the animal for the owner.

Types of Animal Behavior

Communication by Nonhuman Anmials

Different animal species use a range of senses for communicating. They may communicate using hearing, sight, or smell.

- Animals that communicate by making and hearing sounds include frogs, birds, and monkeys. Frogs call out to attract mates. Birds may use calls to warn other birds to stay away or to tell them to flock together. Monkeys use warning calls to tell other troop members that a predator is near.

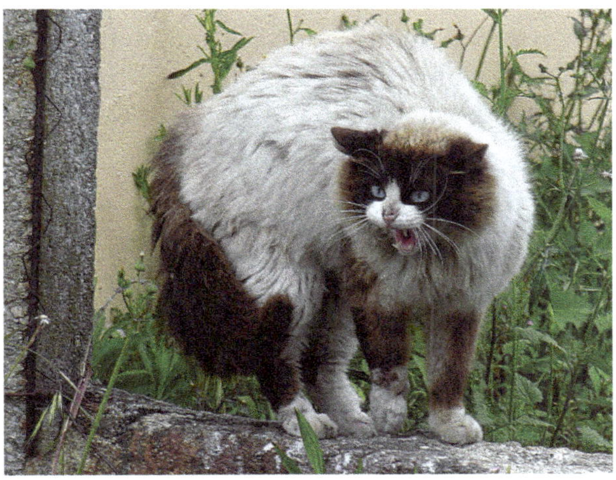

A cat uses body language and a hissing sound as a threat to potential predators.

- Animals may communicate by sight with gestures, body postures, or facial expressions. There's no mistaking the meaning of its arched back, standing hair, and exposed fangs. It's clearly saying "stay away, or else." Bees communicate with a waggle dance. They use it to tell other bees where food is located.
- A wide range of animals communicate by releasing chemicals they can smell or detect in some other way. They include animals as different as ants and dogs. An ant, for example, releases chemicals to mark the trail to a food source. Other ants in the nest can detect the chemicals with their antennae and find the food. Look at the dog in figure below. It's marking its territory with a chemical that it releases in urine. It does this to keep other dogs out of its yard.

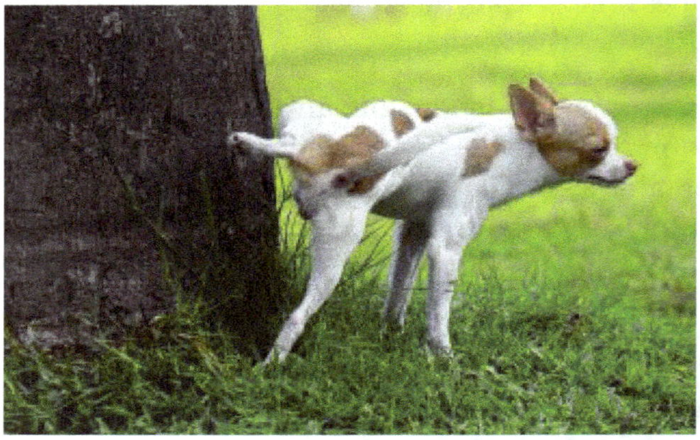

A dog urinates on a tree to mark its territory.

Social Behaviors

Without communication, animals would not be able to live together in groups. Animals that live in groups with other members of their species are called social animals. Social animals include many species of insects, birds, and mammals. Specific examples are ants, bees, crows, wolves, and human beings.

Social Animals

Some species of animals are very social. In these species, members of the group depend completely on one another. That's because different animals within the group have different jobs. Therefore, group members must work together for the good of all. Most species of bees and ants are highly social animals.

Look at the honeybees in figure. Honeybees live in colonies that may consist of thousands of individual bees. Generally, there are three types of adult bees in a colony: workers, a queen, and drones.

- Most of the adult bees in a colony are workers. They cooperate to build the hive, collect food, and care for the young. Each worker has a specific task to perform, depending on its age. Young worker bees clean the hive and feed the offspring. Older worker bees build the waxy honeycomb or guard the hive. The oldest worker bees leave the hive to find food.

- Each colony usually has one queen. Her only job is to lay eggs.
- The colony also has a relatively small number of male drones. Their only job is to mate with the queen.

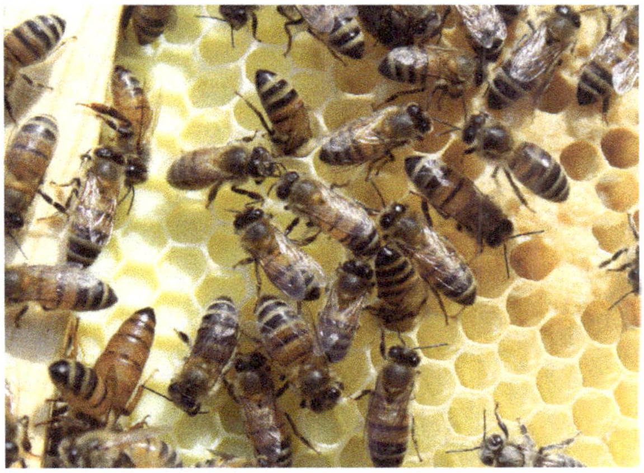

Some of the worker bees in a honeybee colony.

Cooperation

Bees and other social animals must cooperate to live together successfully. Cooperation means working together with others. Members of the group may cooperate by dividing up tasks, defending each other, and sharing food. The ants in figure below are sharing food. One ant is transferring food directly from its mouth to the mouth of another colony member.

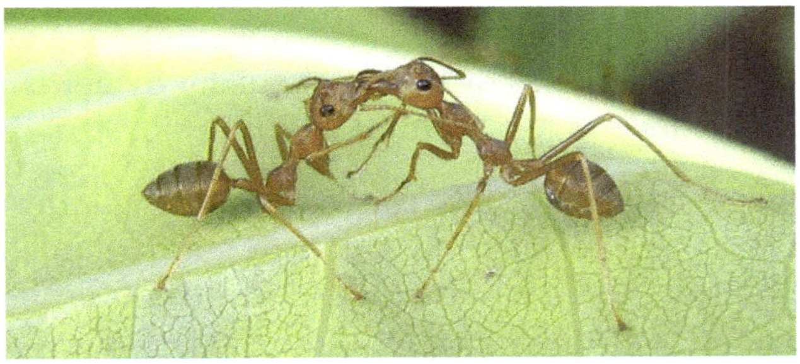

Mouth-to-mouth transfer of food is common in some species of ants.

Besides social insects, animals in many other species also cooperate. For example, in meerkat colonies, young female meerkats act as babysitters. They take care of the baby meerkats while their parents are out looking for food.

Reproductive Behaviors

Some of the most important behaviors in animals involve reproduction. They include behaviors to attract mates and behaviors for taking care of the young.

Courtship and Mating

Mating is the pairing of an adult male and an adult female for the purpose of reproduction. In many animal species, females choose the males they will mate with. For their part, males try to show females that they would be better mates than other males. To be chosen as mates, males may perform courtship behaviors. These are special behaviors that help attract a mate. Male courtship behaviors are meant to get the attention of females and show off a male's traits.

Different species of animals have different courtship behaviors. An example of courtship behavior in birds is shown in figure below. The bird in the picture is a male sharp-tailed grouse, and he's doing a courtship dance. Each year in the spring, as many as two dozen grouse males gather in a grassy area to perform their courtship dance. Female grouse watch the dance and then mate with the males that put on the best display.

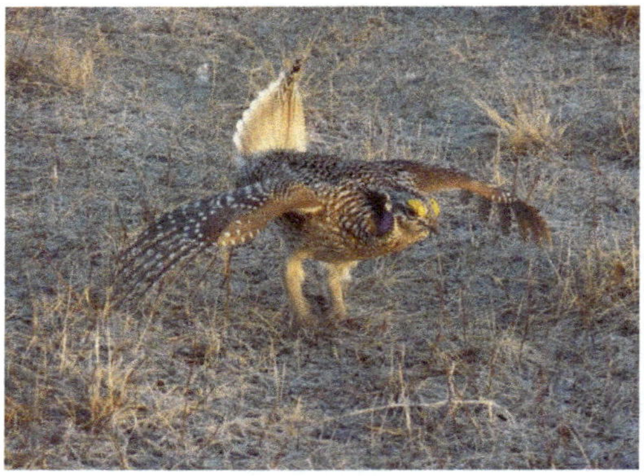

A male sharp-tailed grouse does a courtship dance to attract a female for mating.

Caring for Offspring

In most species of birds and mammals, one or both parents care for the young. This may include building a nest or other shelter. It may also include feeding the young and protecting them from predators. Caring for the young increases their chances of surviving. This, in turn, increases the parents' fitness, so such behaviors evolve by natural selection.

Emperor penguins make great sacrifices to take care of their young. After laying an egg, a penguin mother returns to the sea for two months to feed. Her mate stays behind to keep the egg warm. He balances the egg on top of his feet to keep it warm for the entire time the mother is away. During this time, he goes without food. To survive the cold, he huddles together with other males. If the chick hatches before the mother returns, the father feeds it with a high-protein, high-fat substance he produces just for this purpose. You can see an emperor penguin father feeding his chick in figure below.

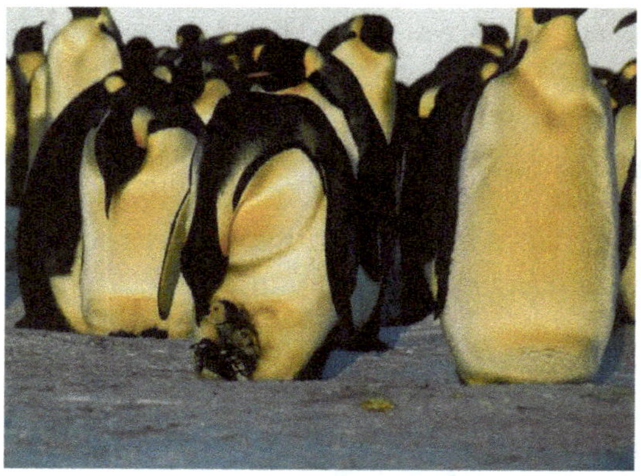

An emperor penguin father feeds his chick.

Defensive Behaviors

Some species of animals are territorial. This means that they defend an area that typically includes their nest and enough food for themselves and their offspring. Animals generally don't fight to defend their territory. Instead, they are more likely to put on a defensive display. For example, male gorillas may pound on their chest and thump the ground to warn other male gorillas to stay away from their territory. This gets the message across without physical conflict, which would be riskier and take more energy.

Behaviors that Happen in Cycles

Many animal behaviors occur in repeated cycles. Some cycles of behavior repeat each year. Other cycles of behavior repeat each day.

Annual Cycles

Examples of behaviors with annual cycles include migration and hibernation. Both are innate behaviors. They are triggered by changes in the environment, such as the days growing shorter in the fall.

- Migration is the movement of animals from one place to another. Migration is most common in birds, fish, and insects. In the Northern Hemisphere, many species of birds, such as finches and swallows, travel south for the winter. They migrate to areas where it is warmer and where more food is available. They return north in the spring. Migrating animals generally follow the same route each year. They may be guided by the position of the sun, Earth's magnetic field, or other clues in the environment.
- Hibernation is a state in which an animal's body processes slow down and its body temperature falls. A hibernating animal uses less energy than usual. This helps it survive during a time of year when food is scarce. Hibernation may last for weeks or even months. Examples of animals that hibernate include some species of bats, squirrels, snakes, and insects.

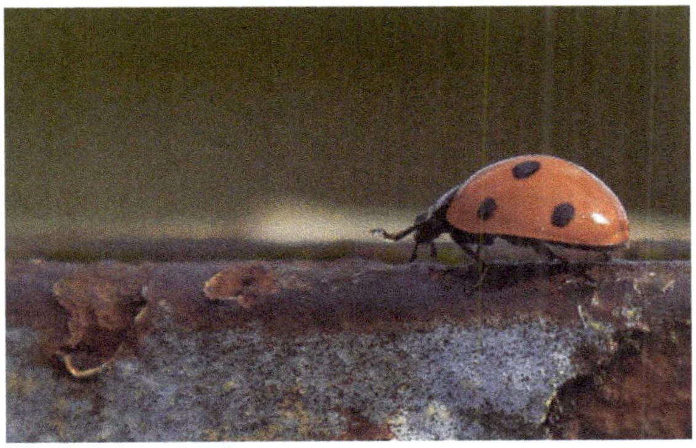

This ladybug is looking for a safe place to hibernate over the winter.

Daily Cycles

Many animals go through daily cycles. Daily cycles of behavior are called circadian rhythms. For example, most animals go to sleep when the sun sets down and wake up when the sun rises. These animals are active during the day and called diurnal. Other animals go to sleep when the sun rises and wake up when the sun sets. These animals are active during the night and called nocturnal. Many owls, like the owls in figure below, are nocturnal. Like some other nocturnal animals, they have large eyes that are specially adapted for seeing when light levels are low.

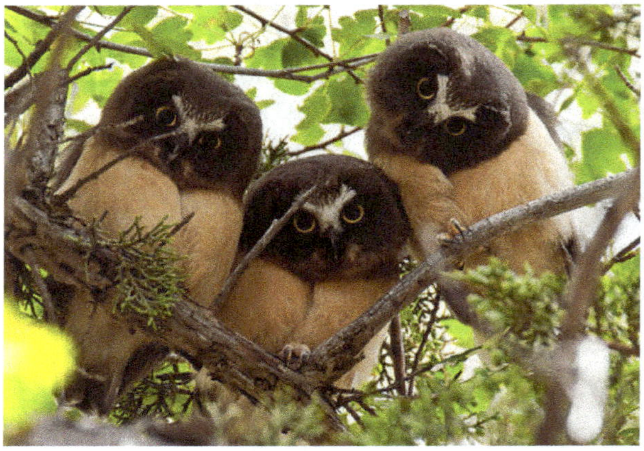

By hunting at night, owls can avoid competing with other hunting birds such as hawks.

In many species, including the human species, circadian rhythms are controlled by a tiny structure called the biological clock. It is located in the hypothalamus, which is a gland at the base of the brain. The biological clock sends signals to the body. The signals cause regular changes in behavior and body processes. The biological clock, in turn, is controlled by changes in the amount of light entering the eyes. That's why the biological clock causes changes that repeat every 24 hours.

Significance of Animal Behavior

Animal behavior is the bridge between the molecular and physiological aspects of biology and the ecological. Behavior is the link between organisms and environment and between the nervous system, and the ecosystem. Behavior is one of the most important properties of animal life. Behavior plays a critical role in biological adaptations. Behavior is how we humans define our own lives. Behavior is that part of an organism by which it interacts with its environment. Behavior is as much a part of an organisms as its coat, wings etc. The beauty of an animal includes its behavioral attributes.

For the same reasons that we study the universe and subatomic particles there is intrinsic interest in the study of animals. In view of the amount of time that television devotes to animal films and the amount of money that people spend on nature books there is much more public interest in animal behavior than in neutrons and neurons. If human curiosity drives research, then animal behavior should be near the top of our priorities.

Research on animal behavior and behavioral ecology has been burgeoning in recent years despite below inflation increases (and often decreases) in research funding.

While the study of animal behavior is important as a scientific field on its own, our science has made important contributions to other disciplines with applications to the study of human behavior, to the neurosciences, to the environment and resource management, to the study of animal welfare and to the education of future generations of scientists.

Animal Behavior and Human Society

Many problems in human society are often related to the interaction of environment and behavior or genetics and behavior. The fields of socioecology and animal behavior deal with the issue of environment behavioral interactions both at an evolutionary level and a proximate level. Increasingly social scientists are turning to animal behavior as a framework in which to interpret human society and to understand possible causes of societal problems.

Research by de Waal on chimpanzees and monkeys has illustrated the importance of cooperation and reconciliation in social groups. This work provides new perspectives by which to view and ameliorate aggressive behavior among human beings.

The methodology applied to study animal behavior has had a tremendous impact in psychology and the social sciences. Jean Piaget began his career with the study of snails, and he extended the use of careful behavioral observations and descriptions to his landmark studies on human cognitive development. J. B. Watson began his study of behavior by observing gulls. Aspects of experimental design, observation techniques, and attention to nonverbal communication signals were often developed in animal behavior studies before their application to studies of human behavior. The behavioral study of humans would be much diminished today without the influence of animal research.

Charles Darwin's work on emotional expression in animals has had an important influence on many psychologists, such as Paul Ekman, who study human emotional behavior.

Harry Harlow's work on social development in rhesus monkeys has been of major importance to theories of child development and to psychiatry. The work of Overmier, Maier and Seligman on learned helplessness has had a similar effect on child development and psychiatry.

The comparative study of behavior over a wide range of species can provide insights into influences affecting human behavior. For example, the woolly spider monkey in Brazil displays no overt aggressive behavior among group members. We might learn how to minimize human aggression if we understood how this species of monkey avoids aggression. If we want to have human fathers be more involved in infant care, we can study the conditions under which paternal care has appeared in other species like the California mouse or in marmosets and tamarins. Studies of various models of the ontogeny of communication in birds and mammals have had direct influence on the development of theories and the research directions in the study of child language. The richness of developmental processes in behavior, including multiple sources and the consequences of experience are significant in understanding processes of human development.

Understanding the differences in adaptability between species that can live in a variety of habitats versus those that are restricted to limited habitats can lead to an understanding of how we might improve human adaptability as our environments change.

Research by animal behaviorists on animal sensory systems has led to practical applications for extending human sensory systems. Griffin's demonstration on how bats use sonar to locate objects has led directly to the use of sonar techniques in a wide array of applications from the military to fetal diagnostics.

Studies of chimpanzees using language analogues have led to new technology (computer keyboards using arbitrary symbols) that have been applied successfully to teaching language to disadvantaged human populations.

Basic research on circadian and other endogenous rhythms in animals has led to research relevant to human factors and productivity in areas such as coping with jet-lag or changing from one shift to another.

Research on animals has developed many of the important concepts relating to coping with stress, for example studies of the importance of prediction and control on coping behavior.

Animal Behavior and Neurobiology

Sir Charles Sherrington, an early Nobel Prize winner, developed a model for the structure and function of the nervous system based only on close behavioral observation and deduction. Seventy years of subsequent neurobiological research has completely supported the inferences Sherrington made from behavioral observation.

Neuroethology, the integration of animal behavior and the neurosciences, provides important frameworks for hypothesizing neural mechanisms. Careful behavioral data allow neurobiologists to narrow the scope of their studies and to focus on relevant input stimuli and attend to relevant responses. In many case the use of species specific natural stimuli has led to new insights about neural structure and function that contrast with results obtained using non-relevant stimuli.

Recent work in animal behavior has demonstrated a downward influence of behavior and social organization on physiological and cellular processes. Variations in social environment can inhibit or stimulate ovulation, produce menstrual synchrony, induce miscarriages and so on. Other animal studies show that the quality of the social and behavioral environment have a direct effect on immune system functioning. Researchers in physiology and immunology need to be guided by these behavioral and social influences to properly control their own studies.

Animal Behavior and the Environment, Conservation and Resource Management

The behavior of animals often provides the first clues or early warning signs of environmental degradation. Changes in sexual and other behavior occur much sooner and at lower levels of environmental disruption than changes in reproductive outcomes and population size. If we wait to see if numbers of animal populations are declining, it may be too late to take measures to save the environment. Studies of natural behavior in the field are vital to provide baseline data for future environmental monitoring. For example, the Environmental Protection Agency uses disruptions in swimming behavior of minnows as an index of possible pesticide pollution.

Basic research on how salmon migrate back to their home streams started more than 40 years ago by Arthur Hasler has taught us much about the mechanisms of migration. This information has also been valuable in preserving the salmon industry in the Pacific Northwest and applications of Hasler's results has led to the development of a salmon fishing industry in the Great Lakes. Basic animal behavior research can have important economic implications.

Animal behaviorists have described variables involved in insect reproduction and host plant location leading to the development of non-toxic pheromones for insect pest control that avoid the need for toxic pesticides. Understanding of predator prey relationships can lead to the introduction of natural predators on prey species.

Knowledge of honeybee foraging behavior can be applied to mechanisms of pollination which in turn is important for plant breeding and propagation. An understanding of foraging behavior in animals can lead to an understanding of forest regeneration. Many animals serve as seed dispersers and are thus essential for the propagation of tree species and essential for habitat preservation.

The conservation of endangered species requires that we know enough about natural behavior (migratory patterns, home range size, interactions with other groups, foraging demands, reproductive behavior, communication, etc) in order to develop effective reserves and effective protection measures. Relocation or reintroduction of animals (such as the golden lion tamarin) is not possible without detailed knowledge of a species' natural history. With the increasing importance of environmental programs and human management of populations of rare species, both in captivity and in the natural habitat, animal behavior research becomes increasingly important. Many of the world's leading conservationists have a background in animal behavior or behavioral ecology.

Basic behavioral studies on reproductive behavior have led to improved captive breeding methods for whooping cranes, golden lion tamarins, cotton-top tamarins, and many other endangered species. Captive breeders who were ignorant of the species' natural reproductive behavior were generally unsuccessful.

Animal Behavior and Animal Welfare

Our society has placed increased emphasis on the welfare of research and exhibit animals. US law now requires attending to exercise requirements for dogs and the psychological well-being of non-human primates. Animal welfare without knowledge is impossible. Animal behavior researchers look at the behavior and well-being of animals in lab and field. We have provided expert testimony to bring about reasonable and effective standards for the care and well-being of research animals.

Further developments in animal welfare will require input from animal behavior specialists. Improved conditions for farm animals, breeding of endangered species, proper care of companion animals all require a strong behavioral data base.

Chapter 5

Veterinary Parasitology

The study of animal parasites which focuses on the relationships between animal hosts and parasites is termed as veterinary parasitology. Some of its sub-disciplines include veterinary entomology and veterinary helminthology. All the diverse aspects related to these branches of veterinary parasitology have been carefully analyzed in this chapter.

Parasites infect the animals and plants we live with and depend on for companionship and food – our pets in the backyard, livestock and crops on our farms, fish in our rivers, lakes and oceans.

Pets

Australians are among the most pet-owning people in the world. As a result the pet care industry is worth somewhere in the order of $3 billion per annum. As pet owners we have a responsibility to manage the wellbeing of the animals we care for.

Fleas on Cats and Dogs

This parasite is the most common flea on dogs but it is also found on cats and is often called the cat flea. It is an ectoparasite, meaning it lives on the exterior or surface of its host.

The adult fleas feed on the blood of the host and in extreme cases can cause anaemia, but more commonly they cause flea allergy dermatitis and secondary skin irritations.

This flea is also the intermediate host of the dog tapeworm Dipylidium caninum. This is known as hyperparasitism, where one parasite is carried by another. Both cats and dogs can become infected with the tapeworm by swallowing infected fleas.

Fleas require a warm damp environment. They can live on cats or dogs for a few months but only survive a few days if not on their host.

The females can produce a few thousand eggs during their life. The eggs are laid on the skin of the host and fall off within a few hours. Those that fall into the host's bedding stand the best chance of developing into adults. The bedding provides a suitable environment with low fluctuations of temperature and humidity. For the larvae that hatch it also provides a ready supply of food, such as dead skin from the host and faecal blood from adult fleas.

Under good conditions the larvae can hatch from the eggs within 2 to 21 days. After pupation, adults emerge to find new hosts.

If no dogs or cats are available, fleas are well known to vary their diet by sampling humans.

Dog Heartworm

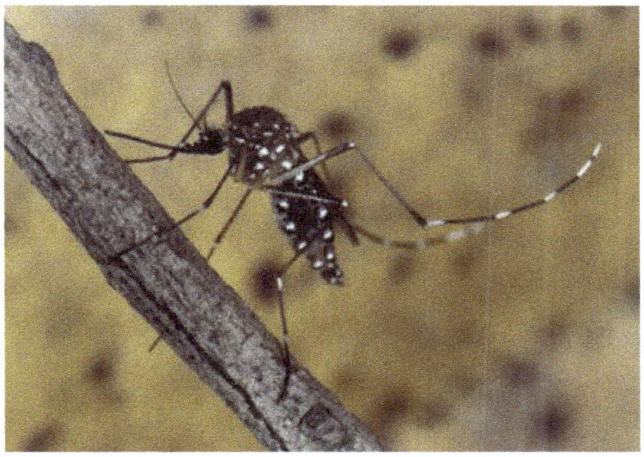

The mosquito, Aedes aegypti is a vector of dog heartworm - it transmits the parasite from one host to another.

Dog heartworm is a dangerous roundworm (nematode) parasite that often results in heart failure and pulmonary artery complications for infected dogs.

Heartworm is prevalent throughout most of Australia and has a broad distribution around the world. Fortunately it is easily treated through the regular application of drugs.

The adult worms in the heart and pulmonary artery of an infected dog produce larvae, called microfilariae, which circulate throughout the bloodstream. These are taken up by a mosquito (typically species of the genus Aedes) when it feeds on the dog and the parasite develops further within the insect.

To complete the lifecycle, the worms migrate to the mouthparts of the mosquito where they escape and enter a new dog host via the wound caused by the mosquito feeding. After several months the juvenile parasites enter the peripheral blood vessels from the tissues of the host, then enter the general circulation and mature in the pulmonary arteries and right side of the heart.

Infections have been detected in humans, who can develop a lung condition called pulmonary dirofilariasis. Fortunately for us, symptoms are generally mild and the parasites are not able to complete their life cycle in humans.

Roundworms in Dogs and Cats

Intestinal roundworms of dogs and cats are ubiquitous and require regular treatment using drugs to control infection.

Unlike the tapeworm Dipylidium caninum, which can infect both cats and dogs, particular species of roundworm, Toxocara canis and T. felis, are exclusive to the dog and the cat respectively. This association is referred to as 'host specificity'.

Signs of infection may include:

- Bloated belly
- Blood or mucus in the stool

- Diarrhoea
- Lethargy
- Loss of appetite
- Vomiting

Severe infection in dogs can create an intestinal obstruction and cause death in puppies.

Adult dogs do show some level of immunity. This immunity is suppressed in bitches when they are whelping and infection can then recur. As a result, the litter of puppies may become infected at a very young age.

Toxoplasmosis in Cats

Cats are infected by eating rodent intermediate hosts harbouring this microscopic parasite.

Toxoplasma infects the cells of the intestine and multiplies (undergoes schizogony). Fertilised eggs (oocysts) are released in the faeces and can then infect rodents or even human intermediate hosts.

White-spot Disease in Fish

Two species of parasites cause white-spot disease in fish:

- Ichthyophthirius multifiliis (also known as 'Ich') in freshwater fish.
- Cryptocaryon irritans in marine fish.

Both species are ciliated, which means they are covered in tiny hair-like projections that they use for locomotion.

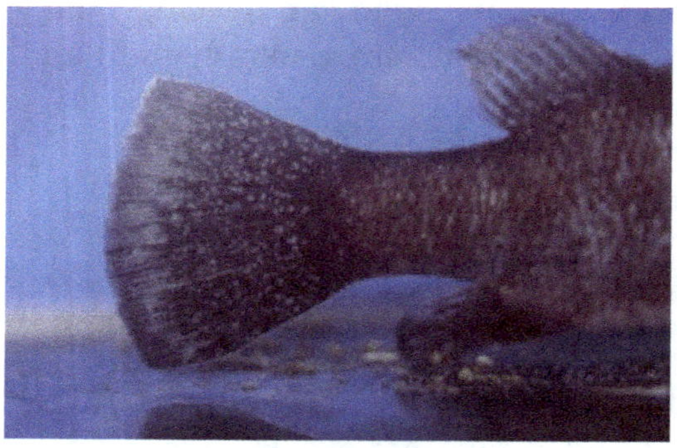

Caudal fin of barramundi, Lates calcarifer, showing the characteristic 'white-spot' appearance due to infection with Cryptocaryon irritans.

They follow similar routes of infection and have very similar lifecycles, as follows:

- Infective stage (theronts): free swimming, actively seek out host fish and burrow into skin.
- Feeding stage (trophonts): feed and grow under upper layer of fish skin.

- Reproductive stage (tomonts): leave fish and fall to bottom, undergo multiple internal divisions, and finally release numerous free swimming infective stages.

The parasites feed on fish host tissue, debris and fluids causing proliferation and swelling of host skin cells (a condition called epithelial hyperplasia).

These feeding stages form the characteristic visible white spots on the skin and gills. Severe infestations can develop rapidly in closed aquarium systems. Where no treatment is provided, the number of parasites on each fish will increase quickly and will generally result in the death of susceptible fish.

Unlike some parasites, white-spot disease can infect and kill many different species of fish. This is known as low host-specificity.

A range of treatments are available through pet stores, but prevention of infection through quarantine of fish and other aquarium material is the best line of defence.

Livestock

As farmers we want to maximise production of our domestic animals and crops, while minimising the costs of production.

Currently it costs around $300 million a year to control blow flies, bot flies and buffalo flies in sheep, cattle and horses; about $220 million per year to minimise the effect of intestinal worms in sheep; and about $200-300 million per year to control plant parasitic nematodes in crops.

Consider that these are only three examples (probably the most significant) of the dollar costs of control of parasites on our domestic animals. Then consider maintaining health in our aquaculture animals and other animal and plant industries - the costs become substantial.

Cattle Ticks

Cattle ticks were introduced to Australia in 1829 with cattle from Indonesia.

They are the most serious external parasites of cattle in Australia. Not only do they cause loss of condition or even death from blood loss, but they can also transmit tick fever (Babesiosis).

Tick fever is itself potentially fatal to cattle. It is caused by the microscopic parasites Babesia bigemina and B. bovis which infect, and eventually kill, the red blood cells of the host cow.

Cattle ticks are 'one-host ticks' which means they complete their development from larvae to nymphs and then to adults on the same host. Adult female ticks engorged with blood from their host, drop onto the pasture and lay thousands of eggs. Larvae hatch from the eggs and if a suitable host comes close enough they will attach, feed and moult, over a period of 3 weeks, to form nymphs and then adults.

Australia's scientists lead the research into Tick Fever in cattle. The Queensland Primary Industries and Fisheries Tick Fever Research Centre has pioneered the development of live vaccines for the control of these diseases.

Coccidiosis

Coccidians are microscopic parasites commonly found in poultry (chickens, ducks, geese and their relatives).

The infective stages (oocysts) are swallowed by the bird. These release small forms (sporozoites) that enter the cells of the intestinal wall and multiply to produce many more parasites (merozoites) that, in turn, invade other intestinal surface cells.

Initially there are no signs of disease, but as the infection progresses birds may appear dull and depressed, show decreased appetite, and have loose or bloody droppings.

After several cycles of build-up of the disease the infective stages develop and pass out with the faeces thereby exposing other birds to infection.

QX Disease in Oysters

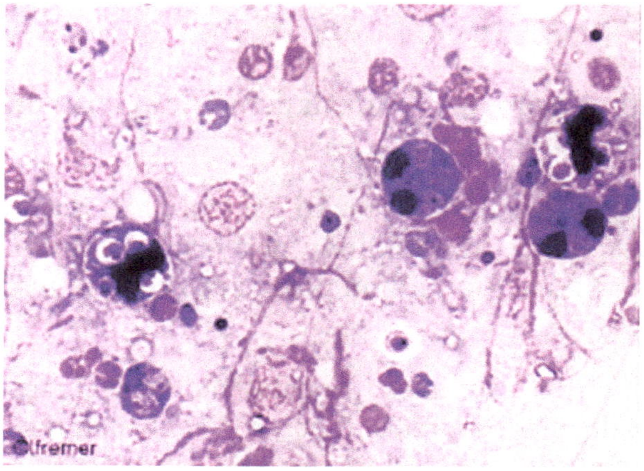

Spores of QX disease as seen under a research microscope at a magnification of 1000 times.

'QX' stands for 'Queensland Unknown', the title given to this disease before scientists discovered the parasitic organism that we now know causes it. In 1976 Marteilia sydneyi was formally described as the cause of QX disease in oysters.

Marteilia sydneyi is a protozoan (single-celled) parasite that belongs to a small group of parasites that mostly affect bivalves (animals with two 'shells', such as oysters, mussels and pipis).

QX disease infects the Sydney rock oyster (Saccostrea glomerata), which is the commercial rock oyster grown along the east coast of Australia from the NSW/Victorian border north to the Great Sandy Strait in southern Queensland.

Infections of oysters usually occur between January and April each year, with many diseased oysters losing condition and dying throughout the winter. This parasite has a life cycle which is thought to involve two hosts, the oyster and a marine worm, but the complete life cycle has yet to be confirmed by scientists.

The parasite enters the oyster through its gills and palps (mouthparts) and migrates to the digestive gland which surrounds the intestine. Here the parasite produces spores and in the process destroys the digestive gland so that the infected oyster can no longer take up nutrients. QX can cause oysters to lose condition quickly (within four weeks in severe cases, longer in others) as they reabsorb their gonads and deplete their stored reserves. Oysters then appear thin and watery (not very inviting as a dinner entree) and infection often continues until the oyster dies - the oyster effectively starves to death. Commercial losses have reached millions of dollars in some oyster growing estuaries.

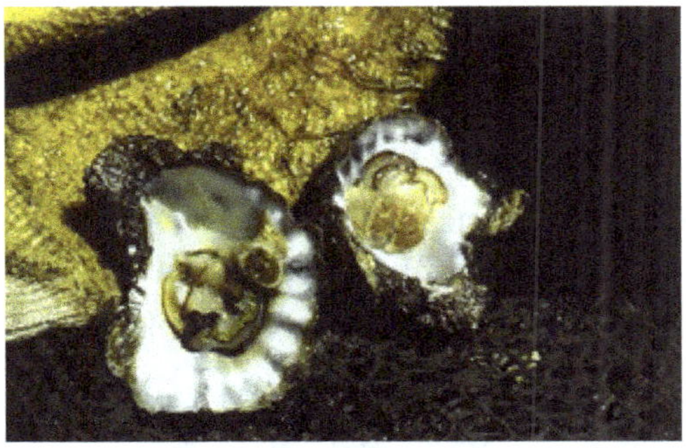

The difference in condition between a healthy oyster (on left) and one infected with QX disease (on right).

Individual spores of QX disease are microscopic and cannot be identified without the use of high power microscopes. However, one indicator of the disease is the light brown to cream colour of the oyster's digestive gland due to the presence of parasite spores. It should be stressed that these gross signs are not specific to oysters with QX disease and can be the result of other environmental and nutritional conditions.

Wildlife

Parasites are a natural part of the environment and can contribute to natural population control of their hosts. If we tried to eliminate parasites we could then interfere with the dynamic balance in natural ecosystems.

The abundance, diversity and even the identity of parasites in much of our wildlife remains largely unknown. Indeed, many invertebrate animals that act as hosts to parasites are yet to be discovered and named by scientists.

Bird Blood Parasites

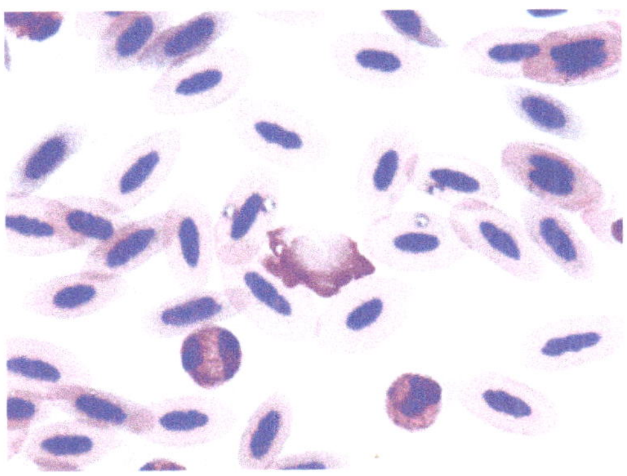

Bird red blood cells infected with Haemoproteus.

Bird blood parasites (avian haematozoa) can cause disease and death of their hosts. It is likely that all species within the genera Haemoproteus, Plasmodium and Leucocytozoon are harmful to a greater or lesser degree, depending the range of hosts they can infect, environmental stress, age, nutrition and the availability of suitable insects (vectors) to transmit disease between birds.

Australia's birds have evolved in relative isolation since the breakup of the southern supercontinent of Gondwana. Australia is now home to more than 700 species of birds, with many groups that are dominant in this country but rare elsewhere (for example parrots, cockatoos, honeyeaters, bowerbirds and kingfishers). Other species migrate seasonally between Australia and northern continents.

Despite the unique nature of our bird fauna and although there is a significant public recreational interest in birds, relatively little is known about their parasitic diseases. In Australia, knowledge of these parasites has been restricted to a few research studies with most reports generally relating to incidental findings of blood parasites.

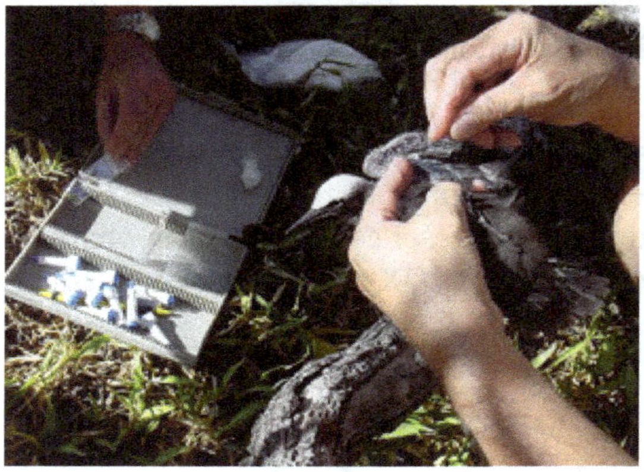

Sampling blood from a Common Noddy at Heron Island.

Research at the Queensland Museum has found that about 10% of birds in southeast Queensland were infected with these parasites but the impacts of such an infection are more difficult to assess. In our built-up areas birds often die from car-strike or from interactions with our pet cats and dogs. It is suspected that parasite-infected birds are more susceptible to meeting such an end even though the actual cause of death may not obviously have been due to the parasitic infection.

International Reference Centre for Avian Haematozoa Collection

In 1995, the Queensland Museum became home to the IRCAH (International Reference Centre for Avian Haematozoa). This collection comprises over 60,000 specimens of bird blood parasites in stained, thin blood smears on glass microscope slides. These include type and voucher specimens from about 45,000 infected birds. The IRCAH is a significant world resource containing samples from over 4,000 species of birds, representing about 150 bird families, collected from 63 countries from all over the globe.

Gordian Worms

Gordian or horse-hair worms belong to the Phylum Nematomorpha. As juveniles they are parasites of land-living arthropods, particularly grasshoppers, mantids, crickets and cockroaches.

The name 'Gordian' is derived from the mythological knot of King Gordius and relates to the ability of these worms to tie themselves in knots when mating.

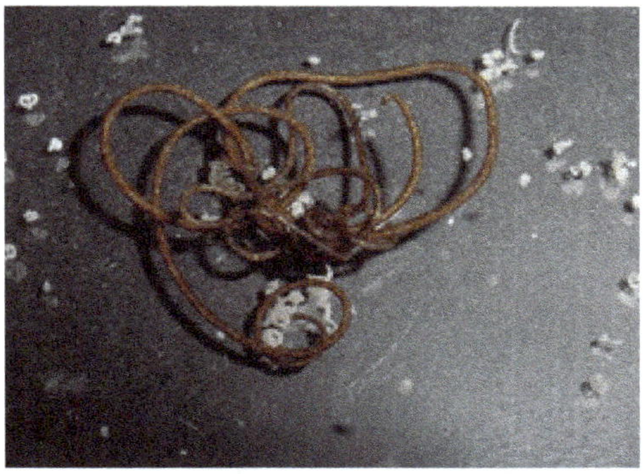

Female Gordian worm with eggs in gelatinous strings.

During spring and summer (September to February) Gordian worms may be found in town water supplies, public and private swimming pools, water tanks, dams and ornamental ponds and even the water bowls of pets. Concerned members of the public or local authorities often contact the Queensland Museum regarding these sightings but by all accounts the worms are harmless to humans, pets or livestock.

Biology and Life Cycle

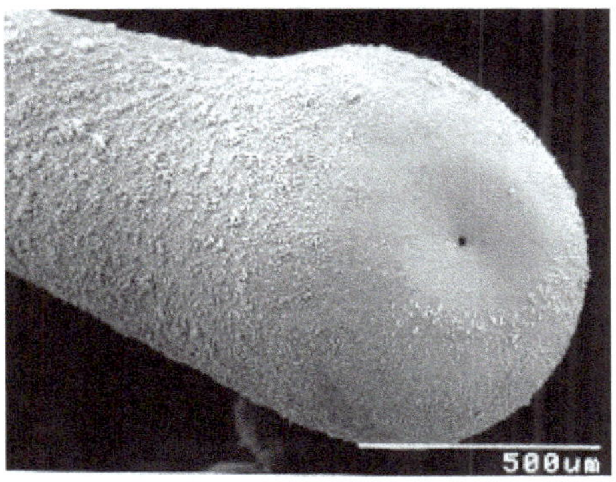

Scanning electron microscope image of rounded posterior of Chordodes sp. female, with cloaca at the end.

Adult worms are relatively long (some can be up to 100 cm), thin (2-3 mm) and rigid rather than limp. Most species of Gordian worms have some bumps or papillae (called areoles) on their surface (cuticle) which may also have projecting spines or filaments.

All nematomorph species have separate sexes, with males and females showing characteristic differences in form. Females have a rounded posterior with the cloaca (common reproductive and intestinal opening) at the end. While in males the cloaca is before the end and males of some species also have a forked posterior.

Mature Gordian worms seek out mates in freshwater and form copulatory tangles. After mating the male dies and the female lays eggs in gelatinous strings. Larvae emerge from the eggs 1-2 weeks later and infective suitable arthropod hosts that ingest them while feeding or drinking. Each larva has a spiny proboscis to allow penetration through the gut wall into the blood system (haemocoel) of the host. It appears that the developing parasite absorbs nutrients directly through its cuticle since the digestive system seems to be non-functional.

After several moults within the host, 'pre-adult' worms may induce their host to move to water, where they emerge (in the process often killing their host) and seek a mate to complete their life cycle.

Identification

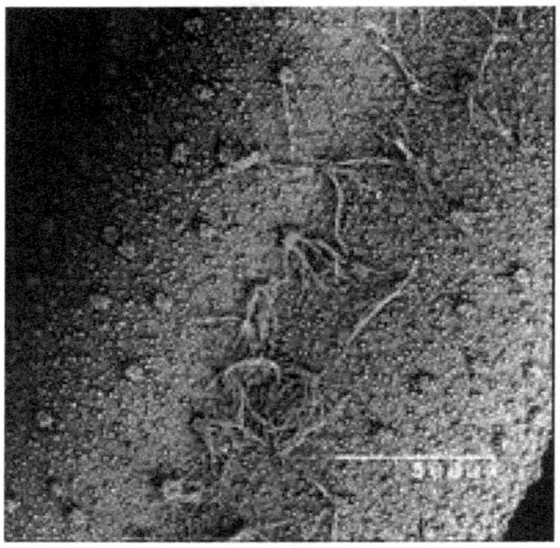

Scanning electron microscope image of the surface of a Gordian worm (genus Chordodes), showing areoles, some with protruding filaments.

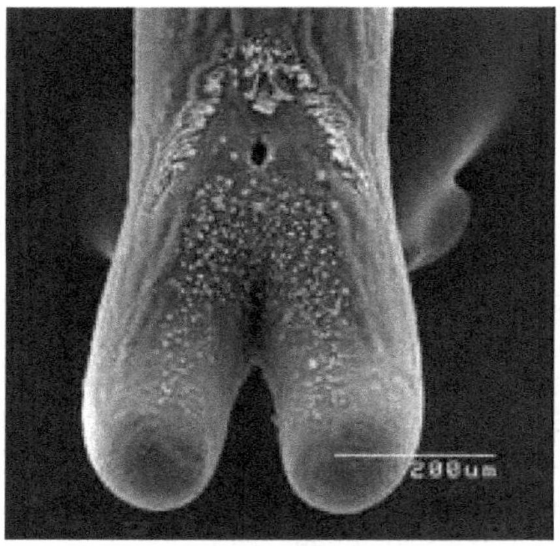

Scanning electron microscope image of forked posterior of Beatogordius sp. male, with cloaca before the end.

To distinguish between the genera of Nematomorpha a range of visible characters are used. These include:

- Colour markings.
- The shape of the anterior and posterior ends.
- The types and patterns of areoles.

The colour of the cuticle can vary from a light creamy brown through to almost black. Some genera (e.g. Chordodes) have a characteristic light and dark mottled appearance while other genera (e.g. Gordius, Gordionus and Beatogordius) have a dark collar with a white tip.

The areoles on the cuticle are an important character and are best observed using a microscope. They range in appearance from simple rounded structures to those with elaborate crowns of protruding filaments. The cuticle may also have tubercles, spines or bristle-fields which, along with the areoles, can be used to distinguish between species.

Other Worms with Similar Lifestyles

Mermithids (Phylum Nematoda) are worms that are superficially similar to the nematomorphs. They also parasitise insects as juveniles and are free-living as adults. They can be distinguished from Gordian worms as female mermithids have no obvious cloaca at the posterior end and male mermithids have 1 or 2 projecting spines (spicules) at the posterior end.

Mermithids have smooth cuticles that lack areoles and are usually pale brown in colour. The cuticle is also much thinner than that of the Gordian worms, so much so that internal structures are visible under microscopic examination.

Myxozoans in Fish

Myxozoans are commonly found parasites that infect both marine and freshwater fishes. They are found principally in the muscle, the brain and the gall bladder of their host fishes.

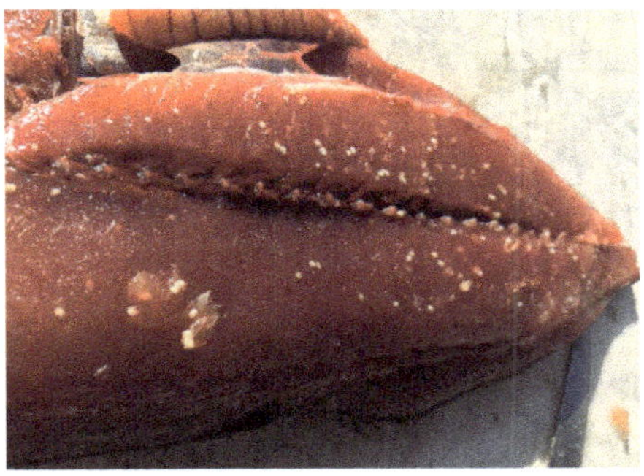

Fish filet with obvious white cysts, in this case a sign of infection with the parasite Kudoa.

Some species of myxozoans can cause death in fish. Non-lethal effects can include the production of small but obvious white cysts in the muscle that make fillets unsightly, unappetising and therefore unmarketable. Some species in the genus Kudoa produce enzymes after their host dies that cause muscle breakdown, making fillets soft and watery. This is known as post mortem muscle liquefaction.

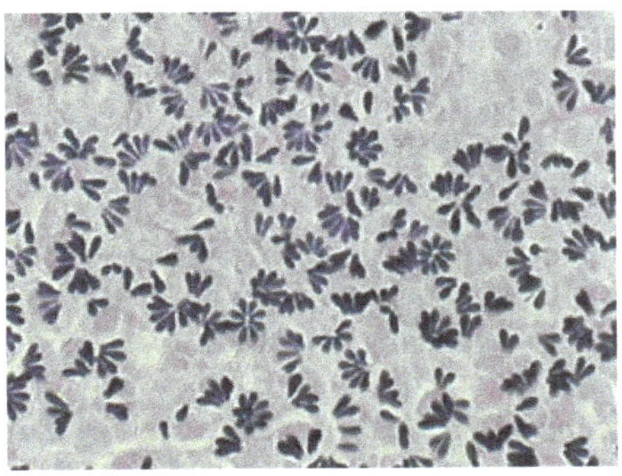

Stained histological section of fish muscle showing numerous Kudoa parasites.

These types of myxozoan infections pose significant challenges in commercial fisheries and are also of concern for aquaculture and Australia's biosecurity.

Taxonomic studies of myxozoans at the Queensland Museum have revealed that they are likely to be far more diverse than their fish hosts. For example, a study of Great Barrier Reef fishes with the parasite Ceratomyxa, found mostly in the gall bladder and just one of the many genera of the Phylum Myxozoa, has shown that there is likely to be almost one species of parasite for every species of fish. This means that Australia's coral reef fish fauna could harbour over 1,500 Ceratomyxa species, of which only 30 (or about than 2%) have actually been discovered by scientists.

Thus, this group is exceptionally rich in coral reef fishes but remains exceptionally poorly known. Knowledge of the identity, range of hosts and geographical distribution of these parasites will increase our understanding of patterns of infection and have specific application when they affect wild harvest and aquaculture fisheries.

Heartworm

Heartworm has been diagnosed in dogs in all parts of the world and is actually very common. This may be due to the fact that heartworm has a virtual 100% prevalence rate in unprotected dogs living in highly endemic areas. Heartworm, also known as Dirofilaria immitis, is transmitted by mosquitoes. The mosquito injects microscopic larvae which grow into an adult worm six to eighteen inches long inside the heart of the affected dog.

The worms can cause mild symptoms, such as coughing, but with time, more severe symptoms such as congestive heart failure, weight loss, fluid build-up in the abdomen, fainting spells, anemia, collapse, and death usually occur.

Luckily we have several excellent medications which can prevent heartworm if given as directed. There are oral medications which need to be given monthly, and which also help protect against some intestinal parasites. There is one topical medication which is also applied monthly. An injectable medication, ProHeart, which is administered every six months, is back on the market after being withdrawn for several years.

Even if a dog has been given preventatives, it is still important to have annual checkups for heartworms by doing a blood test. Many people are not totally compliant about giving the preventive medication on time, and no medication works perfectly. If a dog has heartworms and it is given a dose of preventative, there can be a reaction that is detrimental to the dog, even deadly.

Heartworms were once thought to be rare in cats. Now we know the incidence is anywhere from 10% to 50% of the canine rate. Heartworm disease in cats is different than in dogs. Cats usually test negative on the routine blood test done in the hospital, the worms are smaller and usually do not produce microfilaria which are like baby heartworms that circulate in the bloodstream. Veterinarians have to do different tests, sometimes more than one, to diagnose heartworms in cats.

The symptoms in cats are different also. Cats usually have asthma signs or cough, even vomit. Cats can die acutely. The treatment for adult heartworms in dogs is expensive and potentially harmful to the dog. This is why it is much better to just prevent them in the first place. There is not a treatment for adult heartworms in cats. Many veterinarians are now recommending monthly heartworms preventative for cats in addition to dogs, since heartworm can be such a serious problem.

Hookworms

Hookworms are small, thread-like parasites of the small intestine where they attach and suck large amounts of blood. These parasites are found in almost all parts of the world, being common in dogs, and occasionally seen in cats.

Symptoms are usually diarrhea and weight loss. The parasites can actually suck so much blood that they cause pale gums from anemia, and black and tarry stools. Young puppies can be so severely affected that they die. Infection can be by ingestion of breast milk from an infected mother, by ingestion of infective eggs, or by skin penetration of infective larvae.

Since the adult parasites are so small, they are rarely seen in the stool. Diagnosis of these parasites is by the veterinarian or laboratory finding the microscopic eggs in the stool.

There are a variety of medications that can kill hookworms. The important point to know is that there is no one medicine that will kill all the types of intestinal parasites that exist. Some of the monthly "heartworm preventatives" will also work to treat hookworms.

People exposed to hookworms can develop a rash called cutaneous larval migrans. Infective larvae, usually from contaminated yards, can penetrate human skin and cause red tracts.

Roundworms

There are many types of roundworms, but some of the most common are intestinal parasites of dogs, cats, and raccoons. Puppies are frequently born with roundworms, and kittens can be infected via the mother's milk or feces. Adult roundworms are ivory colored, four to six inches long, and round (not flat) in shape. These parasites can cause diarrhea, vomiting, weight loss, and even coughing in these young patients. In the usual case, the owner will not see the adult roundworms passed in the stool. This is why it is important for the veterinarian to do a laboratory test to check for any parasites that might be present.

It is important to know that animal roundworms can be transmitted to people, and in some cases can cause serious disease. In a recent study, it was reported that almost 14 % of all Americans are infected with Toxocara, the most common roundworm of pets. Although most people infected have no symptoms, the parasite is capable of causing blindness (especially in children) and other systemic illness. The infective agent is the microscopic egg in the animal's stool. It is known that these eggs are very resistant to environmental conditions. They have been shown to live in yards, playgrounds, and fields for up to 10 years.

The most dangerous roundworm is Baylisascaris, a parasite of raccoons that has an affinity for brain tissue. Children infected with this parasite have suffered severe, permanent mental retardation. The majority of raccoons carry this parasite. If wildlife is present on your property, you should patrol the grounds and any raccoon stools should be treated as hazardous waste. Wear disposable gloves to double bag and dispose of the feces. The only thing that will kill the remaining eggs in the soil is fire.

The professional recommends regular deworming of all puppies and kittens to try to reduce the exposure to people. A medication will be dispensed when your puppy or kitten is first seen. Another important measure is monthly parasite preventative, or what we sometimes call "heartworm preventative". Many of these drugs are also effective for roundworms, and are an important part of a wellness program.

Tapeworms

Tapeworms live in the digestive tracts of vertebrates as adults and often in the bodies of various animals as juveniles. In a tapeworm infection, adults absorb food pre-digested by the host, so the worms have no need for a digestive tract or a mouth. Large tapeworms are made almost entirely of reproductive structures with a small "head" for attachment. Symptoms vary widely, depending on the species causing the infection. The largest tapeworms can be 20 m or longer. Tapeworm awareness is importance to humans because they infect people and livestock. Two important tapeworms are the pork tapeworm, and the beef tapeworm.

Veterinary Parasitology

Veterinary parasitology deals with providing comprehensive diagnostic support for the detection and treatment of parasitic infections in animals.

Parasites are all around us—they can be acquired through the environment or via animal vectors such as ticks and flies. Most parasitic infections in animals can also be transmitted to humans, especially children and the elderly. No matter how careful a person may be in taking care of his pets or livestock, they can still be susceptible to subtle parasitic attacks. Parasitic infestations on livestock, for instance, can cause serious consequences in the economy and public health when not properly managed. Thus, it is the fundamental responsibility of the veterinary parasitologist to accurately diagnose these parasitic diseases, and develop methods on how to efficiently protect animals from these threats.

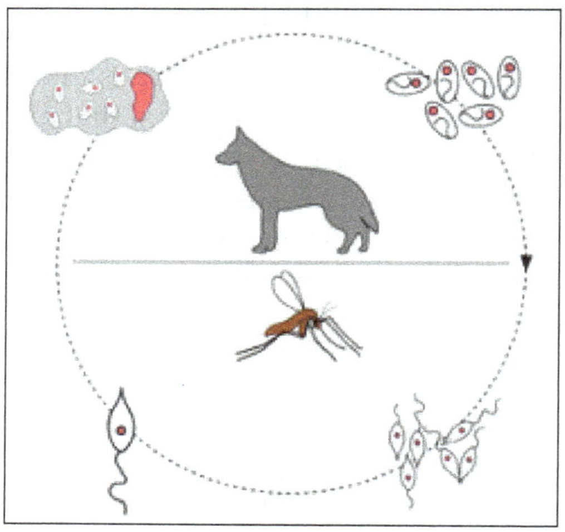

Veterinary parasitology is the study of the origin and development of parasitic infections in animal hosts. It also deals with the taxonomic classification, including morphology, life cycle, and living needs of parasites that can infect both domestic and livestock animals.

Some of the divisions under vet parasitology, include, but are not limited, to:

- Veterinary protozoology (study of unicellular parasites, such as the amoeba).
- Veterinary helminthology (study of roundworms, tapeworms, and flukes).
- Veterinary entomology (study of veterinary-important insect vectors of parasites).

Parasites are organisms that utilize other species such as plants and animals as hosts. These hosts provide the environment that parasites need in order to survive. In fact, the parasitic lifestyle has been extremely successful that the number parasitic species far exceeds the number of free-living species.

Veterinary parasitology is a very dynamic field of study. This is because parasites and their hosts are ever changing—locked into a continuous struggle for survival. Thus, it is essential to understand the mechanics used by both parasite and host to gain advantage against each other.

As a result, veterinary parasitologists not only help in the veterinary practice of improving animal welfare and breeding, but they also contribute significantly to our understanding of how our biological world functions.

Parasites remain one of the most important constraints to animal health, welfare, and productivity. Not only do parasites present an annoyance and discomfort to our pets, they also carry diseases that can prove fatal to both domestic and livestock animals, which may ultimately affect humans as well.

Fortunately, most parasitic infections can easily be diagnosed through physical and laboratory exams, without the need for more invasive procedures.

Veterinarians who specialize in veterinary parasitology are the experts that can detect, identify, and provide support for the treatment of parasitic diseases in animals. They help prevent these harmful diseases from causing disastrous consequences to the economy and public health.

Veterinary Entomology

Veterinary entomology deals with arthropod pests and vectors of disease agents to livestock, poultry, pets, and wildlife. It is T allied with the fields of medical entomology, parasitology, animal sciences, veterinary medicine, and epidemiology. The main pests of veterinary concern are sucking and biting lice, biting flies, nonbiting muscoid flies, bot flies, fleas, and Acari (mites and ticks).

Arthropod Groups

Arthropods that affect animals can be categorized by the intimacy of their host association, and these range from permanent ectoparasites to pests that contact the vertebrate only briefly once every few days.

Permanent Ectoparasites

Some arthropods, such as lice and many parasitic mites, complete their entire life cycle on the host. All stages of sucking lice (Phthiraptera, suborder Anoplura) are mammal parasites and feed on blood. Biting lice (suborders Amblycera and Ischnocera) use either mammal or bird hosts. They feed mostly on skin, hair, and feather debris, but sometimes feed on blood as well. Lice tend to be abundant in cool weather or on animals stressed by poor nutrition or overcrowding. Many lice are specific to one or a few closely related hosts and cannot survive more than one to a few days away from the host. Transmission from host to host is mostly by direct contact.

Parasitic mites (Acari, suborders Mesostigmata, Acaridida, and Actinedida) are found on most groups of birds and mammals. Like lice, most are specific to one host species or a small group of related species. Several genera comprise what are commonly known as "mange mites." Sarcoptes scabei. which causes sarcoptic mange, burrows at the surface of the dermis and exists in a number of races that generally are host specific to swine, dogs, and so on. Demodex mites, causing demodectic mange, live in follicles and can be important especially in immunocompromised hosts. Chorioptes and Psoroptes, causing chorioptic and psoroptic mange, include species of considerable importance for cattle, and wild and domestic sheep. The latter mites complete their development at the skin surface and do not actually burrow in the skin, although mites often are covered by scabs and are frequently called scab mites. Ornithonyssus mites are blood feeders and are especially important for wild and domestic birds, where populations may reach many thousands per host. They occupy fur and feathers, traveling to the skin surface to feed regularly.

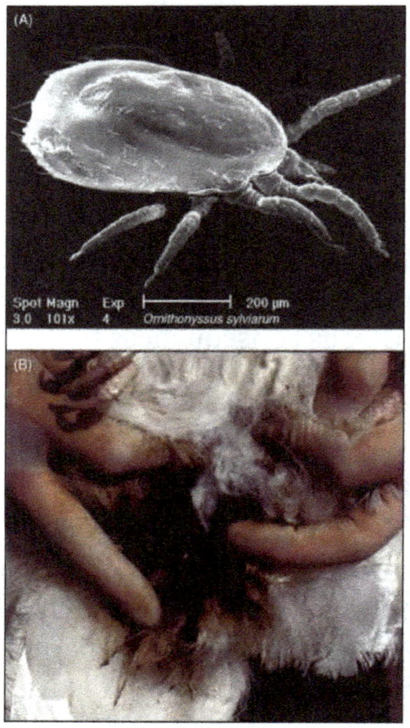

(A) Scanning electron micrograph of the northern fowl mite, O. sylviarum, a permanent ectoparasite of many birds, including domestic chickens. (B) The vent of a chicken, showing the blackened feathers typical of a heavy infestation. This hen has over 20,000 mites.

Some of the more advanced flies are also permanent parasites, and a number of species in three families hardly resemble flies at all because they have secondarily lost their wings (apterous). Members of the dipteran families Streblidae and Nycteribiidae live on bats, whereas members of the Hippoboscidae parasitize various birds and mammals. Some hippoboscids are economically important, such as the sheep ked, Mallophagus ovinus. In all these families, the adult female nurtures a single larva within her body until it is mature; this is a very unusual pattern for insects. After the mature larva exits the female, it promptly pupates on the host or nearby.

Semipermanent Ectoparasites

The semipermanent ectoparasitic arthropods do not complete the entire life cycle on the host, but they do spend at least several days at a time on a vertebrate. The hard ticks (Ixodidae) attach to feed for several days in each of the life stages. Although some, like the cattle tick Rhipicephalus (Boophilus) microplus, complete the entire life cycle on a single host, the most abundant and widespread species tend to use a separate host for each stage. In this case, the engorged tick falls off, molts, and then finds a new host by crawling up on vegetation and waiting for a passing vertebrate to which it attaches. This activity is known as questing. Often the larva hatches from an egg and attaches to a small host such as a rodent, whereas the nymph (the stage after the larval molt) or adult may attach to a larger host such as a deer. An example is the American dog tick Dermacentor variabilis. Adult female hard ticks take a large blood meal, produce a single large batch of eggs (typically several thousand), and then die.

Fleas (Siphonaptera) generally are on a host for most or all of the adult stage, and feed on blood. About 94% of flea species live on mammals, and the rest on birds. Flea eggs fall from the host pelage into a nest environment, where the larvae feed on organic debris and sometimes on excess blood produced by the adults. Fleas thus are often lacking on hosts that do not return to long-term bedding areas or nests.

Bot flies include important species in the dipteran families Oestridae, Gasterophilidae, and Cuteribridae. They spend nearly the entire year as immatures within the vertebrate's body. Eggs, often laid on hairs, hatch and enter the host body.

Horse bot larvae (Gasterophilus) attach to the wall of the gastrointestinal tract for several months before they pass from the host with feces to pupate in soil. Cattle grubs (Hypoderma) migrate through the lining of the esophagus or spinal cord, depending on the species, and eventually form a cyst in the back. After a final period of maturation, larvae exit the cyst and fall into the soil to pupate. Bot fly adults lack functional mouthparts and depend entirely on reserves from the larval stage to sustain them for several days; in this brief time they must find mates and hosts. The invasion of vertebrate tissues by fly larvae is known as myiasis.

Certain other flies also are semipermanent parasites. Among muscoid Diptera, the horn fly, Haematobia irritans, is on cattle most of its adult life, where adults of both sexes take many small blood meals each day. This distinguishes them from the vast majority of blood-feeding flies, which feed far less often. Horn flies leave the host to disperse and to lay eggs in very fresh dung, and then return to the host.

Occasional Parasites

The broad category of occasional parasites includes a range of arthropods. The most intimate host associations in this group include the soft ticks (Argasidae) and some blood-feeding mites such as the bird parasite Dermanyssus gallinae. In both cases, nymphs or adults hide in or near nest areas, sheltered in cracks and crevices or under debris; thus, they are closely associated with animals, although they contact them only periodically. They leave the hiding places, often at night, to feed for periods of 5-30 min, returning to the nest to digest the blood meal. Some soft ticks can withstand dry conditions and years without feeding.

Many serious biting fly pests spend the immature period away from the host, exploiting an entirely different resource base. It is common for larvae to feed on detritus in wet habitats, whereas the adults use plant nectar for energy and blood for egg development. For example, larvae of stable flies live in rotting vegetation, black flies in running water, horse flies and biting midges in swampy mud, or mosquitoes in ponded or slowly moving water. When the adults emerge, they take blood meals at intervals of 1-4 days, but they typically are in contact with the host for only a few minutes at a time. They leave the host to digest the blood in some sheltered resting location. For the higher Diptera (Cyclorrhapha), such as stable flies or tsetse flies, both sexes feed on blood, and multiple blood meals usually are needed to develop a batch of eggs (or, for tsetse, a single mature larva). In the lower Diptera (basal Brachycera and Nematocera) such as horse flies, blackflies, or mosquitoes, only females take blood, and most species require only a single large blood meal to develop an entire batch of eggs numbering 50-300. Some other pests in this general category do not feed on blood but visit the host to take meals of tears or other protein-rich secretions that are also used to develop eggs. A good example is the face fly, Musca autumnalis.

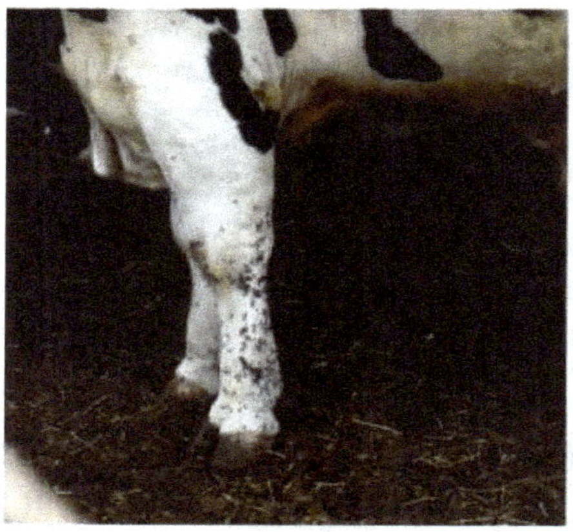

The stable fly, Stomoxys calcitrans may attack animals in high numbers: there are approximately 200 flies feeding on the front leg of this bull. This species is illustrative of the occasional parasites because the adult flies blood-feed for only a few minutes every day or two, and larvae are in rotting vegetation away from the host animal.

Arthropods Cause Damage to Animals

There are several basic ways in which arthropods cause damage to animals, and the different mechanisms interact to impact agricultural production. Arthropod damage to plant crops often is evident to consumers, who react with disgust to cabbage leaves damaged by loopers, corn earworm larvae on an ear of corn, or scale insects on citrus fruit.

In contrast, arthropod damage to animal production tends to be hidden from the consumer because the product is purchased in the form of jugs of milk or wrapped packages of butchered meat. Nevertheless, losses are serious for producers, and costs are passed on to consumers.

Loss of Blood and Tissue Fluids

Many arthropods ingest blood, usually for egg development. Impact of blood loss on the animal reflects the style of feeding and the number of arthropods. Mosquitoes may canulate a vessel, and hosts generally lose only the blood mosquitoes ingest. In contrast, some biting flies macerate the capillary beds of the skin to feed from blood pools. They not only tend to inflict more painful bites, but the bites themselves also lead to a larger quantity of blood loss per feeding insect. For example, horse flies (Tabanidae) may directly remove over 200 ml day^{-1} from a host in a pasture, but blood continues to run from the wound for a period of time, often being fed on by other flies. Many hard ticks (Ixodidae) increase in weight by 100-fold or so as they feed for 7-10 days. Females of very large species of ticks may contain over a milliliter of blood at a time, and hundreds may be attached to a single host animal. Blood or fluids such as lymph are metabolically "expensive" for a vertebrate to produce. Such loss is reflected in reduced feed conversion efficiency, which occurs when animals eat more for a given yield of meat or eggs. Insect feeding also causes significantly lower weight gains or milk production. Losses of 10-20% feed conversion, 0.1-0.2 kg day^{-1} weight gain (cattle), and 5-10% loss in milk yield are not uncommon for animals under heavy attack.

Pain and Interference with Activities

Pain and irritation caused by arthropod attack force animals to alter their feeding or activity patterns and to engage in a number of sometimes vigorous behaviors to defend themselves. There may be economic loss as well, since animals are not feeding normally and must expend energy that might otherwise be directed toward growth or reproduction. For example, stable flies (Stomoxys) and face flies, as well as other biting flies, can cause animals to retreat into groups for refuge. In groups, insect attack rates usually are lower per host (the herd dilution effect), particularly for the animals that occupy the interior of an aggregation. Animals also may enter woods or bodies of water in an apparent attempt to escape insects. Cattle pursued by adults of cattle grubs (Hypoderma) experience no immediate pain from the flies, which cannot bite. The female flies try merely to deposit eggs on the cattle hair at the base of the legs. Still, cattle exhibit an interesting, stereotypical behavior known as "gadding". The animals run at full speed with tails raised straight into the air, which expends energy and may cause accidental injury.

Although pests such as house flies may not cause direct losses to the animals, they are produced near animal operations and thus are a veterinary entomology problem. Excessive numbers of nuisance arthropods cause great annoyance to people living nearby, and thus constitute serious public relations and legal problems for producers. Public health agencies can close facilities unable or unwilling to mitigate such a problem.

Allergic Responses to Saliva

Blood-feeding arthropods possess a potent arsenal of chemicals in their saliva to maintain blood flow (vasodilators, anticoagulants) and sometimes have anesthetics to reduce host defensive response. Like humans, animals can develop allergies to these compounds. Horses commonly react to biting midge (Culicoides) feeding with an allergic reaction called Queensland itch or sweet itch, resulting in skin inflammation and hair loss. Mass emergences of the blackflies Simulium arcticum in Canada and Cnephia pecuarum in the valley of the southern Mississippi River have resulted in the deaths of livestock, probably from allergic responses as well as blood loss. Larvae of sheep blowfly (Lucilia) feed near the skin surface, especially where the wool is wet, and can contribute to a toxic shock-type syndrome fatal to infested sheep. Pets may develop serious allergies to fleas, with resulting hair loss and other symptoms.

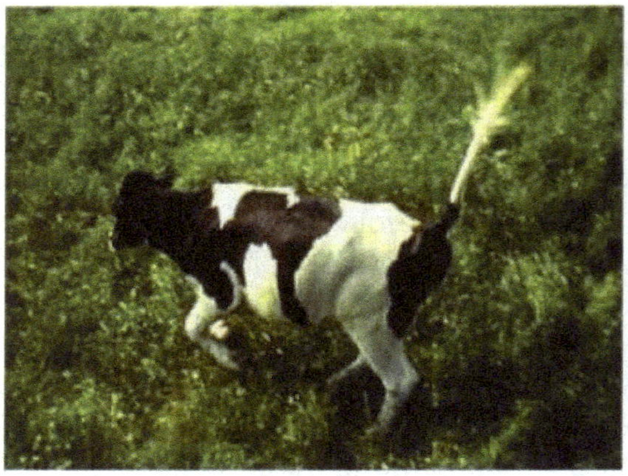

"Gadding" behavior (the tail held up in the air) by a calf being attacked by cattle grub flies (Hypoderma spp.). Vertebrate host behavior can be altered by parasites.

Product Damage

Arthropods sometimes cause direct damage to parts of the animal desired by people. For example, cattle grub (Hypoderma) larvae form large cysts in the backs of cattle. They cut a hole in the skin to breathe, and this skin is the thickest on the animal. Although the holes heal after the larva exits, the scarred skin is less valuable for leather. The presence of larvae also can affect the quality of the meat in this area of the animal, which is the part where the best steaks come from, and damaged meat sometimes must be trimmed at the slaughterhouse. Mites such as Psoroptes and Sarcoptes, as well as many lice, often result in irritation, rubbing, and gross loss or damage to hair and wool.

Cosmetic damage, including rashes or minor hair loss, can be predictably serious to the owner of a pet or a show animal. However, cosmetic damage also can cause losses in animal agriculture out of proportion to actual damage. An example of this is the condition "gotch ear" in cattle caused by the Gulf Coast tick Amblyomma maculatum in the southern United States. Damaged ear cartilage is cosmetic, but causes the animals to be placed in an "odd lot," with per-pound prices less than those of undamaged cattle.

Restricted Trade

Many pests have distinctive distributions, and preventing movement or dispersal into new areas is of paramount importance. Cattle ticks (Boophilus) and screwworms (Cochliomyia hominivorax) were eradicated from the southern United States in the 20th century, but the ticks inhabit Mexico and countries south of it, and screwworms persist on some Caribbean islands and South America.

The U.S. habitat obviously is still suitable. Without complex systems of animal quarantine,treatment, and examination, it is certain these pests would reestablish in the United States.

Exotic arthropods pose a great threat either as direct pests or vectors of disease agents such as those that cause heartwater or African swine fever. The Office International des Epizooties lists diseases of risk for animals worldwide, and one of those on List A (greatest risk) is bluetongue. This viral disease of ruminants, such as cattle and sheep, is transmitted by biting midges, and is endemic in the United States. Trade restrictions from bluetongue cost the U.S. cattle industry many millions of dollars annually, even though cattle themselves do not usually develop obvious disease. Some major trading partners lack bluetongue, and their agricultural authorities fear an impact of bluetongue on their sheep industries, because sheep are more susceptible than cattle are. Western Europe is struggling with trade issues due to a recent, persistent, spreading outbreak of bluetongue extending as far north as northern Germany and England.

Diseases

A number of serious animal disease agents are transmitted by arthropods. The worst of these are tropical, and they cause death and heavy production losses in the affected countries. African trypanosomiasis causes a wasting type disease known as nagana in animals and sleeping sickness in humans, and Theileria parva, called East Coast fever, can cause 90-100% mortality in affected cattle in eastern Africa. People in developed countries tend to underestimate the true value of animals in the developing world. Animals are vital there not only for protein-rich food, but for draft and transportation purposes, and as wealth. They are the basis of many pastoral peoples' economies, and the economic impact of some of these animal diseases can exceed even the impact of similar, serious human pathogens.

Temperate zones also have some rather important arthropod-transmitted animal disease agents, including Anaplasma, dog heart-worm, and equine infectious anemia virus. In the United States and Europe, the direct effects of arthropods on animal production generally exceed losses caused by arthropod-transmitted diseases. However, the role of wild animals as natural reservoirs of pathogens that incidentally infect people is very important in both temperate and tropical zones. Diseases that cycle naturally in animal populations and occasionally infect people are called zoonoses. Zoonoses comprise some of the more notorious arthropod-related human health problems. They include plague (maintained in rodents and transmitted by fleas), Lyme disease (maintained in rodents and transmitted by ticks), and St. Louis encephalitis (maintained in birds and transmitted by mosquitoes). Previously unknown tick-borne ehrlichioses (caused by intracellular bacteria-like organisms in the genus Ehrlichia) have been recently discovered infecting humans in the United States. They are zoonotic in origin and typify a category of "emerging" human diseases that is now of great interest in the medical community.

Veterinary Helminthology

Veterinary helminthology is the study of helminth (worm) parasites of domestic and free-ranging mammals and birds. Some parasitologists would include all vertebrate wildlife. Most attention is focused on species with significant impacts on domestic animal, wildlife or human health, and on the well-being of individuals and communities. While many helminths infect only animals or birds, several species are zoonotic – they are transmissible between animals and people.

Helminth parasites (nematodes, cestodes and trematodes) are ubiquitous among domestic animals and wildlife in ecosystems around the world. Their life cycles depend on close linkages with their hosts and the environment, and transmission for many species depends on amazing behaviors and resilience. Helminths can reduce production (of meat, milk, and wool), can cause clinical disease and death, and many have more subtle effects. The significance of helminths depends primarily on parasite and host species, levels of infection, and the host's overall health status. The detection and identification of many helminths is moving from morphology to molecular biology, but traditional methods remain important. There are four major approaches to the control of helminths: ecological – which depend on shifting the local ecosystem to favor the hosts; chemical – in which drugs are used to treat, and in some cases prevent, helminth infections; genetic – where the aim is to breed livestock with enhanced resistance to important helminths; and immunological – where the goal is safe and effective vaccines. Many helminths are zoonoses – they can transmit between animals and people. Some zoonoses are endemic in animal and human populations, others occur only sporadically in one or both groups. Ecosystem disruptions, including climate change, have the potential to alter patterns of helminth infection and disease, including for some zoonoses. Considerable information is available on helminths of wildlife, but significant knowledge gaps remain for many host species and geographic regions, and for health significance. Critical targets for the future include enhanced control for helminths of domestic animals and for zoonotic species, and increased awareness and understanding of the potential effects of ecosystem disruptions on the occurrence and significance of helminths in all hosts.

Helminths, in veterinary medicine are in four distinct taxonomic groups: nematodes (commonly known as roundworms); cestodes (commonly known as tapeworms); trematodes (commonly known as flukes); and acanthocephalans (commonly known as thorny-headed worms). Globally, acanthocephalans of are of relatively little significance. Species of parasite within each of these four groups share structural, functional and ecological characteristics. Particularly important are: the typical life cycle for each group, involving the production of offspring and their development from immature to adult stages; the locations of immature and adult stages within the organs and tissues of the hosts; the adverse effects these stages have on the hosts; and the ease with which hosts can be treated to remove the parasites and re-infection can be prevented.

While some helminth parasites occur in many parts of the world, others have more restricted distributions. The distributions depend primarily on: 1) History (especially the movement of infected animals, sometimes centuries ago); 2) The current availability of suitable hosts; and 3) A climate supportive of any free-living stages of the parasite, and of other animals (including arthropods and other invertebrates) critical for completion of the parasite's life cycle.

Virtually all domestic animals and wildlife have helminth parasites at some point during their lives, usually as mixed-species infections. In general, the prevalence and abundance of these parasites are higher in young animals than in adults because of variations in inherent resistance, specific immunity, and exposure to the parasites. Also, several helminths have evolved life cycle strategies that enhance the infection of young offspring. For example, egg counts of gastrointestinal nematodes in ewes increase significantly around the time of lambing. This results in large numbers of infective larvae on pastures when the lambs begin to graze.

Helminths: Life Cycles

The life cycle of a helminth is the process by which adult parasites produce offspring, and these develop successfully to infect new and suitable hosts and complete maturation to the adult stage.

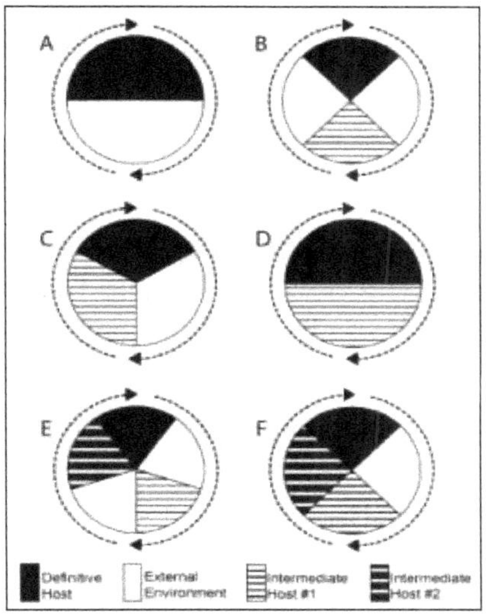

Life cycle patterns of helminth parasites showing species-dependent progress through definitive and intermediate hosts and the external environment. The arrows indicate the direction of parasite progress from adult through immature stages to adult. A – direct life cycle; B-F – indirect life cycles with one (B-D) or two (E-F) intermediate hosts.

The life cycles of parasitic helminths are either direct or indirect. With direct life cycles, characteristic of many nematodes important in veterinary medicine. The adult parasites live and develop only in a mammalian or avian definitive host, in which they undergo sexual reproduction and the parasite, is transmitted among these hosts by free-living stages in the environment. Indirect life cycles, characteristic of other nematodes and of all cestodes, trematodes and acanthocephalans – involve a definitive host, and often the environment, but also require one or more (sequential) intermediate hosts in which immature parasites undergo essential development and may reproduce asexually, but not sexually. Intermediate hosts important in veterinary helminthology include mammals, amphibians, mollusks and arthropods. Completion of the life cycles of several helminth species can also be facilitated by non-essential paratenic hosts – in which there is infection by immature stages but no development, or by transport hosts which simply move immature parasites from place to place on their feet, hair coat or plumage, or in their gastrointestinal tracts.

Helminths and Host Ecology–linkages and Shifts

Anywhere in the world, hosts, parasites and the local environment are intimately linked. Parasites are totally dependent on these linkages for transmission and for persistence in host populations. For example, for helminths with direct life cycles, transmission depends on environmental conditions that support the survival and development of the free-living life cycle stages and host access to these stages. There are the same requirements for helminths with indirect life cycles, but for these the environment must also support the intermediate hosts. For helminths with indirect life cycles transmitted through predator-prey links, relevant food webs must also be maintained.

In many situations, there is balance between the needs of the hosts and of the parasites, but circumstances can shift to favor either the hosts, with a possibility of parasite loss or extinction, or the parasites, with the risk of host morbidity and mortality. For many animal populations, both free-ranging and domestic, these effects on hosts and parasite illustrate the potentially critical role for parasites in the structure and function of local ecosystems, be they savannah, swamp, forest, mountain, or pasture.

Climate change, altered land use, and the search for resources are among the impacts of human activity on ecosystems around the world. A possible result of these impacts is altered patterns of infectious diseases in domestic and free-ranging animals, and in people. For example, for helminth parasites and their hosts the possible effects include shifts in: 1) spatial distributions; 2) host-parasite assemblages and other ecological associations; 3) demographic rates; 4) the seasonal timing of life cycle events for hosts (e.g. mating and birthing) and parasites (e.g. peaks in the availability of infective life cycle stages), and of linkages between these and food supply for the hosts; and 5) patterns of both infection and disease in the hosts. On occasion, and despite the resilience inherent in many ecosystems, these disturbances lead to the emergence of new parasitic diseases, or to the re-emergence of diseases that were common in the past.

Nematodes

Typical adult male and female nematodes are thread-like, have distinct anterior and posterior ends, and vary with species from a few mm to >50 cm in length. Each nematode is essentially a sheath enclosing a bundle of tubular organs for digestion, absorption, reproduction and excretion.

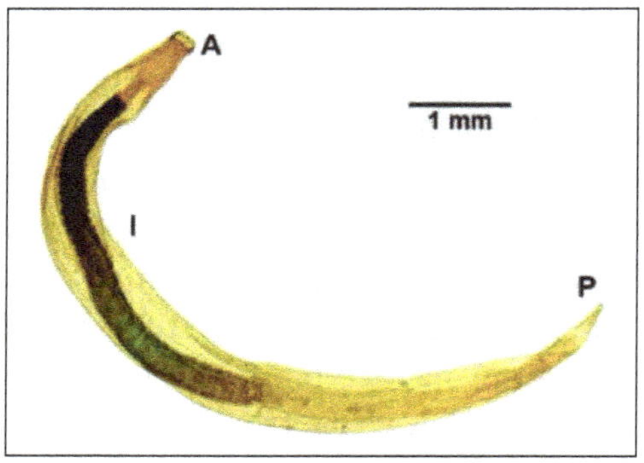

A parasitic nematode – immature female cyathostome from a horse. A – anterior end with mouth; P – posterior end; I – intestine (longitudinal tubular structure with pharynx anteriorly).

Most nematodes have some degree of ecological specificity: each species is found in only one or a few host species; the life cycle stages of each species in the host are almost always in the same organ and tissue; and the life cycle of individuals within a species follow the same basic pattern. Worldwide, probably the most important nematodes of domestic animals and wildlife are those with adults infecting the gastrointestinal system. Considering nematodes as a group, however, adult and immature parasites can live successfully in almost any organ or tissue in any mammalian or avian host. Other parasitic nematodes are found in amphibians, reptiles, fish, and arthropods. There are also nematode species that parasitize plants, and many are free-living in terrestrial, freshwater and marine environments.

The life cycles of all nematodes include adults and four larval stages. Females of most species produce eggs, but some produce first-stage larvae. The larval (immature) stages are miniature, sexually immature versions of the adults and proceed from one larval stage to the next by molting (growing a new sheath beneath the existing sheath, which is then shed). Each nematode species has a larval stage that is infective for its definitive hosts. These infective stages include first- and third-stage larvae free in the environment, first and second stage larvae within eggs, and larval stages in intermediate and paratenic hosts. For almost all nematodes important in veterinary medicine, one egg or larva becomes only a single adult of the next generation.

Cestodes

Adult cestodes are hermaphrodite, have the appearance of a segmented ribbon, and vary with species from a few mm to a meter or more in length. All adult cestodes are parasitic, and the adults of most species live only in the intestinal tract of their definitive hosts. Adults have a distinct anterior holdfast organ (the scolex) which anchors the parasite to intestinal mucosa. The body of a tapeworm consists of a ribbon of connected segments that are produced behind the scolex. Each segment contains one or two sets of reproductive organs, depending on species.

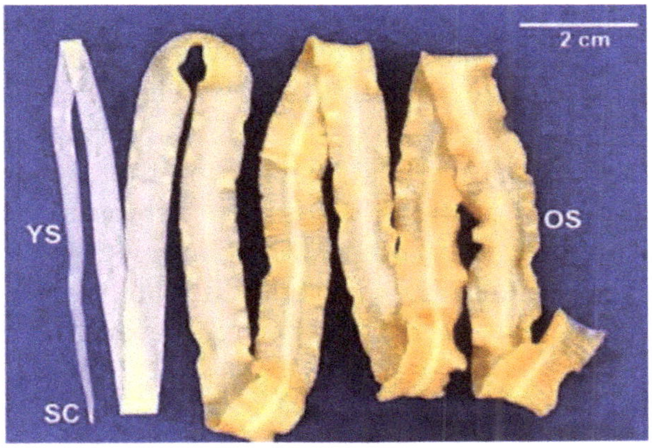

An adult cestode – Diphyllobothrium species from a dog. SC – scolex; YS – younger segments (close to the scolex); OS – older segments (distant from the scolex).

Cestodes lack an anatomical gut, and nutrients are absorbed through the body covering. Cestodes have ecological specificities similar to those of nematodes. All cestodes important in veterinary helminthology have indirect life cycles with a single intermediate host. Depending on parasite species, suitable intermediate hosts include arthropods, gastropods and mammals. Many cestodes can utilize several similar species of these hosts. Infection of intermediate hosts is by ingestion of tapeworm eggs in the feces of the definitive host. Each cestode species has a specific larval stage that is infective for the definitive host, and among cestodes as a group these stages show considerable morphological diversity. For many cestode species, one egg produced by an adult can become only a single adult of the next generation, but with some species there is asexual reproduction by the larvae in the intermediate hosts, and for these one egg can become several adults of the next generation.

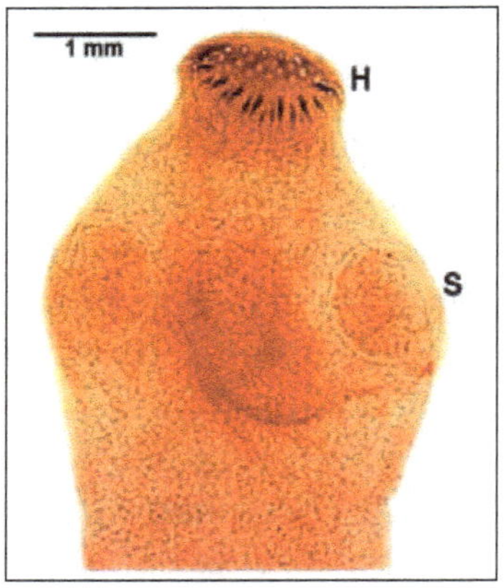

A cestode scolex – Taenia species from a cat. H – hooks on the rostellum (retractable and helps to keep the parasite attached to the host); S – muscular suckers on the scolex (helps to keep the parasite attached to the host).

Trematodes

All adult trematodes are parasitic and the adults of species important in veterinary helminthology are hermaphrodite, leaf-shaped, and vary with species from a few mm to a few cm in length. All have a prominent muscular sucker surrounding the apical mouth, and another on their ventral surface. Trematodes have an anatomical gut.

Adults of most trematodes live in the gastrointestinal system, including the liver, gall bladder and bile ducts. Other species parasitize the lungs, the vascular system or the urinary tract. All trematodes have an indirect life cycle. Depending on species, there may be one or more intermediate hosts, and sometimes paratenic hosts. The first intermediate host is always a snail. Subsequent intermediate and paratenic hosts depend on the trematode species, and include amphibians, fish and mammals. For the larval stages of trematodes in snails there is a consistent sequence of development through the various larval stages to the infective stage, and each stage is morphologically distinct. Asexual reproduction in the snail intermediate hosts is a feature of all trematodes, and thus one egg can become several adults of the next generation.

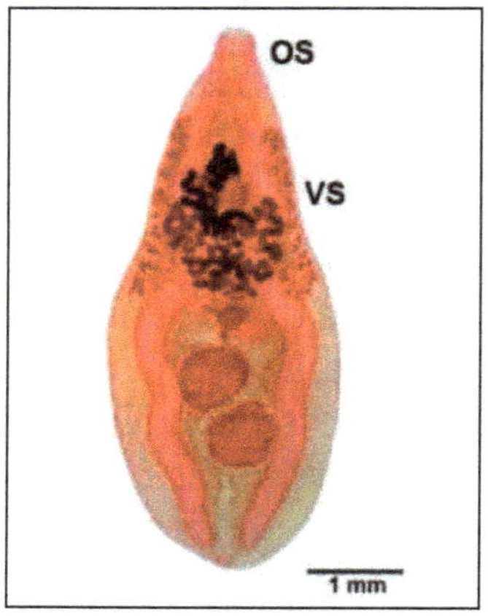

An adult trematode – Metorchis conjunctus from a dog. OS – oral sucker (surround mouth); VS – ventral sucker (partly obscured by the dark, coiled uterus).

Helminths and Disease Mechanisms

Many domestic animals and wildlife infected with helminths rarely if ever show obvious evidence of the parasites. In many of these situations the parasites are probably having adverse effects, but these are subtle and not detected by current clinical and laboratory-based evaluations. Obvious morbidity and mortality among hosts can result, however, when the balance within the ecosystem favors the parasites. Among the many factors precipitating disease and death in such situations are: 1) parasite species that are particularly pathogenic; 2) large numbers of parasites; 3) hosts that are unable to resist, mitigate and curtail the infections: and 4) absence of adequate preventative, anti-parasite and host-supportive interventions. Another key factor in the host-parasite balance is the ubiquity of simultaneous infections with several species of parasite (polyparasitism), as well as with other pathogens such as fungi, bacteria and viruses. Acting together, these multiple pathogens might have additive or synergistic effects on the hosts.

The various life cycle stages of helminth parasites within their hosts can causedamage by several means including: 1) physical and functional disruption of the organs and tissues through which they migrate and in which they establish as adults; 2) interference with appetite and with the digestion, absorption and utilization of key nutrients, potentially causing loss of body mass or reduced growth, reduced wool growth or milk production, and a reduced capability to resist parasites and other pathogens; 3) stimulation of immune responses that are harmful to the host; and 4) alteration in the condition and behavior of hosts that might affect their reproductive success. Some helminth species (e.g. Haemonchus contortus in sheep, Fasciola hepatica in cattle, Oxyuris equi in horses, and Ancylostoma caninum in dogs) are capable of producing distinct disease syndromes in their hosts. These and other species can also act together to suppress host health and productivity. In these situations it can be difficult to precisely identify the relative significance of the various parasite species.

References

- Animal-parasites: qld.gov.au, Retrieved 5 July, 2019
- Parasites-worms, common-pet-health-issues, pet-care: ardmoreah.com, Retrieved 31 January, 2019
- Veterinary-parasitology: all-veterinary-schools.com, Retrieved 28 June, 2019
- Veterinary-entomology-insects, insects: what-when-how.com, Retrieved 8 February, 2019

Chapter 6

Different Types of Veterinary Surgical Procedures

There are numerous surgical procedures which are used in the field of veterinary medicine. Some of these are surgical sterilization, cardiac surgery and ophthalmological surgical procedures. This chapter closely examines these key veterinary surgical procedures to provide an extensive understanding of the subject.

Veterinary surgery is a type of surgery which is performed on animals by veterinarians. It is divided into three primary categories. These categories are orthopaedics (bones, joints, and muscles), soft tissue surgery (skin, body cavities, cardiovascular system, respiratory tracts) and neurosurgery. It is like a practice or a service that provides health care for animals. Veterinary Surgery means the art and science of veterinary medicine and surgery including the diagnosis of diseases in animals and injuries to animals, performing tests on animals for diagnostic purposes, giving advice based on diagnosis and the medical or surgical treatment of animal and performing surgical operations on animals.

Surgical Sterilization

Surgical sterilization has been the cornerstone of efforts to curb pet overpopulation. While undoubtedly effective in preventing reproduction in individual animals, surgical techniques are far from ideal tools for the simple reason that they are expensive. Many owners cannot afford or choose not to spend the money to "neuter" their pets. Additionally, the procedures require general anesthesia and invasive surgery, which, while generally very safe, imposes some risk to the animal. Nonetheless, surgical sterilization remains a valuable means of blunting increases in populations of pets.

Gonadectomy

The most widely used techniques for surgical sterilization of pets involve removal of the gonads (gonadectomy). Terminology and procedures differ between the two sexes:

- In males, each testis with attached epididymis is removed in a procedure commonly referred to as "neutering" or castration. In dogs, both gonads are usually removed through a single incision made just anterior to the scrotum and the incision is sutured closed. Typically in cats, an incision is made into each side of the scrotum and left open to heal.
- In females, the uterus is removed in concert with both ovaries in a procedure called "spaying"

or ovariohysterectomy. This procedure is usually performed through an incision in the mid-ventral abdomen, although some veterinarians prefer a flank incision. The reason for removal of the uterus is to eliminate the possibility of uterine disease following the sterilization.

Each of these procedures is performed under general anesthesia, which presents a small but finite risk to the animal. As with any surgical procedure, there are occasional complications, including bleeding, infection, or dehiscence (breakdown of the suture line, sometimes from the animal chewing), and postoperative observation is clearly warranted.

In addition to eliminating animals from the breeding pool, gonadectomy has a number of beneficial effects on the animal's health, and from the viewpoint of most owners, on the animal's behavior.

Castration and spaying are most commonly performed on dogs and cats that are 6 or more months old. This practice is at odds with efforts to control pet populations because many animals enter or are approaching puberty by that time, and even a short delay can result in the animal producing offspring. Clearly, it would be advantageous to sterilize most pets well before puberty, and a significant body of research now supports the safety and efficacy of early spay-neuter programs for dogs and cats.

Other Techniques for Surgical Sterilization

Surgical techniques not involving the removal of gonads have been applied, though not commonly, to dogs and cats. Vasectomy (cutting the vas deferens) in males and tubal ligation (tying off and cutting the oviducts) in females are not significantly easier to perform that gonadectomy. Although these procedures eliminate the animal from the breeding population, they do not provide the other benefits to animal and owner that are obtained with gonadecomy and are not widely practiced.

Orchiectomy in Dogs

An orchiectomy is a form of castration in male dogs, in which the veterinary surgeon removes the male reproductive organs known as the testicles. Unlike a castration (also referred to as a neuter), an orchiectomy can be either unilateral or bilateral, meaning one or both of the testicles can be removed in this type of surgical procedure. Veterinarians commonly recommend an orchiectomy procedure to male dogs that have been diagnosed with cryptorchidism, but it can also be recommended for dogs at risk of developing health problems specific to male canines. Orchiectomy is a relatively quick procedure, which means the total amount of time the dog spends receiving anesthetic is very short and cost effective for the owner.

Prior to conducting an orchiectomy surgery, the veterinarian will run an overall assessment exam of the patient to insure he is healthy enough to undergo surgery. If cancer or other disease of the prostate or testicles is suspected, diagnostic imagery may also be taken prior to the surgery. The canine will be placed under a general anesthetic and prepped for surgery. The patient will require shaving of the fur around the scrotal and abdominal area before being aseptically scrubbed. The vet will make an incision in the scrotum and above the location of the undescended testicle. Once the testicles are removed, bleeding will be controlled and the incision site will be closed with an absorbable suture material.

Efficacy of Orchiectomy

Orchiectomy in dogs is a highly effective surgical procedure for canines affected by cryptorchidism, testicular cancer, prostate disease, and hormone dependent conditions and is an effective form of castration. The technique used in an orchiectomy surgery greatly benefits the canine as the risk for accidentally cutting the urinary structures and hemorrhage are eliminated.

Orchiectomy Recovery

A dog that has undergone an orchiectomy surgery will be able to return home on the same day as the surgery. At home, physical activities will be restricted and the veterinarian will ask that the owner give the canine a soft, secluded area in the house to rest for the next couple days. An Elizabethan collar will likely be worn to prevent the canine from manipulating the surgical site and medications to prevent an infection, as well as pain, are given. Post-surgical swelling is a possibility, which can be treated at home with cold pack applied directly to the site of swelling in 5 to 15 minute intervals.

Dog Orchiectomy Considerations

Postoperative drainage causing swelling of the scrotum is a common occurrence for canines after surgery. The issue is short-lived and can be prevented with a scrotal wrap. However, if the area appears red or abnormally large, surgical help may be required for the canine.

Orchiectomy Prevention

The need for an orchiectomy cannot be prevented, as the conditions associated with cryptorchidism pose too high of risk to not perform this type of castration surgery. A dog that is diagnosed with undescended testicles should not be allowed to reproduce, as the condition can easily be passed down to offspring.

Surgical Oncology in Small Animals

Cancer is one of the major causes of morbidity in veterinary patients, and surgical removal of tumors is one of the most common surgical procedures performed by veterinarians.

In human surgical oncology, 60% of human patients battling cancer are cured by surgery alone. Likewise, in veterinary medicine, surgery is considered the most important component of treatment in dogs and cats suffering from solid tumors because, in many cases, surgery offers the best chance for improving patients' quality of life.

To help assure a positive outcome, the veterinarian needs a thorough understanding of the basic principles of surgical oncology, including:

1. Characteristics of specific tumor being treated;

2. Surgical options available;
3. Potential need for adjunctive treatments, such as chemotherapy or radiation therapy.

Regardless of the treatment options sought, the overall goal of the therapeutic plan is to improve the patient's quality of life.

Patient Evaluation

The patient's treatment plan should be based on:

1. Complete history;
2. Thorough physical examination;
3. Diagnostic imaging;
4. Clinical pathology with cytology;
5. Histopathology, when appropriate.

Tumor Identification

The annual physical examination plays a key role in detecting neoplasia, either directly via palpation or through paraneoplastic syndromes, which may be found on routine blood and urine analysis. The physical examination allows detection of possible tumor presence and identification of concurrent conditions that may influence the treatment plan.

When a tumor is identified, record its size, location, and gross appearance, and palpate regional lymph nodes. If the lymph nodes are enlarged, firm, or immovable, the suspicion of a metastatic neoplasm rises; however, normal lymph node palpation does not guarantee lack of metastasis. Therefore, some form of lymph node biopsy is recommended in most cases.

Tumor Evaluation

Histopathologic analysis of tissues obtained by biopsy allows definitive diagnosis of:

1. Tumor type (hyperplasia, metaplasia, or neoplasia);
2. Biological behavior (malignant or benign);
3. Aggressiveness;
4. Tumor grade.

There are 4 main types of tumor biopsy techniques:

1. Fine-needle aspiration (FNA) is a cost-effective, minimally-invasive procedure that is useful for differentiating non-neoplastic from neoplastic diseases and, in many situations, obtaining a definitive diagnosis.

- FNA is usually reserved for cutaneous and subcutaneous masses; some tumors, such as mast cell tumors and lymphoma, are readily identifiable on most needle aspirates.

- Intracavitary structures (especially splenic and hepatic masses) may be sampled with ultrasonography or computed tomography guidance.
- However, FNA is generally the least diagnostic biopsy technique due to the minimal amount of tissue sampled and lack of organized tissue architecture, which prevents tumor grading.
- Certain tumor types, such as sarcomas, may not exfoliate cells well, leading to false-negative results. Interpret negative aspirates or aspirates with questionable results with caution, and utilize more aggressive biopsy techniques when clinically appropriate.

2. Needle-Core biopsy is more invasive than FNA but has proven to be highly diagnostic, with an accuracy of 100% for epithelial cell tumors and 94% for mesenchymal cell tumors.

- Needle-core biopsy includes 2 main techniques:
  - Tru-cut needle-core biopsy (soft tissue).
  - Jamshidi needle-core biopsy (ossified tissue).
- Typically, sedation and local anesthesia provide sufficient analgesia for biopsy collection. Caution should be used to avoid infiltrating anesthetic agents into the tumor to prevent distortion of the collected tissues.
- Collecting multiple tissue samples increases the accuracy of biopsies.

3. Incisional biopsy is utilized when less invasive techniques fail to yield a diagnosis.

- Wedge and punch biopsies are examples of incisional biopsy techniques; they are:
  - Especially useful for diagnosis of soft, friable, inflamed, and necrotic tumors.
  - Commonly used to sample peripheral lymph nodes and masses located on the extremities.
- For most cases, include the border between normal healthy tissue and abnormal tissue, which allows the pathologist to determine extent of tumor invasion into normal tissue.

4. Excisional biopsy allows the identified tumor to be removed in its entirety, with or without additional surgical margins.

- While this is a common approach for mass removal in veterinary medicine, it remains controversial:
  - It may provide a diagnosis and, therefore, a therapeutic plan, but the mass is removed without knowing the tumor type.
  - It is also often impossible to excise the mass without contaminating clean tissue planes or complicating future surgical procedures.
- A less invasive biopsy procedure is generally recommended to guide the surgeon in choosing the appropriate method of surgical resection.

- Excisional biopsy is best reserved for cases in which adequate surgical margins are easily achievable with biopsy alone (e.g., small cutaneous mass on trunk of a dog).

Biopsy Procedure

Carefully plan the biopsy procedure to prevent spread of neoplastic cells to unaffected tissues and allow removal of biopsy tracks or scars during surgical excision of the tumor. When obtaining a biopsy from a vascular organ, such as the liver or spleen, coagulation testing should be considered.

Although a presurgical biopsy is not always required, it is essential when the:

- Surgical plan will be affected by tumor characteristics.
- Tumor location will make closure of the surgical site difficult without reconstructive surgery (i.e., skin flaps, grafts).
- Owner's willingness to treat may be altered based on diagnosis.

Once the biopsy is collected and properly preserved, have it processed and evaluated by a histopathologist.

Grading and Staging

Tumor Grading

Tumor grade is the histopathologic assessment of the tumor's aggressiveness, and includes information, such as the mitotic index, invasiveness into surrounding tissues, and degree of differentiation. This information is valuable when the surgeon is developing a treatment plan for the patient.

For some tumor types, the grading scheme may also include features, such as percent necrosis; for these neoplasms, a grade may not be accurately assessed by incisional biopsy.

Tumor Staging

If the tumor is suspected to be malignant, tumor staging establishes to what extent the tumor has invaded local, regional, or distant (systemic) tissues.

Method of tumor metastasis is highly dependent upon the tumor type: Carcinomas and round cell tumors tend to spread via lymphatic routes, while sarcomas tend to spread via hematogenous routes. Common areas where metastatic disease is identified include the lungs and lymph nodes.

In most cases, the following diagnostics are recommended:

- Three-view thoracic radiographs.
- Regional lymph node palpation.
- Biopsy (lymph node palpation does not guarantee lack of metastasis).

Additional diagnostics, such as abdominal ultrasound, may be needed depending on the biologic behavior of the tumor. Other modalities, such as computed tomography or magnetic resonance, may help increase the sensitivity of detecting metastatic disease and more accurately determine the local extent of the tumor in an effort to determine prognosis and help guide resection.

Surgical Intervention

There are 4 levels of surgical aggressiveness, or surgical "dose," to classify the extent of surgical resection. The most common surgical mistake is use of a surgical dose that is too low, which results from concerns about the ability to close the resultant defect. However, if the diagnosis of malignancy has been confirmed, it may be better to manage an open wound than leave tumor cells behind.

Surgical Planning

Careful surgical planning should be performed, as the first surgery is often the surgeon's best chance for achieving a positive outcome.

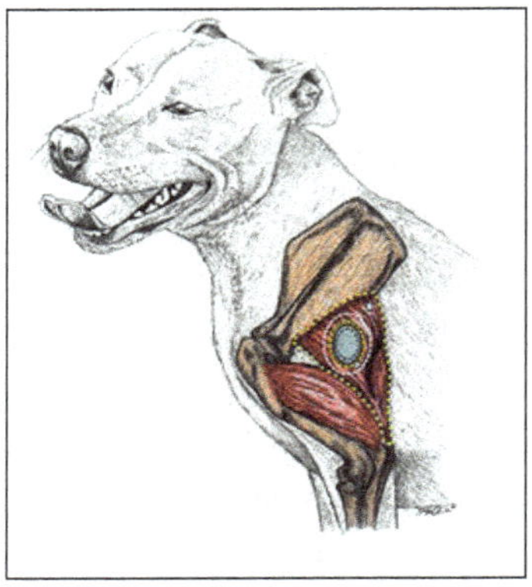

Figure shows a representation of a primary soft tissue tumor (blue), tumor pseudocapsule, and surrounding reactive zone (yellow), along with two satellite tumors (light blue); the lateral margins of the 4 levels of surgical resection are depicted (dotted lines): intralesional (inner most black dotted line), marginal (black dotted line at the level of the pseudocapsule), wide (white), and radical excision (chartreuse).

Multiple factors should be considered when determining aggressiveness of surgery:

- Type of tumor;
- Short- and long-term prognosis;
- Ability to achieve desired surgical margins, with an acceptable level of morbidity;
- Concurrent disease;
- Owner wishes;
- Availability of adjunctive therapy, if needed following surgery.

Surgical Doses

- Intralesional, or debulking, surgery is incomplete resection of a tumor (inside the pseudocapsule) with residual gross disease; it is rarely an acceptable treatment for neoplastic diseases, whether benign or malignant. This technique leaves a tumor cell burden that is often too large to result in a positive outcome even with adjunctive treatments, such as radiation therapy and chemotherapy.

- Marginal resection is defined as removing the majority of the tumor just outside the tumor's pseudocapsule. This approach works well with lipomas and other benign tumors; however, it tends to fail with malignant neoplasms because satellite tumors are often left behind. In some cases, marginal resection can be combined with adjuvant therapies, such as radiation or chemotherapy, to provide an optimum outcome. Excisional biopsy of a malignant tumor, without prior knowledge of tumor type, is essentially an unplanned marginal resection and should be avoided in most cases. Marginal resection of malignant tumors can complicate subsequent surgical interventions, which may require a more aggressive approach, as the remaining neoplastic cells are usually poorly defined.
- Wide resection is a form of curative-intent surgery: The intent is to resect macroscopic (primary tumor) and microscopic (satellite cells) tumor burdens, including biopsy tracks. This surgical dose is recommended over intralesional and marginal resections for treatment and management of solid tumors.
- Radical resection is removal of an entire tissue compartment. Examples include removal of a complete organ, such as splenectomy to remove a splenic hemangiosarcoma or limb amputation to treat appendicular osteosarcoma. Depending on tumor location, type, and size, radical resection is occasionally needed to completely excise the primary tumor and its surrounding pseudocapsule and satellite tumor cells.

In some cases, adequate surgical margins may be too disfiguring, painful, or expensive; minimally advantageous; or simply incompatible with life. Therefore, when planning radical resections, strongly consider patient quality of life.

Determining Surgical Margins

In order to achieve a wide resection, excise a normal tissue margin en bloc with the gross tumor. Determine the width of the surgical margins by:

- Tumor type and grade, if appropriate (eg, mast cell tumors);
- Biologic behaviour;
- Anatomic location;
- Barrier provided by surrounding tissues (tumor resistant fascial layers).

It is imperative to remember that margins are 3-dimensional:

- Lateral margin width is determined by tumor type and biologic behavior.
    - Benign tumors and most malignant carcinomas can be completely resected with 1 cm lateral margins.

- Soft tissue sarcomas can be resected with 3 cm lateral margins.
- Mast cell tumors are typically resected with at least 2 cm lateral margins, although grade 1 tumors may be adequately excised with 1 cm margins.

- Deep margins tend to be the hardest to predict, and are universally determined by natural tissue barriers if deep margins (1–3 cm) are not possible.
    - Fat, subcutaneous tissue, muscle, and parenchymal tissue do not provide adequate barriers to tumor invasion or suffice as deep margins.
    - Connective tissues, including muscle fascia, cartilage, and bone, are resistant to neoplastic invasion, proving a natural tissue barrier.

In order to accurately achieve the desired lateral margin, use of a surgical marking pen and ruler is advisable.

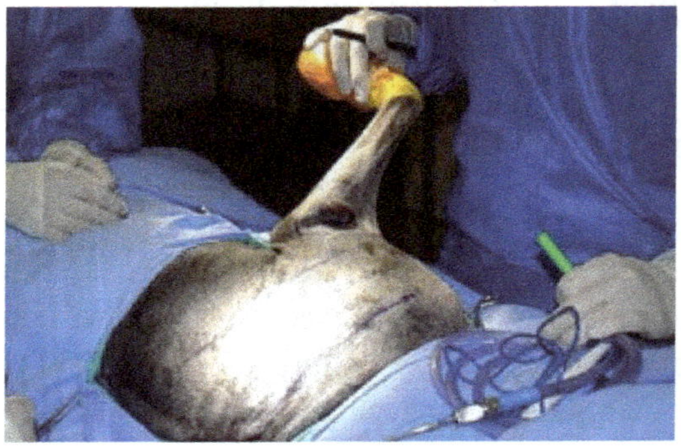

Mark the lateral surgical margins with a surgical marking pen; for this soft-tissue sarcoma, the edge of the visible tumor is first marked, followed by marking a 3-cm lateral margin.

Because of this protective barrier, deep margins should include removal of at least 1 fascial plane; however, vaccine-associated sarcomas require removal of at least 2 fascial planes.

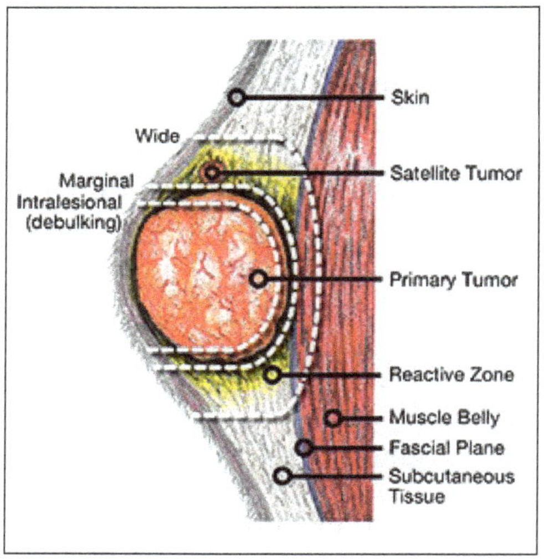

Figure shows deep surgical margins are dependent upon the tissue layers and fascial planes, not actual measured depth. The intralesional margin is an incomplete resection inside the surrounding pseudocapsule (black line), marginal resection is dissection exterior to the surrounding pseudocapsule within the reactive zone (yellow), and wide margin resection removes both microscopic and macroscopic disease, including at least 1 fascial layer.

Tissue Handling

Careful tumor handling is required to prevent exfoliation of cells and local recurrence. To minimize seeding of neoplastic cells, avoid direct handling of the tumor and change surgical gloves and instrument packs between tumor excision and closure.

Surgical Closure

For some large defects in areas that can be easily bandaged (e.g., extremity, trunk), consider leaving the wound open while awaiting the biopsy report. If the margins are not clean, resect additional tissue until a clean margin is obtained; then close the wound. This is particularly useful when the wound requires major reconstructive surgery, such as an axial pattern flap or skin graft.

Make the decision to use a surgical drain during closure carefully, and avoid if possible. Placement of a drain may increase the chance of seeding neoplastic cells and complicate future resections, if the primary resection was incomplete.

Tissue Analysis

Resected tissue should be properly prepared for analysis:

- If the resection is marginal, it is helpful to "pin" the tissue on cardboard, which prevents shrinkage during fixation.
- Marking the surgical margins with ink (e.g., India ink) or suture strands helps the pathologist determine the extent of tumor resection.
- With large tumors, making several partial thickness slices (i.e., "loafing") with a scalpel blade ensures the entire sample is adequately fixed.
- Tissue should be promptly placed in formalin at a ratio of 10 parts formalin to 1 part tissue.

Dirty Margins

Despite the surgeon's best efforts, biopsy analysis following resection occasionally reveals that the tumor was inadequately resected. Treatment of choice for most dirty margins is additional surgery to excise the surgical scar and an additional margin of normal tissue (at least 1 cm). If additional resection is not feasible due to tumor location, adjuvant therapy, such as radiation, may further eliminate the local tumor burden and decrease the chance for recurrence.

General Rules for Collecting Diagnostic Tissue Biopsies

- Substantial tissue biopsies yield better diagnostic results.
- Multiple tissue samples increase the overall understanding of the sampled site.

- When handling tissue samples, take great care to avoid iatrogenic artifacts.
- Always submit tissue samples to a pathologist along with pertinent, detailed information about the patient and tissues biopsied.
- Remove any biopsy tracks or scars during tumor excision.
- Fix tissue samples from needle-core, incisional, and excisional biopsies in 10% buffered formalin at a ratio of 10:1 (formalin: tissue).

Cardiac Surgery in Animals

Cardiac surgery includes procedures performed on the pericardium, cardiac ventricles, atria, venae cavae, aorta, and main pulmonary artery. Closed cardiac procedures (i.e., those that do not require opening major cardiac structures) are most commonly performed; however, some conditions require open cardiac surgery (i.e., a major cardiac structure must be opened to accomplish the repair). Open cardiac surgery necessitates that circulation be arrested during the procedure by inflow occlusion or cardiopulmonary bypass. Venous inflow occlusion provides brief circulatory arrest, allowing short procedures (less than 4 minutes) to be performed. Longer open cardiac procedures require establishing an extracorporeal circulation by cardiopulmonary bypass to maintain organ perfusion during surgery.

Preoperative Management

Animals requiring cardiac surgery often have prior cardiovascular compromise that should be corrected or controlled medically when possible before anesthetic induction. Congestive heart failure (CHF), particularly pulmonary edema, should be managed with diuretics (e.g., furosemide) and angiotensin-converting enzyme (ACE) inhibitors (e.g., enalapril, benazepril, lisinopril) and an inodilator (pimobendan) before surgery. Cardiac arrhythmias should be recognized and treated . Other antiarrhythmic drugs to consider include sotalol and amiodarone. Lidocaine is effective for management of ventricular tachyarrhythmias during and immediately after surgery. Supraventricular tachycardia may require digoxin, β-adrenergic blockers (e.g., esmolol, propranolol, atenolol), or calcium channel–blocking drugs (e.g., diltiazem) before surgery. Atrial fibrillation should be controlled before surgery with a β-blocker or a calcium channel blocker with or without digoxin to lower the ventricular response rate to below 140 beats per minute. Alternatively, amiodarone may be used to control the ventricular response rate, and in a small percentage of cases, to convert atrial fibrillation to normal sinus rhythm. Animals with bradycardia should undergo an atropine or glycopyrrolate response test before surgery. If bradycardia is not responsive to atropine or glycopyrrolate, temporary transvenous pacing or constant intravenous infusion of isoproterenol may be required.

All animals should undergo a complete echocardiographic evaluation before cardiac surgery; an incomplete or inaccurate diagnosis can have devastating consequences. With the advent of Doppler echocardiography, cardiac catheterization is no longer routinely necessary before cardiac surgery.

Anesthesia

Anesthesia of the patient with cardiac compromise has risks that vary depending on the cause of the underlying disease. For example, the anesthetic protocol that is safest for the patient with mitral regurgitation can be dangerous for the patient with aortic stenosis. The pathophysiology of the patient's cardiac condition needs to be fully understood. Likewise, the practitioner needs to have a working knowledge of the pharmacology of the drugs used to manipulate heart rate and blood pressure. Although cardiac surgery is typically performed at veterinary teaching hospitals and referral institutions, veterinarians from a variety of practices are required to anesthetize the patient with heart disease.

Table: Cardiovascular Parameters for Patients with MR, SAS, or Tamponade.

Parameter	Mitral Regurgition	Subaortic Stenosis	Cardiac Tamponade
LV preload	Normal to ↑	↑	↑
Heart rate	↑	Slow normal to	↑
Rhythm	Maintain NSR	Maintain NSR	Maintain NSR
Contractility	Maintain	Maintain	Maintain
SVR	↓	Modest ↑	↑
PVR	Avoid ↓	Avoid ↓	Maintain

LV, Left ventricular; MR, mitral regurgitation; NSR, normal sinus rhythm; PVR, pulmonary vascular resistance; SAS, subaortic stenosis; SVR, systemic vascular resistance.

Preanesthetic medication is appropriate for most animals undergoing cardiac surgery. Parenteral opioids (i.e., hydromorphone, butorphanol, buprenorphine, and fentanyl) induce sedation with minimal cardiovascular effects; however, all opioids can produce respiratory depression and bradycardia. α2-Agonists (e.g., demedetomidine) and acepromazine should be avoided in cardiac patients owing to significant alterations in hemodynamic parameters associated with their administration. Anticholinergics (i.e., atropine and glycopyrrolate) should be administered only as needed. Carefully consider whether an elevated heart rate will assist or hinder forward flow of blood in the individual patient. Benzodiazepines (e.g., diazepam 0.2 mg/kg, midazolam 0.2 mg/kg) have minimal cardiopulmonary effects and enhance sedation when given alone or combined with opioids. Some patients may have an unpredictable behavioral response (e.g., excitation, aggressiveness) to benzodiazepine administration. Therefore, they are often used in combination with an opioid.

Induction of anesthesia should be undertaken with caution in animals with cardiopulmonary compromise. Thiobarbiturates should be avoided in patients with significant cardiac disease because they result in dose-dependent cardiac depression and are arrhythmogenic. Propofol (Diprivan or Rapinovet) produces rapid induction but causes essentially the same cardiovascular compromise as thiobarbiturates. The addition of fentanyl decreases propofol requirements in healthy dogs with minimal alteration in cardiovascular parameters. Ketamine combined with diazepam may be appropriate for induction of compromised patients. It should be avoided in animals with mitral insufficiency because it increases the regurgitant fraction by increasing peripheral vascular resistance. However, it is the induction agent of choice in animals with pericardial constriction. Opioids can be used for induction of very sick and compromised dogs; however, opioids do not induce hypnosis, so intubation may be difficult. Etomidate is not arrhythmogenic, maintains cardiac output, and offers rapid induction, although it is associated with longer and poorer recoveries. Mask induction is discouraged in all patients with cardiopulmonary disorders because the patient's reduced cardiac output will cause an increased time to achieve adequate induction. Additionally, inhalants cause marked hypotension, which is often undesirable. A balanced anesthetic approach using benzodiazepine, opioids, and modest amounts of inhalant is generally much safer. Atracurium is a short-acting muscle relaxant that is not dependent on metabolism or excretion to terminate its action; it may be used if further muscle relaxation is needed (it must be used with intermittent positive-pressure ventilation [IPPV]).

Thoracic surgery always requires controlled ventilation. Controlled ventilation can be achieved by manually squeezing the reservoir bag or by attaching a mechanical ventilator to the anesthetic machine. Ideally, mechanical ventilation should achieve a tidal volume of 6 to 10 ml/kg of body weight at an inspiratory pressure of less than 20 cm of water. Ensuring adequate ventilation is accomplished by optimizing tidal volume, inspiratory pressure, and respiratory rate to achieve ventilation with the least risk of causing pulmonary injury or cardiovascular compromise. Ultimately, the goal of mechanical ventilation is to maintain normocapnia. Ventilation can be monitored by measurement of end-tidal CO_2 by capnography, or of arterial CO_2 by blood gas analysis.

Successful inflow occlusion requires meticulous anesthesia. Intraoperative and postoperative care may be complicated and may require multiple vasoactive medications. Balanced anesthetic techniques that minimize inhalation anesthetic agents are indicated (e.g., fentanyl citrate plus atracurium besylate combined with isoflurane). Administration of a single dose of dexamethasone after induction may be beneficial in reducing cardiac damage and improving postoperative outcomes. Mild hypothermia (32 °C to 34 °C) reduces basal metabolic rate, allowing lengthening of occlusion time; however moderate hypothermia (<32 °C) is associated with spontaneous ventricular fibrillation. Animals should be hyperventilated for 5 minutes before inflow occlusion. Ventilation is discontinued during inflow occlusion and is resumed immediately upon reestablishment of blood flow. Drugs and equipment for full cardiac resuscitation must be available immediately after inflow occlusion. Gentle cardiac massage may be necessary after inflow occlusion to reestablish cardiac function. Digital occlusion of the descending aorta during this period helps direct available cardiac output to the heart and brain. If ventricular fibrillation occurs, immediate internal defibrillation is necessary as soon as inflow occlusion is discontinued. Constant intravenous infusion of lidocaine should be initiated before inflow occlusion and continued as necessary. Epinephrine, administered as a constant rate infusion, should be given as the animal is being weaned off inflow occlusion or a pump. If long-term inotropic support is necessary, dobutamine or amrinone should be given.

Transesophageal echocardiography (TEE) can be an invaluable tool for assessing both cardiac function and volume status in the cardiac patient. Its use intraoperatively and immediately postoperatively can guide the choice of pharmacologic intervention and can assist in assessing the effectiveness of therapy. Central venous pressure measurements have been shown to poorly correlate with volume status. When TEE is used, ventricular filling can be visualized and volume replacement modified accordingly.

Antibiotics

Perioperative antibiotics are indicated for cardiac procedures lasting longer than 90 minutes. First-generation cephalosporins (e.g., cefazolin, cephapirin) can be administered intravenously at induction and repeated once or twice. For cardiac procedures involving circulatory arrest or cardiopulmonary bypass, intravenous cefoxitin should be administered before surgery and continued for 24 hours after surgery owing to impairment of humoral host defenses associated with these procedures.

Surgical Anatomy

The heart is the largest mediastinal organ. It generally extends from the third rib to the caudal border of the sixth rib; however, variations have been noted among breeds and between individuals. The heart base (i.e., the craniodorsal aspect [from where the great vessels originate]) faces dorsocranially, whereas the apex (i.e., formed by muscles of the left ventricle) points caudoventrally. Except for a portion of the right side of the heart (cardiac notch), most of its surface is covered by lung. The right ventricular wall accounts for approximately 22% of the total heart weight; the left ventricular wall accounts for nearly 40%.

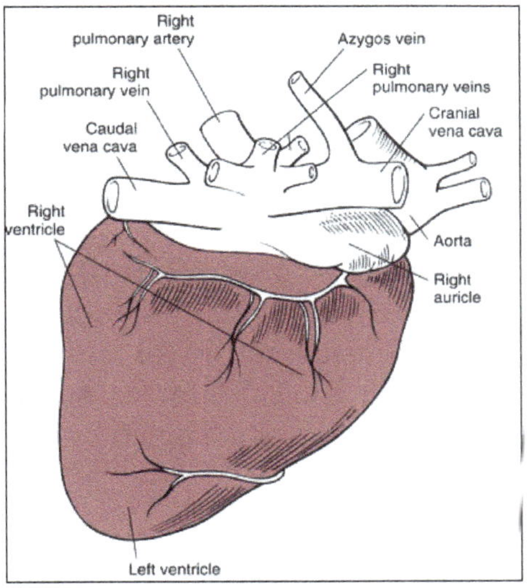

Cardiac anatomy as viewed from the right side.

The right atrium receives blood from the systemic circulation. The coronary sinus enters the left caudal aspect of the atrium, ventral to the caudal vena cava. The caudal vena cava returns blood from the abdominal viscera, the pelvic limbs, and a portion of the abdominal wall. The cranial vena cava returns blood to the heart from the head, neck, thoracic limbs, and ventral thoracic wall, and from a portion of the abdominal wall. The azygos vein usually enters into the cranial vena cava; it carries blood from the lumbar regions and the caudal thoracic wall. The brachycephalic trunk is the first large artery from the aortic arch. The common carotid arteries usually arise from it as separate vessels. The left subclavian artery arises from the aortic arch distal to the brachycephalic trunk (the right subclavian is a branch of the brachycephalic trunk). The vertebral arteries, costocervical trunk, internal thoracic arteries, and axillary arteries branch from the subclavian vessels.

The pericardium is a thick, two-layer sac composed of outer fibrous and inner serous layers. The pericardial cavity is located between two layers (visceral and parietal) of serous pericardium and normally contains a small amount of fluid. The fibrous pericardium blends with the adventitia of the large vessels, and its apex forms the sternopericardiac ligament. Phrenic nerves lie in a narrow plica of pleura adjacent to the pericardium at the heart base. Complete pericardiectomy requires that these nerves be elevated to avoid incising them. The vagus nerves lie dorsal to the phrenic nerve. They divide to form dorsal and ventral branches that lie on the esophagus in the caudal thorax. The left recurrent laryngeal nerve leaves the vagus and loops around the aortic arch distal to the ligamentum arteriosum to run cranially along the ventrolateral tracheal surface.

Surgical Technique

Cardiac surgery is not fundamentally different from other types of general surgery, and similar principles of good surgical technique (i.e., atraumatic tissue handling, good hemostasis, and secure knot tying) apply. Consequences of poor surgical technique are often devastating. Cardiac surgery differs from other surgeries in that motion from ventilation and cardiac contractions adds to the technical difficulty of performing these procedures. Approaches that provide limited access to dorsal structures require that surgeons incise, suture, and ligate structures located deep within the thorax. Ligature placement using hand ties is useful in such situations, and the ability to place hand-tied knots should be considered a fundamental skill for cardiac surgeons. Secure knot tying is critically important for successful cardiac surgery. Hand tying of knots is fast and produces tighter and more secure knots than instrument tying. The one-handed knot tie technique is best suited to the fine sutures used in cardiac surgery. Tight knots are facilitated by throwing the first two or three throws in the same direction before finishing with square knots for security.

Closure of cardiovascular structures requires precise suturing techniques and good instrument handling skills to minimize hemorrhage. Using fine suture with swaged-on atraumatic needles and carefully following the needle contour when suturing (to minimize the size of needle tracts) are important. "Palming" of needle holders is a good skill for fast suturing but should be avoided when suturing inside the thoracic cavity. Finer control is gained by grasping instruments with fingers placed in the instrument rings.

Inflow Occlusion

Inflow occlusion is a technique used for open heart surgery in which all venous flow to the heart is temporarily interrupted. Because inflow occlusion results in complete circulatory arrest, it allows limited time to perform cardiac procedures. Ideally, circulatory arrest in a normothermic patient should be less than 2 minutes, but it can be extended to 4 minutes if necessary. Circulatory arrest time can be extended up to 8 minutes with mild, whole-body hypothermia (32 °C to 34 °C). Temperatures below 32 °C may predispose to spontaneous ventricular fibrillation and should be avoided. The advantage of inflow occlusion is that it does not require specialized equipment; however, the limited time available to perform the surgery requires that the procedure be well planned and executed with speed and expertise.

Depending on the cardiac procedure that is being done, perform a left or a right thoracotomy or a median sternotomy. With a right thoracotomy or median sternotomy, occlude the cranial and caudal vena cava and the azygos vein with vascular clamps or Rumel tourniquets. Make a Rumel tourniquet by passing umbilical tape around the vessel, then thread the umbilical tape through a piece of rubber tubing that is 1 to 3 inches long. When the umbilical tape has been adequately tightened to occlude the vessel, place a clamp above the rubber tubing to hold it securely in place. Take care to prevent injuring the right phrenic nerve during placement of the clamps or tourniquets. For left thoracotomies, pass separate tourniquets around the cranial and caudal venae cavae. Then, while dissecting dorsal to the esophagus and aorta, occlude the azygos vein by placing a tourniquet around it.

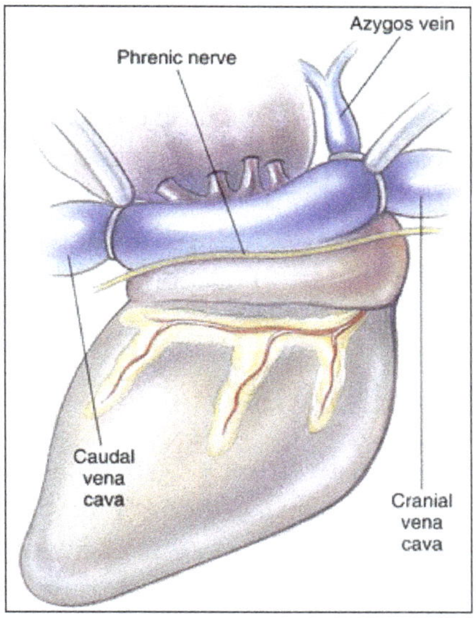

To occlude cardiac inflow from the right side of the thorax, pass tapes around the caudal vena cava and the common drainage of the azygos veins and the cranial vena cava.

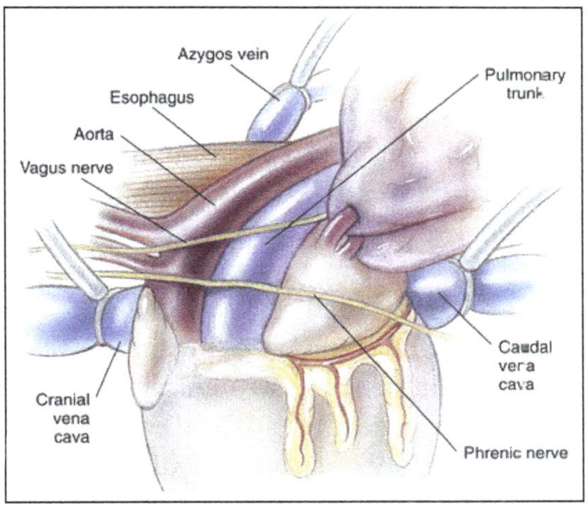

During inflow occlusion from the left side of the thorax, pass tapes around the cranial and caudal vena cava and the azygos vein. Fashion tourniquets for inflow occlusion by passing the tapes through rubber tubing.

Cardiopulmonary Bypass

Cardiopulmonary bypass is a procedure whereby an extracorporeal system provides flow of oxygenated blood to the patient while blood is diverted away from the heart and lungs. This greatly extends the time available for open cardiac surgery. Several advances (i.e., development of membrane oxygenators, improved methods of myocardial protection, increased availability of monitoring technologies, and improved veterinary critical care) have made cardiopulmonary bypass increasingly feasible in dogs. Cardiopulmonary bypass can be used to treat dogs with congenital or acquired cardiac defects.

Healing of Cardiovascular Structures

Vascular structures heal quickly, forming a fibrin seal within minutes. Epithelialization and early endothelial regeneration occur in veins used for grafts. Thrombosis commonly occurs in small veins that have been traumatically occluded for short periods of time; however, thrombosis of large veins occluded during inflow occlusion or cardiac bypass procedures has not been a clinically recognized problem. To prevent thrombosis of vascular structures, they should be handled gently, because trauma may lead to the deposition of platelets, fibrin, and red cells on the intimal surface. If the torn intima is lifted upward, a flap may develop that partially or completely occludes the distal lumen. This in turn can lead to accumulation of blood within the vessel wall, vascular sludging, and thrombosis.

Suture Materials and Special Instruments

Polypropylene (Prolene, Surgipro) and braided polyester (Ticron, Mersilene) suture are the standard sutures used for cardiovascular procedures. The sizes most commonly used are 3.0, 4.0, and 5.0, although smaller sizes may be needed for vascular anastomoses. Sutures should be available with swaged-on taper-point cardiovascular needles in a variety of sizes. Some procedures require that the suture be double-armed (i.e., with needles at both ends). Teflon pledgets are useful for buttressing mattress sutures in ventricular myocardium or great vessels.

Successful cardiac surgery requires proper surgical instrumentation. Most of the basic instruments required for general surgery can be used for cardiac surgery; however, a few specialized instruments are desirable for thoracic surgery. The standard thoracic retractor is a Finochietto retractor. It is helpful to have retractors of at least two sizes to accommodate animals of different sizes. Self-retaining orthopedic retractors can substitute as thoracic retractors in small dogs and cats. The standard tissue forceps for thoracic surgery is a DeBakey tissue forceps. At least two DeBakey forceps should be available, and it is helpful if one has a carbide inlay for grasping suture needles. Metzenbaum scissors are the standard operating scissors for cardiac surgery. Curved Metzenbaum scissors are more versatile than the straight design. Potts scissors (45-degree angle) are desirable for some cardiac surgery procedures. Needle holders should be long and available in different sizes to accommodate a variety of suture needle sizes. Mayo-Hegar, Crile-Wood, and Castroviejo needle holders represent a good selection of sizes for thoracic surgery in animals. Angled thoracic forceps are an important instrument for cardiac surgery and should be available in a variety of sizes. Vascular clamps are noncrushing clamps used for temporary occlusion of cardiovascular and pulmonary structures. They come in a variety of sizes and shapes, including straight, angled, curved, and tangential. The most versatile shape for most cardiac surgery procedures is a medium-width tangential clamp.

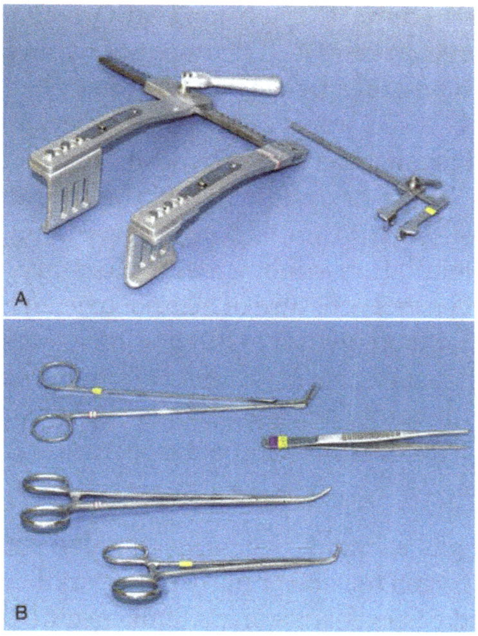

Instruments for cardiovascular surgery. A. Large and small Finochietto retractors. B. (from top to bottom) Potts scissors, DeBakey tissue forceps, angled thoracic forceps (45 and 90 degree).

The 90-degree forceps is also called a right-angle or Mixter forceps; the 45-degree forceps is also called a Julian thoracic artery forceps or Mixter forceps.

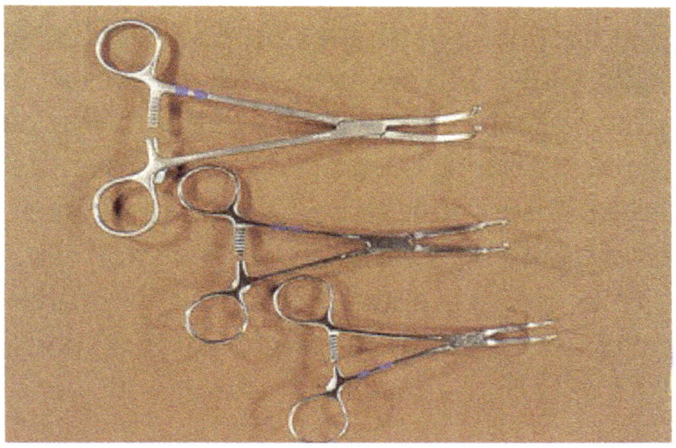

Tangential (Satinsky) vascular clamps.

Postoperative Care and Assessment

Patient monitoring and postoperative care are the cornerstones of successful cardiac surgery. The level of supportive care required for cardiac surgeries depends on the patient and the surgical procedure performed. A working knowledge of cardiopulmonary function and good patient observation skills are as important to successful patient management as advanced monitoring devices.

Evaluation of ventilation is important after any thoracic surgery. Poor ventilatory efforts may first be noted in the period after surgery, when the influence of anesthetic drugs is still present but ventilatory support has been discontinued. Hypoventilation may also result from uncontrolled pain. Total ventilation can be assessed directly by measuring the volume of expired gas with a respirometer. Tidal volume should be at least 10 ml per kg of body weight. Ultimately, the best measure of alveolar ventilation is arterial CO_2 tension ($PaCO_2$). Alveolar hypoventilation is present when $PaCO_2$ is increased to above 40 mmHg. Treatment of hypoventilation should be directed at correcting its underlying cause if possible. Drugs that are known to depress ventilation (i.e., opioids and muscle relaxants) should be used with caution in the perioperative period, and the risk of ventilatory depression weighed against the risk of hypoventilation due to pain. Pleural air or fluid should be evacuated if present. Injury or dysfunction of the neuromuscular ventilatory apparatus should be corrected, if possible. If hypoventilation is severe and the cause is not immediately correctable, positive-pressure ventilation is indicated. If necessary, keep the animal intubated and ventilated postoperatively until partial pressure of arterial oxygen (PaO_2), partial pressure of arterial carbon dioxide ($PaCO_2$), pH, blood pressure (BP) and heart rate (HR) indicate that the patient is stable enough to extubate. Constant-rate infusions of fentanyl and propofol can assist in keeping the patient comfortable until complications such as significant ventilation/perfusion ($\dot{V}/\dot{Q}$) mismatch or acidosis have improved. If necessary, vasopressors may be administered to correct hypotension caused by propofol.

Under physiologic conditions, gas exchange between the alveolus and the pulmonary capillary blood is efficient, and alveolar oxygen tension (PAO_2) and arterial oxygen tension (PaO_2) are nearly equal. In patients with impaired gas exchange, hypoxemia occurs because PAO_2 and PaO_2 are not equal. The most common cause of impaired pulmonary gas exchange in the postoperative setting is ventilation/perfusion ($\dot{V}_A/\dot{Q}$) mismatch with formation of pulmonary shunts secondary to alveolar collapse. The importance of ($\dot{V}/\dot{Q}$) ratios relates to how well the lungs resaturate venous blood with O_2 and eliminate CO_2. During procedures involving circulatory arrest or cardiopulmonary bypass, ventilation is temporarily ceased and the remaining oxygen is absorbed, resulting in collapsed alveoli (absorption atelectasis). With reperfusion of collapsed pulmonary tissues, blood passes through the lungs without becoming oxygenated. The result can be large shunts of deoxygenated blood returning to the left side of the heart. Patients with shunts are not responsive to higher concentrations of oxygen. Instead, they need assisted ventilation and positive end-expiratory pressure (PEEP). Therefore, response to supplemental oxygen therapy must be evaluated for each individual patient, preferably by arterial blood gas analysis. The therapeutic goal of supplemental oxygen should be to keep PaO_2 above 80 mmHg. Ventilation and PEEP are indicated for patients with severe gas exchange impairment that is not responsive to supplemental oxygen therapy alone.

Maintaining an adequate PaO_2 in a patient is important because it is the soluble oxygen that crosses membranes. Total oxygen content of the blood is the sum of the oxygen in solution (PaO_2) plus that carried by hemoglobin. The major determinant of hemoglobin oxygen saturation (SaO_2) is hemoglobin. SaO_2 can be measured by pulse oximetry. The therapeutic goal should be to maintain SaO_2 at or above 90%. Oxygen content of the blood is a function of SaO_2 and hemoglobin concentration. Thus maintenance of adequate oxygen content requires not only adequate pulmonary function, but also an adequate hemoglobin concentration. Maintenance of the packed cell volume above 30% is an important therapeutic goal for animals undergoing cardiac surgery, especially if cardiopulmonary compromise is present.

Systemic blood pressure is directly proportional to cardiac output and systemic vascular resistance. Measurement of blood pressure provides a good assessment of cardiovascular function, especially during and immediately after surgery. Indirect techniques for measuring blood pressure include the oscillometric method, which serves as the basis of monitors such as the Dinamap, or

Doppler, method. Doppler technique provides only systolic pressure but is useful for evaluating blood pressure trends during and after surgery. Indirect methods of blood pressure assessment are less invasive, but are also less accurate than direct measurements. Direct measurement of blood pressure requires placement of an arterial catheter. Arterial catheters have the additional advantage of providing access for arterial blood gas analysis. An arterial catheter can be placed percutaneously into a dorsal pedal artery. Direct blood pressure measurement also requires a pressure transducer and a monitor, or a manometer. The therapeutic goal is to maintain a mean blood pressure above 65 mmHg and systolic blood pressure above 90 mmHg. Blood pressure can be elevated by increasing cardiac output or systemic vascular resistance. In many instances (depending on the cause), a more appropriate therapeutic strategy to correct hypotension is to improve cardiac output. Maintenance of adequate vascular volume is the most important aspect of maintaining adequate cardiac output. Central venous pressure should be maintained at between 5 and 10 cm of water. If echocardiography is available, evaluation of ventricular filling is a more reliable way to detect hypovolemia. Indications for arterial pressor therapy are rare. Inotropic and pressor support can be obtained by constant intravenous infusion of epinephrine. Long-term inotropic support is maintained with dobutamine.

Monitoring the electrocardiogram for disturbances in cardiac rhythm is important for animals undergoing cardiac surgery. Sinus tachycardia is the most common rhythm disturbance in surgery patients. Therapy for sinus tachycardia should be directed at correction of its underlying cause (e.g., hypovolemia, pain, anxiety, acidosis, hypotension, anemia, hypoxemia, drug-induced) and improvement in cardiac output. Ventricular dysrhythmias, including premature ventricular complexes (PVCs) and nonsustained or sustained ventricular tachycardia, are frequently encountered during and after cardiac surgery. Frequent PVCs, particularly when they occur with a short coupling interval (i.e., R-on-T phenomena), and rapid ventricular tachycardia should be suppressed in the perioperative period. Continuous intravenous infusion of lidocaine is effective in most instances. Ventricular fibrillation is a form of cardiac arrest that requires immediate electrical defibrillation. If cardiac surgery is performed, equipment for defibrillation should be available.

Complications

The major complication associated with cardiac surgery is hemorrhage. Severe hemorrhage may be encountered intraoperatively or postoperatively. Materials for blood transfusion should be available. Fresh whole blood should be collected as close as possible to the time that it is needed and should not be cooled because this may reduce platelet content. If possible, a compatible donor should be identified by cross-matching the patient before surgery. Cell Saver autologous blood recovery systems (Haemonetics, Braintree, Mass.) are available for collection and processing of blood for procedures in which rapid bleeding or high-volume blood loss may occur. They can also be used to sequester platelets and plasma from a patient immediately before surgery, thereby reducing the need for donor blood.

Special Age Considerations

Most animals undergoing surgery for congenital cardiac defects are young. Special care must be given to these animals during and after surgery. Young animals should not have food withheld for longer than 4 to 6 hours before surgery and should be fed as soon as they are fully recovered from anesthesia. If they cannot be fed, blood glucose concentration should be maintained by adding glucose to intravenous fluids; blood glucose concentrations should be monitored intraoperatively. Hypothermia is common in young patients during thoracotomy and is protective during cardiac procedures. However, the temperature should be monitored closely, and patients should be actively rewarmed postoperatively.

Ophthalmology Surgical Procedures

Veterinary Ophthalmology is the branch of veterinary medicine that deals with the anatomy, physiology and diseases of the eyeball of animals. Veterinary Ophthalmologist is a specialist person who can solve medical and surgical eye related problem of animals. A number of diseases and different types of conditions can be diagnosed from the eye itself only. Some conditions such as entropion, ectopic cilia and protrusion of the nictitans gland occur much more frequently in younger animals whereas neoplasia occurs much more commonly in older animals. Medications can influence the eye. People sometimes give their pet's old eye medicines which initially prescribed for other pets or for themselves. This can cause problems such as bacterial contamination of a corneal ulcer or may cause changes such as atropine dilating the pupil.

Many of the surgeries below are performed under an operating microscope due to the delicate nature of the surgery. Surgical lasers including the carbon dioxide laser and diode laser are commonly used for ophthalmic surgery.

Eyelid

- Entropion and ectropion correction;
- Ectopic cilia removal;
- Distichia cryoepilation;
- Medial canthoplasty;
- Tumor excision with adjunct reconstruction, chemotherapy, laser ablation, cryotherapy or photodynamic therapy (pdt);
- Eversion of scrolled cartilage.

Lacrimal System

- Repositioning of prolapsed nictitans gland (cherry eye).
- Parotid duct transposition (pdt) for end stage dry eye.

Cornea

- Reconstructive surgeries (tissue grafts, corneal grafts).

- Dermoid, sequestrum and foreign body removal.
- Tumor excision with adjunct laser ablation or cryotherapy.
- Grid and diamond burr keratotomy (outpatient).
- Corneal intrastromal injection for fungal keratitis (outpatient).

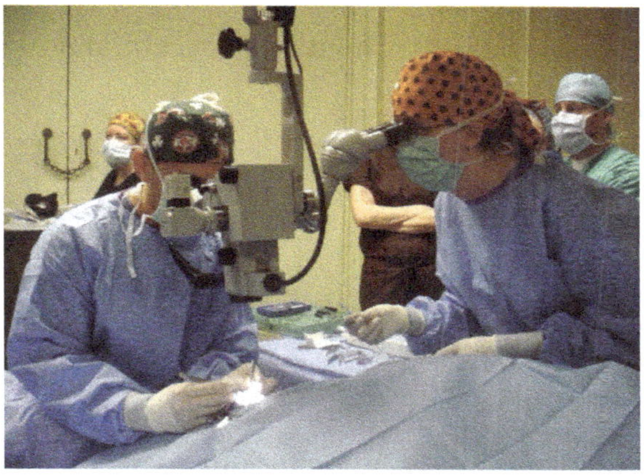

Cataract surgery being performed on a horse.

Cataract/Lens

- Cataract surgery with intraocular lens implants.
- Lens removal for lens luxation.

Glaucoma

- Endolaser and transscleral laser ciliary body ablation valve placement.

Intraocular

- Foreign body removal.

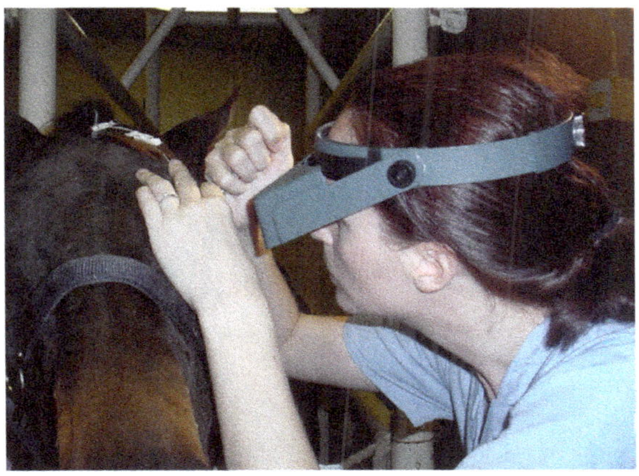

Intracorneal injections on a horse with a fungal infection of the cornea.

Retina

- Laser retinopexy for retinal detachment.

Globe and Orbit

- Prosthesis surgery (evisceration with intraocular prosthesis).
- Eye removal (enucleation) with or without an intraorbital prosthesis.
- Exenteration for orbital tumor.
- Orbital eploratory surgery.

References

- Surgical: colostate.edu, Retrieved 14 March, 2019
- Orchiectomy: wagwalking.com, Retrieved 17 August, 2019
- Fundamentals-of-surgical-oncology-in-small-animals: todaysveterinarypractice.com, Retrieved 7 May, 2019
- Surgery-of-the-cardiovascular-system: veteriankey.com, Retrieved 20 July, 2019
- Surgical-procedures, ophthalmology: okstate.edu, Retrieved 27 January, 2019

Permissions

All chapters in this book are published with permission under the Creative Commons Attribution Share Alike License or equivalent. Every chapter published in this book has been scrutinized by our experts. Their significance has been extensively debated. The topics covered herein carry significant information for a comprehensive understanding. They may even be implemented as practical applications or may be referred to as a beginning point for further studies.

We would like to thank the editorial team for lending their expertise to make the book truly unique. They have played a crucial role in the development of this book. Without their invaluable contributions this book wouldn't have been possible. They have made vital efforts to compile up to date information on the varied aspects of this subject to make this book a valuable addition to the collection of many professionals and students.

This book was conceptualized with the vision of imparting up-to-date and integrated information in this field. To ensure the same, a matchless editorial board was set up. Every individual on the board went through rigorous rounds of assessment to prove their worth. After which they invested a large part of their time researching and compiling the most relevant data for our readers.

The editorial board has been involved in producing this book since its inception. They have spent rigorous hours researching and exploring the diverse topics which have resulted in the successful publishing of this book. They have passed on their knowledge of decades through this book. To expedite this challenging task, the publisher supported the team at every step. A small team of assistant editors was also appointed to further simplify the editing procedure and attain best results for the readers.

Apart from the editorial board, the designing team has also invested a significant amount of their time in understanding the subject and creating the most relevant covers. They scrutinized every image to scout for the most suitable representation of the subject and create an appropriate cover for the book.

The publishing team has been an ardent support to the editorial, designing and production team. Their endless efforts to recruit the best for this project, has resulted in the accomplishment of this book. They are a veteran in the field of academics and their pool of knowledge is as vast as their experience in printing. Their expertise and guidance has proved useful at every step. Their uncompromising quality standards have made this book an exceptional effort. Their encouragement from time to time has been an inspiration for everyone.

The publisher and the editorial board hope that this book will prove to be a valuable piece of knowledge for students, practitioners and scholars across the globe.

Index

www.ingramcontent.com/pod-product-compliance
Lightning Source LLC
LaVergne TN
LVHW080705210926
848485LV00003B/424